Sharon Moore

~ *Contents* W9-CSM-953

● Weight control is not just a weight issue but a **lifestyle issue.** A truly effective weight control program should incorporate: ▲Sensible dieting ▲Regular exercise ▲Behavior changes to control over-eating or bingeing; ▲Motivation and positive thinking.

● **Self-Esteem:** How you think about yourself affects whatever you want to achieve in life.

Enhancing your self-esteem will boost motivation to control your weight; and to adopt a more positive and brighter outlook on life.

● **Arrange Moral Support:** The support of family, friends and work-mates, is vital to your success. You will feel more committed and they will be less likely to sabotage your efforts. You might also join a support group.

● **Be patient!** Weight control is a life-time project — not one that you win or lose over a 2-week or even 2-month period. **Perseverance** usually wins out. (See notes on *Weight Plateaus* — p. 18)

● **Do not dwell on past failures.** Think only of achieving positive results. **Write down your goals,** both short-term and long-term. Plan carefully what you need to do — day by day, hour by hour — to achieve your goals. **Set realistic, attainable goals.**

MEDICAL CHECK-UP

Before you commence your program, **see your doctor** for a medical check-up. Have the doctor confirm that your overweight state is not glandular. If you have any medical ailment, get your doctor's approval.

Note: Persons with deep-seated emotional problems and eating disorders require expert counselling.

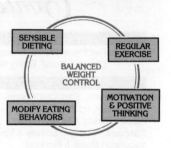

SENSIBLE DIETING		REGULAR EXERCISE
	BALANCED WEIGHT CONTROL	
MODIFY EATING BEHAVIORS		MOTIVATION & POSITIVE THINKING

The 4 basic components of a balanced weight control program.

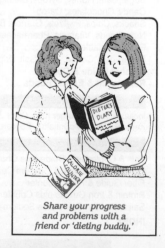

Share your progress and problems with a friend or 'dieting buddy.'

● **Counting calories** takes the guess-work out of dieting. It enables you to make calorie-saving choices. Planning calorie-controlled meals also becomes much easier.

● Commence with a calorie-controlled diet that allows a **moderate weight loss** of ½-1 lb per week. Initial weight losses may be larger due to fluid losses.
See *Sample Diet Plans* — Pages 10-11.
Also see *Ten Dieting Hints* — Page 9.

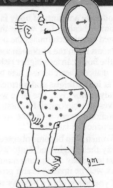

Weighing each day will remind you that weight control is a daily event.
See extra notes on Body Weight Variations (p. 18)

SUGGESTED CALORIE LEVELS

		CALORIES
Women:	Sedentary —	**1000-1200**
	Active —	**1200-1500**
Men:	Sedentary —	**1200-1500**
	Active —	**1500-1800**
Children:	—	**1200-1500**
Teenagers:	—	**1200-1800**

EXERCISE DAILY FOR WEIGHT CONTROL

Exercise can mean the difference between success and failure. Regular exercisers lose more fat and keep it off. They also feel better, look better, and can eat more food.
(Extra Notes & Walking Program — See Pages 12-13.)

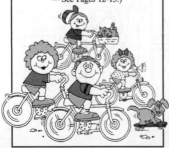

KEEP A DIARY OF FOOD & EXERCISE

Persons who keep a food and exercise diary **lose more weight** and **keep it off.** Recording forces you to focus on your eating habits and make wiser choices. It also **keeps you honest** and helps prevent 'calorie amnesia.'
(Extra Notes — See Page 15.)

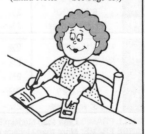

3

BODY FAT DISTRIBUTION & HEALTH

Moderate amounts of body fat do not compromise health. Just where the body fat is stored largely determines the health risk.

Excess fat in the **abdomen and upper part of the body** carries a **higher risk of ill-health**; e.g. diabetes, heart disease, high blood pressure.

Fat in the thighs and buttocks has a relatively minor risk. The fat in women's thighs serves the biological function of an energy storehouse were a famine to occur during pregnancy or lactation.

Women who become obsessed with dieting away their thighs and buttocks on an otherwise lean body, are fighting mother nature and may well be inviting health problems.

If you are within a healthy weight range, it is better to exercise regularly to maintain body shape, rather than to be constantly dieting and lacking in energy. **Accept the situation** and focus on enjoying life.

Excess fat in the abdomen and upper body carry a higher risk of ill-health.

HIGHER HEALTH RISK

MINOR HEALTH RISK

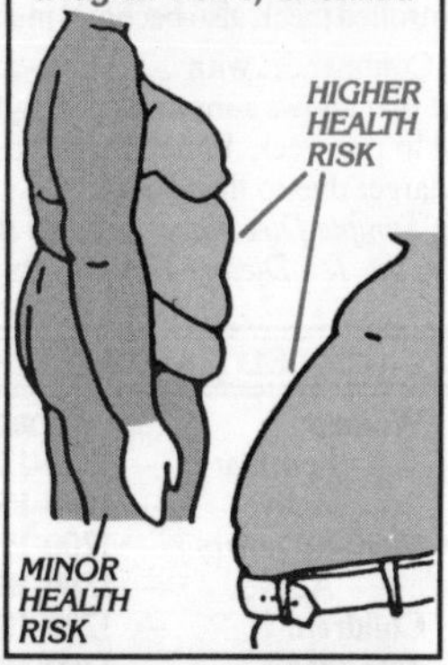

GUIDE TO BODY FRAME SIZE

ESTIMATION OF MEDIUM BODY FRAME SIZE

	HEIGHT (No Shoes)	ELBOW BREADTH
W O M E N	4'9" – 4'10"	2½ – 2⅞"
	4'10" – 5'2"	2⅝ – 2⅞"
	5'3" – 5'6"	2¾ – 3"
	5'7" – 5'10"	2¾ – 3⅛"
	5'11" and over	2⅞ – 3¼"
M E N	5'1" – 5'2"	2¼ – 2½"
	5'3" – 5'6"	2¼ – 2½"
	5'7" – 5'10"	2⅜ – 2⅝"
	5'11" – 6'2"	2⅜ – 2⅝"
	6'3" and over	2½ – 2¾"

HOW TO ESTIMATE ELBOW BREADTH

1. Place thumb and index finger on the 2 prominent bones in either side of the bent elbow.

2. Measure space between **inside of the 2 fingers.**

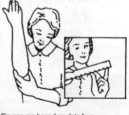

Figures are based on data from Metropolitan Life Insurance Company.

SMALL FRAME: *Less than* Medium Elbow Breadth
LARGE FRAME: *More than* Medium Elbow Breadth

CALCULATING CALORIES IN FOOD

The **calorie** value of any food is a measure of the energy available to the body — just like the foot is a measure of length. The calorie is also a measure of the energy used by the body, or 'burned' (as in exercise).

The calorie (actually the kilocalorie) is the amount of heat required to raise the temperature of one liter of water (approx. 1 quart) by 1° centigrade.

CALORIES IN FOOD

Calories in food food are derived from 3 nutrients — **protein, fat, carbohydrate**.

Vitamins, minerals and water provide no calories even though they are vital in the body's production of energy.

Proteins: 4 Calories per gram
Carbohydrates: 4 Calories per gram
Fats: 9 Calories per gram
Vitamins and Minerals: Nil Calories
Water: Nil Calories
Alcohol: 7 Calories per gram

Note that **fats** have over double the energy value of protein and carbohydrate. Thus the higher the fat (or oil) content of food, the higher the calories.

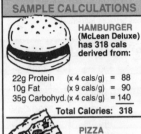

SAMPLE CALCULATIONS

HAMBURGER (McLean Deluxe) has 318 cals derived from:

22g Protein	(x 4 cals/g)	= 88
10g Fat	(x 9 cals/g)	= 90
35g Carbohyd.	(x 4 cals/g)	= 140
	Total Calories:	**318**

PIZZA 2 slices (16") **Combo Deluxe** has 520 cals derived from:

27g Protein	(x 4 cals/g)	= 108
20g Fat	(x 9 cals/g)	= 180
58g Carbohyd.	(x 4 cals/g)	= 232
	Total Calories:	**520**

CALORIE BALANCE & BODY WEIGHT

Your body uses energy (calories) for every activity whether at work or play and even when sleeping. The heavier you are, the more energy that is used — similar to a large car using more petrol than a small car. Food is the 'fuel' that provides energy to the body.

Note: Excess calories whether from fats, carbohydrates or protein are stored as body fat.

To **maintain weight**, food calories should balance with calories used by the body. To **lose weight** more calories should be used than consumed.

To lose **1 pound** of body fat/week, a **deficit** of around 3,500 calories (500 calories/day) is required — from eating less food, or exercising more.

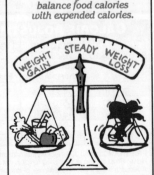

For weight control balance food calories with expended calories.

5

• **Different people** require different amounts of calories — even between 2 people of the same age, weight and physical activity.

• Allow up to 400 calories above or below the figures below, for normal variations between individuals.

• The **charts below** are for persons with sedentary occupations of very light (average) activity. Any **extra calories** required for moderate or strenuous activity, and for pregnancy and lactation, **must be added** to these figures.
(See *Calorie Adjustments Chart* below.)

WOMEN

	18-35 Years	36-55 Years	56 Years
100 lbs	1760 Cals	1570 Cals	1430 Cals
110 lbs	1860 Cals	1660 Cals	1500 Cals
120 lbs	1950 Cals	1760 Cals	1550 Cals
133 lbs	2050 Cals	1860 Cals	1600 Cals
143 lbs	2150 Cals	1960 Cals	1630 Cals
155 lbs	2250 Cals	2050 Cals	1660 Cals
165 lbs	2400 Cals	2150 Cals	1720 Cals

MEN

	18-35 Years	36-55 Years	56 Years
130 lbs	2480 Cals	2300 Cals	1900 Cals
143 lbs	2620 Cals	2400 Cals	2000 Cals
155 lbs	2760 Cals	2480 Cals	2100 Cals
165 lbs	2900 Cals	2560 Cals	2200 Cals
175 lbs	3050 Cals	2670 Cals	2300 Cals
190 lbs	3200 Cals	2760 Cals	2400 Cals
200 lbs	3500 Cals	3000 Cals	2600 Cals

CALORIE ADJUSTMENTS FOR ACTIVITY

BODY WEIGHT (Pounds)	INACTIVE Bedridden Subtract from Charts Above	LIGHT/MODERATE ACTIVITY Skilled Trades, Housework Add to Charts Above	STRENUOUS OR HEAVY ACTIVITY Worker, Sportsperson Add to Charts Above
90-110	-480 Cals	+240 Cals	+480 Cals
111-130	-570 Cals	+290 Cals	+570 Cals
131-150	-670 Cals	+340 Cals	+670 Cals
151-170	-760 Cals	+380 Cals	+760 Cals
171-200	-860 Cals	+430 Cals	+860 Cals

PREGNANCY: Add 300 calories (from 4th month). **LACTATION:** Add up to 500 calories.
Note: Strict dieting during pregnancy is not recommended.
Adequate weight gain lessens risk of low birth weight baby.

CALORIES USED IN EXERCISE

LIGHT 4 Cals/Minute	MODERATE 7 Cals/Minute	HEAVY 10 Cals/Minute
Walking, slow	Walking, brisk	Walking (power), Jogging
Calisthenics	Aerobics, light	Aerobics, advanced
Cycling, light	Cycling, moderate	Cycling, vigorous
Gardening, light	Swimming, crawl	Swimming, strenuous
Golf, social	Weight-training, light	Weight-training, heavy
Tennis, doubles	Tennis, singles	Wrestling/Judo, advanced
Housework, Cleaning	Racket Sports	Racket Sports, advanced
Rebounding, light	Rebounding, moderate	Skipping
Canoeing	Football/Grid Iron	Boxing
Table Tennis	Basketball	Basketball (Pro)
Horse-riding	Volleyball, advanced	Climbing Stairs
Ice Skating	Snow Skiing (downhill)	Skiing (cross country)
Roller Skating	Aquarobics, light	Aquarobics, advanced
Skate Boarding	Dancing, Jazzercise	Dancing, strenuous

NOTES

1. Above calorie figures are for a 140 pound person. Add or subtract 10% of calories for each 14 lbs above or below 140 lbs. The heavier the person, the more energy expended.

2. Only those sports or activities that are sustained over a period of time (e.g. jogging) qualify for heavy exercise. Stop-start sports such as tennis are 'moderate' on average.

3. Calories required for **basal metabolism** (e.g. while sleeping):
   Women: Approx. 1400 calories/day (for 130 lb person).
   Men: Approx. 1800 calories/day (for 155 lb person).

CHILDREN & ADOLESCENTS
DAILY CALORIE NEEDS

AGE GROUP		AVERAGE WEIGHT	CALORIE NEEDS (with range)
Infants:	0-6 months	(13 lbs)	50 Cals (45-60) per lb
	6-12 months	(20 lbs)	45 Cals (40-55) per lb
Children:	1-3 years	(30 lbs)	1300 Cals (900-1800)
	4-6 years	(45 lbs)	1700 Cals (1300-2300)
	7-10 years	(62 lbs)	2400 Cals (1650-3300)
Boys:	11-14 years	(100 lbs)	2700 Cals (2000-3700)
	15-18 years	(145 lbs)	2800 Cals (2100-3900)
Girls:	11-14 years	(100 lbs)	2200 Cals (1500-3000)
	15-18 years	(120 lbs)	2100 Cals (1400-3000)

7

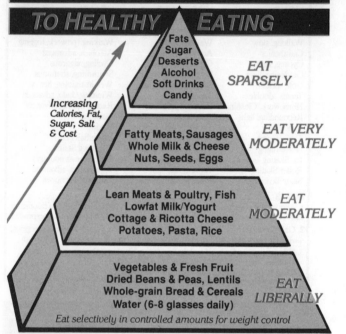

THE PYRAMID GUIDE TO HEALTHY EATING

**Fats
Sugar
Desserts
Alcohol
Soft Drinks
Candy**

EAT SPARSELY

*Increasing
Calories, Fat,
Sugar, Salt
& Cost*

**Fatty Meats, Sausages
Whole Milk & Cheese
Nuts, Seeds, Eggs**

EAT VERY MODERATELY

**Lean Meats & Poultry, Fish
Lowfat Milk/Yogurt
Cottage & Ricotta Cheese
Potatoes, Pasta, Rice**

EAT MODERATELY

**Vegetables & Fresh Fruit
Dried Beans & Peas, Lentils
Whole-grain Bread & Cereals
Water (6-8 glasses daily)**

EAT LIBERALLY

Eat selectively in controlled amounts for weight control

The Pyramid Guide encompasses the 2 sets of guidelines that help to select a nutritious diet:

(a) The *Five Food Groups* group together foods with similar nutrients. Daily selection from each group helps to ensure good nutrition:

1. Breads/Cereals/Rice/Pasta
2. Vegetables
3. Fruits
4. Meats/Poultry/Fish/Eggs; Dry Beans & Peas/Nuts
5. Milk/Yogurt/Cheese

(b) The *Dietary Guidelines for Americans* complement the 5 Food Groups and focus on other issues:
- Eat a variety of foods.
- Maintain a healthy weight.
- Choose a diet low in fat, saturated fat, and cholesterol.
- Choose a diet with plenty of vegetables, fruits, and grain products.
- Use sugars only in moderation.
- Use salt and sodium only in moderation.
- If you drink alcoholic beverages, do so in moderation.

1. Avoid fad diets. They don't re-educate your eating habits. Eat 3 moderate meals daily that are nutritionally balanced. (See *Sample Diet Plans* following.)

2. Carefully plan each meal rather than just grabbing haphazardly whatever comes into your line of vision.

3. Don't skip meals — you are more likely to snack on high calorie foods.

4. Use minimal amounts of fat and oil. Trim fat from meat, and skin from poultry. Use lowfat dairy products and low calorie salad dressings. Use fat-free cooking methods.

Avoid fried foods, high-fat snacks and high-fat fast foods, cookies, cakes, and icecream. Limit nuts. (Extra Notes — See Pages 149-151.)

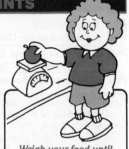

Weigh your food until you can accurately estimate food portion sizes. Better control of calories will result.

5. Avoid sugar and foods high in sugar such as soft drinks, fruit drinks, jams, chocolate, cookies, cakes, donuts, icecream and ice-confections. Use artificial sweeteners and artificially sweetened diet products.

6. Eat adequate fresh fruits, vegetables, and whole-grain cereal products. They also help to prevent **constipation.** (See *Fiber Guide & Constipation* — Pages 158-163)

7. There is no food that cannot occasionally be eaten; e.g. chocolate, cake, dessert, wine. It is the quantity that is critical.

8. Avoid alcohol when dieting (See *Alcohol Guide* — p. 100). **Avoid** regular **soft drinks**; use sugar-free diet drinks. **Limit fruit juice.**

9. When dining out, avoid fried and sauce-laden dishes as well as pastries, salad dressings and desserts. Eat moderately. Quench your thirst on water or mineral water.

10. Take a multi-vitamin and mineral supplement daily when dieting — particularly if tired and irritable.

Additionally, keep track of your calories with a food diary.

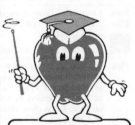

Eating a high-fiber breakfast gives you a good start to the day . . . and helps prevent high calorie snacking.
Desirable lower calorie snacks include apples, oranges, carrot sticks and plain popcorn.

BREAKFAST
1 small Fruit **or** ½oz Dried Fruit

Plus Cereal: 1½oz Dry (high fiber)
or 1 cup cooked, e.g. Oatmeal

Plus Milk (from daily allowance)

BREAKFAST — CHOICE 2
1 small Fruit
Plus 1 Egg (no added fat)
or ¾oz Cheese
or 2oz Cottage Cheese
or ¼ cup Baked Beans
Plus 1 Toast **or** ½ Muffin (low-fat)

MILK ALLOWANCE (160 Calories)
2 cups Skim Milk **or** 1½ cups Fat-Reduced Milk
or equivalent Yogurt, Cheese, Soy Milk, Tofu

FAT ALLOWANCE (140 Calories)
4 tsp Fat **or** 6-8 tsp Diet Margarine **or** 3 tsp Oil
or 1½ Tbsp Mayonnaise **or** ½ medium Avocado
or 1½ Tbsp Peanut Butter **or** 1oz Nuts/Seeds

 LUNCH
2 slices Bread (2oz) **or** 1 Bagel **or** 4 Crispbreads

Plus 2oz lean Meat, Chicken or Turkey
or 3½oz Tuna (in water) **or** 2½oz Salmon
or 1oz Cheese **or** 3oz Cottage Cheese
or 2½oz Ricotta Cheese (part-skim)
or 1 cup (8oz) Fruit Yogurt (low or non-fat)
or ¾ cup (4oz) Bean Salad (no-oil dressing)

Plus Large Salad (low calorie dressing)
Plus 1 small fruit **or** ½oz Dried Fruit

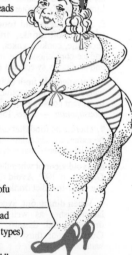

DINNER
Soup (low calorie, fat-free)

Plus 3oz lean Meat (cooked weight)
or 4oz Chicken Breast (no skin)
or 3oz Chicken Thigh/Leg (no skin)
or 5oz Fish (grilled, no fat)
or 1 cup Beans (Soy, Haricot etc)/Lentils/Tofu
or 1 serving Low Calorie Entree

Plus 1 small Potato **or** ½ cup Rice/Pasta **or** 1 Bread

Plus 2-3 servings Vegetables/Salad (lower calorie types)
Plus 1 small Fruit + Gelatin Dessert (sugar-free)

BETWEEN MEALS: Water, Coffee, Tea, Milk from Allowance,
Fruit from main meals; Raw vegetable pieces
Note: Take a multivitamin/mineral supplement daily while dieting.

For extra flexibility in meal planning, or to meet special dietary requirements,
seek referral to a registered dietitian through your doctor.

BREAKFAST
1 medium Fruit **or** 1oz Dried Fruit

Plus Cereal: 1½oz Dry (high fiber)
or 1 cup cooked, e.g. Oatmeal

Plus Milk (from daily allowance)

Plus 1 slice Bread **or** ½ Muffin (plain)
or extra Cereal

BREAKFAST — CHOICE 2
1 medium Fruit

Plus 1 Egg (no added fat)
or ¾oz Cheese
or 2oz Cottage Cheese
or ¼ cup Baked Beans

Plus 2 Toast/Bread
or 1 Muffin (low-fat)
or 1 Toast + small Cereal

MILK ALLOWANCE (160 Calories)
2 cups Skim Milk **or** 1½ cups Fat-reduced Milk
or Equivalent Yogurt, Cheese, Soy Milk, Tofu

FAT ALLOWANCE (175 Calories)
5 tsp Fat **or** 8-10 tsp Diet Margarine **or** 4 tsp Oil
or Equivalent Avocado, Peanut Butter, Mayonnaise

 LUNCH
2 slices Bread (2oz) **or** 1 Bagel **or** 6″ Pita

Plus 2oz Lean Meat, Chicken **or** Turkey
or 3½oz Tuna (in water) **or** 2½oz Salmon
or 1oz Cheese **or** 3oz Cottage Cheese
or 2½oz Ricotta Cheese (part-skim)
or 1 cup (8oz) Fruit Yogurt (low or nonfat)
or ¾ cup (4oz) Bean Salad (no-oil dressing)

Plus Large Salad (low calorie dressing)
Plus 1 small Fruit **or** ½oz Dried Fruit

 DINNER
Soup (low calorie, fat-free)

Plus 3oz lean Meat (cooked weight)
or 4oz Chicken Breast (no skin)
or 3oz Chicken Thigh/Leg (no skin)
or 5oz Fish (grilled, no fat)
or 1 cup Beans (Soy, Haricot etc)/Lentils/Tofu
or 1 serving Low Calorie Entree

Plus 1 large Potato **or** 1 cup Rice/Pasta **or** 2 slices Bread

Plus 2-3 servings Vegetables/Salad (lower calorie types)
Plus 1 small fruit + Gelatin Dessert (sugar-free)

EXTRAS (100 Calories)
1 small Fruit, Raw Vegetable pieces, 1 cup Popcorn
Water, Coffee, Tea, Bouillon, Milk from Allowance

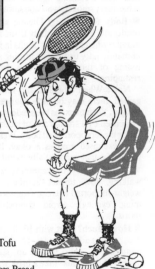

- Persons who exercise regularly **lose more weight** and keep it off longer than non-exercisers.

- Exercise also improves general health and well-being. **Confidence and self-esteem** are enhanced by a sense of control and accomplishment.

- **Exercise increases the metabolic rate** of the body even for hours after exercise — a good way to 'wake-up' a sluggish metabolism. **Exercise compensates for any decrease in metabolic rate** with increasing age and also in some heavy smokers who stop smoking.

- **Body Re-Shaping:** Dieting alone results in a loss of both fatty tissue and muscle, whereas exercise results in loss of mainly fatty tissue. The firming and toning of muscles also aids **body reshaping.**

   Note: When fat is lost and muscle gained, there may be **little change in weight.** Yet fatness has been reduced as evidenced by a smaller size of clothing fitting the reproportioned body. Weight from exercised muscles is okay. It is surplus fat that is potentially harmful.

- **Avoid injury** by beginning with walking, low impact aerobics, or weight-supported exercise (e.g. swimming, cycling). Avoid competitive sports.

- **How Much?** Start with 10-20 minutes/day and progress to 30-45 minutes/day. Also walk up stairs instead of using lifts. Take a brisk walk at lunch. Use an exercise bike when watching T.V.

- **How Often?** While aerobic fitness requires only 3-4 sessions weekly, weight control is a **daily** event which requires daily exercise.

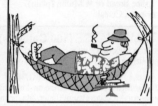

Middle-age spread has little to do with getting older. Too little exercise is the main culprit.
Regular exercise and sensible eating can prevent middle-age spread.

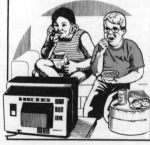

T.V. CAN BE FATTENING
Many children and adults watch over 20 hours T.V. per week and indulge in high calorie snacks — potent contributors to obesity!
Don't become a 'couch potato'. Limit T.V. hours and plan healthy physical activities.
Parents need to set the example!

WALKING — Ideal for Weight Control

Regular brisk walking is ideal exercise for unfit or overweight people. Walking is less likely to cause injury and more likely to become an enjoyable **daily** habit.

As your fitness improves you will be able to walk faster and for longer periods. Try the walking program outlined below.

EXTRA HINTS

- Spend 5 minutes doing gentle stretching before you start your walk.
- Walk with a comfortable long stride. Shuffling along uses fewer calories.
- Wear comfortable walking shoes. In hot weather wear a hat and drink plenty of water. In cold weather, protect yourself from the rain and wind.
- Aim to achieve 250-500 calories of exercise daily.

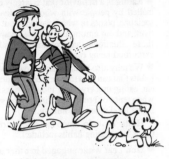

Brisk walking each day is a safe and effective way to keep trim and fit. Try it — you'll like it!

WALKING PROGRAM			
Weeks	Distance To Walk	Time Taken	Calories Used (140lb Person)
Weeks 1-2	1 mile	20 mins	110 calories
Weeks 3-5	1½ miles	28 mins	160 calories
Weeks 6-8	2 miles	35 mins	200 calories
Weeks 9-10	2½ miles	44 mins	250 calories
Weeks 11+	3½ miles	60 mins	340 calories

EXERCISE CALORIES USED EACH 30 MINUTES					
Activity Weight	120 lbs	140 lbs	160 lbs	180 lbs	200 lbs
Slow walk, 2 mph	85	100	110	125	140
Brisk walk, 4 mph	150	170	195	220	250
Jogging, 5.5 mph	260	300	340	385	425
Cycling, 5.5 mph	120	140	160	180	200
Swimming, moderate	230	270	300	335	370
Aerobics - beginners	210	240	270	300	330
- advanced	300	350	390	430	470

● **Eating is a behavior** that is largely controlled by people with whom we live or socialize, places in which we carry out our lives, and our emotions. **Become aware** of those situations that commonly lead to extra food being eaten.

● We may also be unaware of 'bad' eating habits that can lead to excess calorie intake; e.g. eating quickly, large mouthfuls, eating when tense or bored, finishing a large serving of food when not hungry.

Hints to help uncover and correct those 'bad' eating habits include:

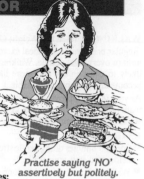

Practise saying 'NO' assertively but politely.

● **Don't eat while engaged in other activities;** e.g. watching TV, reading. Eat only at the table, not at the fridge or while standing.

● **Don't eat quickly.** Chewing slowly allows time to register a feeling of fullness. Don't use fingers, only utensils. Cut food into smaller pieces. Don't load your fork until the previous mouthful is finished.

● **Don't purchase problem high calorie foods.** Shop from a set list to prevent impulse buying. Avoid shopping with children. Plan meals in advance. Stick to a set menu.

● **Plan a strategy** to avoid uncontrolled eating and drinking at social events, or when your emotions urge you to binge.

Rehearse repeatedly in your mind exactly what you will do in such situations. Remind yourself several times each day that you are in charge of your actions and that you can be strong-willed. Seek counselling or coaching on various strategies.

● **Promise yourself** that when you feel the urge to snack, you will engage in some activity that will distract you away from food (e.g. go for a walk, brush your teeth, phone a friend.)

If you eat out of **boredom**, find some new hobby or interest that gets you out of the house; even enrol in an adult education class.

Note: Persons with deep-seated emotional problems and eating disorders require counselling.

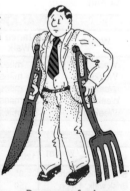

Do you use food as an emotional crutch? If so, professional counselling may be helpful.

The food diary is the most powerful proven aid for dieters. Here are some of the reasons:

● Recording your eating and exercise habits, jolts you into realizing just what you do eat and drink each day; and also whether you exercise sufficiently.

● **Helps you identify problem foods and drinks** with excessive calories.

● **Helps identify moods, situations and events** that lead to excessive eating of unwanted calories. You can then plan to overcome or avoid them.

● **Prevents 'calorie amnesia,'** the forgetfulness that leads to rebound weight gain after successful weight loss. Recording puts you back on the right track.

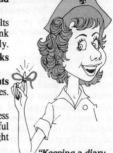

● **Helps you develop greater self-discipline.** You will think twice about over-indulging if you have to record it — especially if you have arranged for someone to check your diary regularly. It certainly keeps you honest!

● **Motivates you to plan your meals and exercise** regularly. Even the ritual weighing each morning serves as a reminder that weight control is a daily event.

● **Serves as a check system** for your doctor, dietitian or counsellor to assess your progress and make recommendations.

"Keeping a diary gives me feedback on exactly what I eat each day.

It helps prevent 'calorie amnesia' and reminds me to exercise each day.

It's a must for successful weight control!"

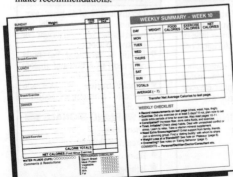

Sample pages from *The Pocket Dieter's Diary* — a 10-week diary to record food and exercise.

At end of day, exercise calories are deducted from food calories.

Includes Weekly Summary Page plus Food Exchanges Checklist.

Some **12 million** Americans have diabetes, almost half of whom don't even realize it. Around **70% are overweight** at the time they develop diabetes. Many of these overweight people may well have prevented diabetes developing. Certainly, **weight control** can lessen the severity of diabetes; and for some, it may even be a 'cure.'

WHAT IS DIABETES?

Diabetes is a disorder in which the body cannot make proper use of carbohydrates (sugar and starches).

After digestion, sugar and starches are changed into **glucose** — the simplest form of sugar that is vital to body cells for energy and growth.

Insulin is the hormone which acts like a key that opens the doors to body cells for the glucose to enter.

Without sufficient insulin, unused glucose builds up in the blood and passes into the urine. This produces symptoms of frequent urination, continual thirst and tiredness.

Untreated diabetes increases the risk of damage to nerves and blood vessels.

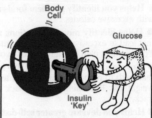

Insulin acts like a key. It opens the door to body cells and allows glucose to enter.

Some persons with diabetes (Type 1) have too few or no keys and require insulin injections.

Others (Type 2) have ample keys but 'mis-shapen' keyholes (insulin resistant) — particularly if obese.

TYPE 1 DIABETES	TYPE 2 DIABETES
Insulin Dependent Diabetes	**Non-Insulin Dependent**
• Occurs in 15% of diabetes cases. • Usually children and young adults. • Pancreas gland produces little or no insulin. Daily insulin injections are necessary, plus: • Regular meals with even carbohydrate distribution to match insulin dosage. Regular exercise and weight control are also important.	• Occurs in 85% of diabetes cases. • Occurs mainly in adults — particularly in overweight or inactive persons. • Insulin is produced but body cells resist its action and glucose cannot enter cells. • Usually treated with diet and exercise. Sometimes requires medication.
■ WARNING SIGNALS ■	**■ WARNING SIGNALS ■**
• Constant urination • Continual thirst • Rapid weight loss • Unusual hunger • Excessive weakness/fatigue • Nausea, vomiting, irritability	• Drowsiness • Excessive fatigue • Blurred vision • Itching • Skin infection with slow healing

INSULIN RESISTANCE & OVERWEIGHT

Persons with diabetes who are overweight may in fact have insulin levels much higher than normal. It's just that the insulin does not efficiently perform its task.

As the fat cells in the overweight person enlarge, they may resist in varying degrees the efforts of insulin to allow glucose to enter the cell. Glucose subsequently builds up in the bloodstream. The **pancreas gland** responds by producing larger amounts of insulin in an attempt to continue storage of the glucose in the body's cells. With continued weight gain, insulin resistance may further increase and lead to symptoms of diabetes.

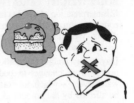

A 'cure' for many overweight persons with diabetes (Type 2) is simply losing weight and exercising regularly.

This condition **can often be corrected simply by restricting calories** to a level sufficiently low to allow weight loss. Within several weeks, the tissue cells can lose their resistance and become sensitive once again to the effects of insulin. Insulin production and blood glucose levels may become normal and any former symptoms of diabetes may disappear.

Regular testing of blood sugar levels should confirm the effectiveness of weight loss.

Thus, diet alone can control the symptoms of many persons with Type 2 diabetes. A diet rich in fiber and complex carbohydrates; and low in sugar, fat and calories can stabilize blood sugar levels and maximize weight loss.

An individualized diet plan from a dietitian is recommended. Proper instruction and regular supervision is important for success.

Exercise is also an important aid to diabetes control. It assists weight control and may improve sensitivity of body cells to insulin.

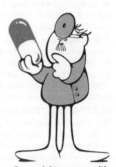

Overweight persons with diabetes (Type 2) should give diet a fair trial before trying drug therapy.

BODY WEIGHT VARIATIONS

Misinterpretation of weight changes is a constant source of frustration amongst dieters. Weight changes are rarely the result of changes only in fatty tissue.

Day to day weight fluctuations result mainly from changes in body fluid/water levels — which, for example, can be affected by the amount of salt, carbohydrate or water in the diet, by hormonal changes (e.g. monthly period), or the amount of exercise.

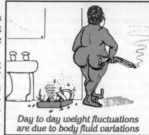

Day to day weight fluctuations are due to body fluid variations

Weight change over several weeks is more likely to reflect changes in body levels of fat and muscle. Unfortunately, the scales do not distinguish between weight changes from water, fat or muscle.

While weekly weighing may eliminate this dilemma, many people find the daily weighing ritual a reminder that weight control is a daily event that requires daily attention. Weigh at much the same time of day and in similar clothing or nude — and on the same scales.

When dining out, be aware that the extra pound or two that might show on the scales the next morning, is not necessarily the result of a **small** dietary indiscretion. It is more likely due to **fluid retention** resulting from the more highly seasoned and salted food — or a **large** dietary indiscretion! Of course, it is important to drink adequate water when thirsty. When dining out, a glass of wine is fine but quench your thirst on water, mineral water, or diet soda.

PLATEAUX — THE DIETER'S BAIN!

The 'plateau' is possibly an example of how the body adapts to a famine situation. In spite of much lowered calories, weight may be static for several weeks. The body's metabolism slows down in order to preserve as much body mass as possible — a welcome situation in a famine, but not appreciated by the dieter!

So, treat it as a period of rest for the body to adjust to the weight loss. **Self-discipline and perseverance** are the keys to success during plateaux. The longer the plateau, the closer you are getting to the next phase of weight loss. Now, that's positive thinking!

Regular exercise is important. If you have not been exercising, now is an excellent time to start. It could make all the difference.

Note: Weight on the scales does not tell the complete story, particularly as you approach your ideal weight. Fatty tissue losses from increased exercise may be cancelled on the scales by lean tissue gains — a healthy situation. Weight can be static even though you are still losing inches and reproportioning your body.

(Also see Exercise Notes — Page 12)

NOTES, ABBREVIATIONS, MEASURES

● Calorie and fat values have been **rounded off** for easier use.

Calories – to the nearest 5 or 10 calories.

Fat – to the nearest gram.

Note: Trace amounts of fat (less than 0.3 gram), have been treated as zero; and between 0.3-1.0 gram as <1.

● Because manufacturers' figures on labels are rounded off, figures in this book may differ slightly from the label. Serving sizes in this book may also vary from that on the label.

● **Food product formulations change** from time to time, and hence the need to regularly update this type of publication. Many products also come and go. Check the food label for any changes.

● **Calorie variations** between this book and other calorie books may be quite reasonable. For example, no two pieces of meat ever have exactly the same calories or fat content. (A mere 5 grams of extra fat can add an extra 45 calories.)

● Feedback Welcome: Please contact the author directly with your queries, and suggestions for foods to be included in future editions. (Ideally, enclose the label with the manufacturer's name and address.)

ABBREVIATIONS	
tsp	= teaspoon
Tbsp	= Tablespoon
oz	= ounce(s)
c	= cup
fl.oz	= fluid ounce(s)
g	= gram(s)
CALS	= Calories
n.a.	= not available
<1	= less than 1

VOLUME MEASURES	
3 tsp	= 1 Tbsp
2 Tbsp	= 1 fl.oz
½ cup	= 4 fl.oz
1 cup	= 8 fl.oz
	or 16 Tbsp
2 cups	= 1 Pint
2 Pints	= 1 Quart

(All measures are level)

Note: 8 oz weight is not the same as 8 fl.oz volume (space occupied). Dense foods weigh more per set volume.

For example:
1 cup popcorn weighs ½ oz
1 cup milk weighs 8½ oz
1 cup pudding weighs 10 oz

METRIC CONVERSION	
1 oz	= 28.4 grams
1 fl.oz	= 30 mls
1 Calorie	= 4.18 Kilojoules

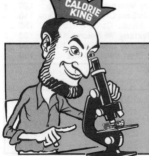

SOURCES OF INFORMATION

● U.S. Dept. of Agriculture
● Food manufacturers
● Food Industry Boards & Councils
● Independent laboratory analysis
● Scientific publications
● Overseas food composition tables
● Author extrapolations

MILK & MILK DRINKS

COW'S MILK

	CALS	FAT
Whole (3.5% fat):		(g)
2 Tbsp, 1 fl.oz	20	1
1 Glass, 6 fl.oz	110	6
1 Cup, 8 fl.oz	150	8
1 Pint, 16 fl.oz	300	16
Lowfat (2% fat):		
2 Tbsp, 1 fl.oz	15	<1
1 Glass, 6 fl.oz	90	4
1 Cup, 8 fl.oz	120	5
1 Pint, 16 fl.oz	240	10
Lowfat (1% fat):		
2 Tbsp, 1 fl.oz	10	<1
1 Glass, 6 fl.oz	75	1
1 Cup, 8 fl.oz	100	2
1 Pint, 16 fl.oz	200	4
Skim (Nonfat):		
2 Tbsp, 1 fl.oz	10	0
1 Glass, 6 fl.oz	60	0
1 Cup, 8 fl.oz	90	0
1 Pint, 16 fl.oz	180	0
Fortified Milk: Per Cup		
Lowfat, 2%, protein fort.	140	5
Skim, protein fortified	100	1
Borden Hi-Calcium	150	8
Condensed: ½ Cup, 4 fl.oz	480	14
Canned, 2 Tbsp, 1 fl.oz	120	4
Evaporated: Per 4 fl.oz		
Whole, ½ cup	170	10
Skim, non-fat, ½ cup	100	<1
Lowfat, ½ cup	110	3
Dried: Whole, ¼ cup, 1 oz	150	9
Skim: ¼ cup, 1 oz	110	<1
Made-up, 1 cup, 8 fl.oz	80	<1
Buttermilk, dry, ¼ cup, 1 oz	100	1
Malted: Reg./Flav., 1 oz	120	2

OTHER MILKS — Per Cup

Acidophilus (Borden), 1% fat	100	2
Buttermilk: Cultured, 1 cup	100	2
Dry/Sweet Cream, 1 Tbsp	25	0
Lowfat (Borden), 1½%	120	4
Lactaid, 1 cup, 8 fl.oz	100	0
Goat's Milk, 1 cup, 8 fl.oz	170	11
Human Milk, 1 cup, 8 fl.oz	170	11
Whey, average, 8 fl.oz	60	1
Dry, ¼ cup	130	<1

FLAVORED MILKS

	CALS	FAT
Chocolate Milk: Average		
Whole Milk, 1 cup, 8 fl.oz	210	8
Lowfat (2% fat), 1 cup	180	5
Lowfat (1% fat), 1 cup	160	3
Skim/Nonfat, 1 cup	140	<1
Hershey's, 8 fl.oz box	150	2
Eggnog, 1 cup, 8 fl.oz	320	18
Milkshakes: Average all flavors		
Whole Milk, 10 fl.oz	325	12
Lowfat, 10 fl.oz	270	7
Cocoa/Coffee/Tea: Page 96		

SOY & RICE DRINKS

Soy Milk, Powdered:		
(1 oz dry makes 1 cup, 8 fl.oz)		
Soyagen, ¼ cup, 1 oz	130	6
Soyamel, ¼ cup, 1 oz	130	7
Ah Soy: Original, 6 fl.oz pouch	110	5
Carob; Chocolate; Vanilla	160	5
Vanilla Creme, 8 fl.oz	140	5
Cocoa Creme, 8 fl.oz	170	6
Amazake (Sweet Rice Drink):		
Original Flavor, 8 fl.oz	203	<1
Almond Shake, 8 fl.oz	272	7
Eden Soy, average, 8 fl.oz	150	4
Ener-G, dry: Soy Quik, 2 Tbsp	60	2
Nut Quik, 2 Tbsp, ½ oz	110	9
Malted (Westbrae): Per 6 fl.oz Pouch		
Almond; Vanilla	250	11
Carob; Cocoa-Mint, Java	270	11
Rice Dream: Almond, 8 fl.oz	240	3
Carob, Chocolate, 8 fl.oz	225	3
Soy Moo (Hlth Valley): 1 cup	120	6
Vita Soy: Creamy Orig., 6 fl.oz	110	5
Vanilla; Carob, 6 fl.oz	150	4
Westsoy, 'All Natural', 8 fl.oz	150	5
Westsoy Lite: Cocoa, 8 fl.oz	140	2
Plain; Vanilla, 8 fl.oz	100	2

MAXIMUM DESIRABLE DAILY FAT INTAKE

1200 Calories — 30 grams	
1500 Calories — 40 grams	
2000 Calories — 60 grams	
2500 Calories — 80 grams	
3000 Calories — 100 grams	

YOGURT

	CALS	FAT (g)
Average All Brands, Per 8 oz		
Plain Yogurt: Whole, 8 oz	180	7
Lowfat	140	4
Nonfat	110	0
Fruit Flavored: Whole, 8 oz	250	6
Lowfat	230	3
Nonfat, regular	150	0
Nonfat, no sugar added	120	0
Goat's Milk Yogurt — Same as Regular.		

YOGURT BRANDS

	CALS	FAT
Borden: Light, 8 oz	120	<1
Lite-Line: Plain, 8 oz	140	2
Fruit Flavors, 8 oz	240	2
Lowfat, fruit, 8 oz	225	4
Breyers: Average, 8 oz	270	5
Colombo: Per 8 oz		
Fruit on the Bottom: Reg.	230	6
Nonfat, average	190	<1
Whole Milk: Plain	160	8
French Vanilla	215	7
Strawberry	210	8
Nonfat Lite: Plain	110	<1
Fruit, average, 8 oz	180	<1
Minipack, 4.4 oz	100	0
Dannon: Light, 8 oz cup	100	0
Minipack, 4.4 oz	60	0
Plain, lowfat, 8 oz	140	4
Plain, nonfat, 8 oz	110	0
Fruit on the Bottom:		
Lemon; Vanilla, 8 oz	200	3
Other flavors, 8 oz	240	3
Knudsen: Cal 70, all flav., 6 oz	70	<1
Light n' Lively (Nonfat):		
Fruit Flavors, aver., 8 oz	90	0
Minipack, 4.4 oz	50	0
Meadow Gold: Per 8 oz		
Lowfat, plain	160	5
Lowfat, flavors, aver.	250	4
Mountain High: Honey Light	190	<1
Fruit Flavors, aver., 8 oz	220	6
Yoplait: Breakfast, aver., 6 oz	230	3
Original: Plain, 6 oz	120	3
Fruit flavors, aver., 6 oz	190	3
Minipack, 4 oz	120	3
Vanilla, 6 oz	180	3
Light, fruit flavors, 6 oz	90	<1
Fat Free 150, 6 oz	150	0
Custard Style, aver., 6 oz	190	4

	CALS	FAT (g)
Weight Watchers:		
Nonfat: Plain, 8 oz	90	<1
Fruited, 8 oz	150	<1
Ultimate 90, 8 oz	90	0

FROZEN YOGURT

	CALS	FAT
Per ½ Cup, 4 fl.oz		
Borden: Average of flavors	100	2
Colombo: Peanut Buttercup	130	7
Bavarian Choc Chunk	130	4
Vanilla Dream; Strawberry	120	2
Rasp. Chs/ck; Carml/Pec.	120	2
Mocca Swiss; Heath Bar Cr.	125	5
Soft Serve: Lowfat, ½ cup	110	2
Colombo Diet, ½ cup	60	0
Dannon: Lo-fat, plain	90	1
Lo-fat Chocolate	140	2
Lo-fat Strawberry/Vanilla	110	2
Nonfat Strawberry/Vanilla	100	0
Nonfat Chocolate/Lemon	110	0
Dreyer's/Edy's: Choc. Chip	135	1
Cookies 'N' Cream	135	1
Marble Fudge	135	1
Other flavors, average	110	1
Elgin: Soft Serve	100	<1
I Can't Believe It's Yogurt:		
Original, small, 6¾ fl.oz	185	5
Nonfat, small	135	0
Sugar-free, small	115	0
Sealtest: Fruit flavors	100	2

21

CHEESES

	CALS	FAT
Average of Natural Hard Cheeses		
(Cheddar, Colby, Coon, Gouda, Swiss)		
1 oz piece	110	9
8 oz package	880	72
16 oz (1 lb) package	1760	144
Cubes: 1" cube, ½ oz	55	5
1¼" cube, 1 oz	110	9
Diced: 1 cup, 4½ oz	500	40
Grated: 1 Tbsp, ¼ oz	27	2
Shredded: ¼ cup, 1 oz	110	9
1 cup, 4 oz	440	36
Sliced: 1 thin (3½" sq.), ¾ oz	85	7
Rectangular (7"x4"x⅛"), 1½ oz	165	14
Round (3¼" diam. x ⅛"), ¾ oz	85	7
Semi-circular, 1¼ oz		
(5½" long, 3½" radius, ⅛" thick)	140	11
Cholesterol Content: 30mg per 1 oz		
Sodium Content: 180mg per 1 oz		

NATURAL CHEESES

Per 1 oz, unless indicated

	CALS	FAT
Babybel/Bonbel (Laughing Cow)		
Mini-cheese: Reg., ¾ oz	70	6
Reduced Calorie, ¾ oz	45	3
Bakers (skim milk), 1 oz	35	<1
Blue/Bleu	100	8
Brick	105	8
Brie	95	8
Camembert: Average, 1 oz	85	7
Caraway	105	8
Cheddar: Regular, average	110	9
Kraft Light Naturals, Mild	80	5
Chedda Delite (Dorman's)	90	7
Cheddar Jack (Dorman's)	90	7
Lorraine Lites	90	6
Weight Watchers	80	5
Chesire	110	9
Colby: Regular	110	9
Churny Lite; Wt Watchers	80	5
Colbi-Lo (Alpine Lace)	80	5
Kraft Lite Naturals	80	5
Cottage Cheese:		
Creamed: 2 Tbsp, 1 oz	30	1
½ cup, 4 oz	120	45
w/fruit, ½ cup, 4 oz	140	4
Lowfat (2%), 2 Tbsp, 1 oz	25	<1
½ cup, 4 oz	100	2

	CALS	FAT
Cottage Cheese (cont.):		
Lowfat (1%), 2 Tbsp, 1 oz	20	<1
½ cup, 4 oz	80	1
Borden Dry Curd (0.5%), 4 oz	80	1
Lite-Line (1.5%), 4 oz	90	2
Light 'n Lively (S'test), 4 oz	90	1
Weight Watchers (1%), 4 oz	90	1
(2%), 4 oz	100	2
Cream Cheese: 2 Tbsp, 1 oz	100	10
Philadelphia: All types	100	10
w/Chvs/Pimento/On./Frt.	90	9
Light Philadelphia	60	5
Edam	100	8
Emmenthal	110	9
Feta (sheep's milk), 1 oz	75	6
½ cup, crumbled, 2½ oz	190	15
Fontina	110	9
Gammelost (skim milk)	60	4
Gjetost	130	9
Gorgonzola	110	9
Gouda	100	8
Gruyere	115	9
Havarti (Casino/Kraft)	120	11
Jarlsberg	105	8
Kanter: Regular	90	7
Lowfat	70	5
Kefir, 2 Tbsp, 1 oz	60	4
½ cup, 4 oz	240	16
Lancashire, Leicester	110	9
Leyden: Regular	90	7
Lowfat	65	5
Liederkranz (Borden)	90	7
Limburger	95	8
Monterey Jack: Average	105	9
Kraft/Casino, with Peppers	110	9
Kraft Light	80	5
Lorraine Lites	90	6
Monti-Jack-Lo (Alpine)	80	5
Slim Jack (Dorman's)	90	7
Mozzarella: Regular, 1 oz	80	6
Low Moisture	90	7
Part Skim, Low Moisture	80	5
Low Sodium (Dorman's)	80	5
Weight Watchers	70	4
Muenster: Regular	110	9
Dorman's, Low Sodium	110	9
Neufchatel	75	7

CHEESES (CONT)

NATURAL CHEESE (CONT)

	CALS	FAT
Parmesan: Hard/Block, 1 oz	110	7
Grated, packaged, 1 oz	140	9
1 rounded Tbsp	35	2
½ cup, 1¾ oz	245	15
Shredded, ½ cup, 1½ oz	170	11

Grated and shredded Parmesan have more calories than block Parmesan, due to a lower moisture content.

Port Salut	100	8
Provolone: Regular	100	5
Dorman's, Low Sodium	90	7
Ricotta Cheese:		
Whole Milk, 2 Tbsp, 1 oz	50	3.5
½ cup, 4½ oz	215	16
Part Skim, 2 Tbsp, 1 oz	40	2
½ cup, 4½ oz	170	10
Lite, red. fat, ½ cup, 4½ oz	110	4
Romano: Block/Hard, 1 oz	110	8
Grated: Kraft, 1 oz	130	9
1 Tbsp, ¼ oz	33	2

(Grated has higher calories than Block due to lower moisture content of grated.)

Rondele, semi-soft: Plain, 1 oz	110	9
Spiced/Herbs, 1 oz	105	9
Roquefort (sheep's milk)	105	9
Sage: Whole Milk	110	9
Part Skim	80	7
Stilton	120	10
Swiss: Average	110	8
Churny Lite	90	5
Dorman's No Salt	100	8
Kraft Light	90	5
Kraft Low Sodium	110	8
Swiss-Lo (Alpine Lace)	100	7
Weight Watchers	90	5
Taco (Kraft)	110	9
Tilsit, Tilsiter	95	8
Wensleydale	110	9
Yogurt Cheese	100	8

CHEESE-NUT BALL LOG

Cracker Barrel: Per 1 oz		
Port W./Shrp/Smky, w/alm.	90	9
Sargento: Swiss, w. almonds	95	9
Cheddar/Port Wine w/alm.	100	10
Wispride: Mini Cheese Balls:		
Ched. & Alm., 1 ball, ½ oz	50	5

PROCESS. CHEESEFOOD & SUBSTITUTES

BORDEN, FISHER, LITELINE

	CALS	FAT
Process Cheese: Per 1 oz		
American: Slices	110	9
Cheese Food	90	7
Light American Singles	70	5
Process Swiss	100	8
Cheese Substitutes: Per 1 oz		
Cheeztwo, 1 oz	90	6
Fisher: Ched-O-Mate	90	7
Pizza Mate	90	7
Sandwich Mate	90	6
Lite-Line, Low Cholesterol	90	7
Lite-Line Cheese Product:		
Amer/Mozz/Ched/Swiss	50	2

CHEEZ-OLA

(Diet & Health, Lima, Ohio)
Low Cholesterol Cheese Product

Cheez-ola: Regular, 1 oz	90	6
Sodium Red. (160mg/1 oz)	90	6
Count Down (Imitation)	40	<1

(Cholest. – Negl; Sodium – 2mg/1 oz)

DELICIA (CHURNY)

American Cheese Substitute	80	6
Colby Imitation Cheese	80	6

FORMAGG

Pizza/Salad Topper; Other var.	75	5
American Flavor	70	5

HEART BEAT (NUCOA)

Heart Beat Process, 1 oz	50	2

KRAFT

Process Cheeses: Swiss	90	7
American; Old English	110	9
Cheese Food: American	90	7
Grated American	130	7
Cracker Barrel, all types	90	7
Velveeta, shredded	100	7
Other varieties	90	7
Golden Image (Imitation):		
Cheddar; Colby	110	9
Light 'n Lively: American	70	4
Kraft Free:		
(Nonfat chs. product), 1 oz	45	0
Spreadery Chse. Snack: 1 oz		
Cheddar; Mexican; Port W.	70	4
Neufchatel varieties	70	6

Continued Next Page

LAND O'LAKES

Process Cheese:	CALS	FAT
American; Cheddar/Bacon	110	9
Sharp American; Cheddar	100	9
Jalapeno Jack	90	8
Cheese Food: Average	90	6
Individual Slices: ¾ oz	70	5
⅔ oz	60	4
Golden Velvet Spread	80	6

LAUGHING COW

Process: Regular, 1 oz	70	6
Reduced Calorie, 1 oz	50	3
Low Calorie, 1 oz	35	2

LO-CHOL (DORMAN'S)

Lo-Chol American, 1 oz	90	7
Lo-Chol Colby	90	6
Lo-Chol Muenster/Swiss	100	7

SOY TOFU SUBSTITUTES

Soy Curd Cheese, 1 oz	40	2
Tofutti Brand: Per 1 oz,		
'Better than Cream Cheese'	80	8
(No cholesterol.)		

WEIGHT WATCHERS

American Slices, 1 oz	50	2
Cheddar Slices; Swiss Slices	50	2

CHEESE SPREADS

Alouette/C'est Light:		
Herb & Garlic, 1 oz	70	6
Garden Vegetables, 1 oz	75	7
French Onion; Garlic, 1 oz	95	9
Kraft: Old English (Per 1 oz)	80	7
Cheese Whiz: All types	80	6
American; Bacon; Garlic	80	6
Mohawk Valley; Limburger	70	6
Squeez-A-Snak: All types	80	7
Velveeta: Mex.; Pimento	80	6
Land O'Lakes: Gld Velv., 1oz	80	6
Laughing Cow: Per 1 oz		
American; Blue; Provolone	72	6
Gruyere, reduced calorie	46	2
Nabisco: Per 1 oz		
Easy Cheese: All varieties	80	6
Weight Watchers: Per 1 oz		
Port Wine/Sharp Chedd. Cup	70	3

DIPS

Per 2 Tbsp (Approx. 1 oz)	CALS	FAT (g)
Avocado/Guacamole Dip, 1 oz	50	4
Baba Ghannouj (Eggplant/Sesame)	70	6
Cheese Base Dips, flavored:		
Cream Cheese: Regular	100	10
Whipped	70	6
Philadelphia Light	30	2
Cottage, creamed	30	1
Neufchatel	75	7
Ricotta	40	2
Cream Base Dips, flavored:		
Half & Half	40	4
Sour Cream	60	6
French Onion, average	50	4
Hummus, 2 Tbsp	50	3
Mayonnaise: Regular	200	24
Light/Calorie Reduced	100	12
Pate, Chicken Liver, aver.	60	4
Skordalia (Greek Potato/Olive)	40	4
Taco Dip, average	12	<1
Tahini (Sesame Seed Butter)	180	8
Taramosalata (Fish Roe Puree)	70	6
Tzatziki (Cucumber/Yogurt)	40	3
Yogurt Base Dip, flavored	40	2

BRAND-NAME DIPS

Per 2 Tbsp (Approx. 1 oz)		
Eagle: Bean Dip	35	2
Frito-Lay: Cheese	45	3
French Onion	60	5
Hain: Taco Dip	12	<1
Bean varieties	35	<1
Kraft, Premium: Per 2 Tbsp, 1 oz		
Avocado (Guacamole) Dip	50	4
Bac.&Onion; Horseradish	50	5
Blue Cheese; Clam	45	4
Creamy; French Onion	45	4
Jalapeno; Nacho; Clam	50	4
Nalley: Avocado; Guacamole	110	12
French Onion	105	11
Jalapeno	110	12

*"Be sure to stay healthy.
You can kill yourself later!"*
(Yiddish Proverb)

ICECREAMS & ICES

Icecream: Average all flavors	CALS	FAT (g)
Reg. (10% fat): 3 fl.oz scoop	105	5
½ Cup, 4 fl.oz	140	7
1 Pint, 16 fl.oz	640	28
½ Gallon	2200	110
Rich (16% fat): 2½ fl.oz scoop	160	9
½ Cup, 4 fl.oz	260	14
½ Gallon	4160	224
Soft Serve, ½ cup	180	9
Ice Milk: Average all flavors		
Hard (4% fat), ½ cup	100	3
Soft Serve (3% fat), ½ cup	110	2
Icecream Cones/Cups: Average		
Regular Cone	20	<1
Sugar Cone	40	<1
Vanilla Cup	15	<1
Waffle Cone	100	<1
Waffle Bowl	60	<1

BASKIN-ROBBINS

Deluxe Ice Cream: Per 1 Scoop		
Choc; Jamoca Almond Fudge	270	14
Chocolate Chip	260	15
Daiquiri Ice; Red Rasp. Sorbet	140	0
French Vanilla	280	18
Pralines 'n Cream	280	14
Rainbow Sherbet	160	2
Rocky Road	300	14
Vanilla	240	14
Very Berry Strawberry	220	10
World Class Chocolate	280	14
Intl. Cr: Choc.Raspb. Trifle	310	17
Low-Lite: Banana, ½ cup	100	1
Cones: Sugar Cone	60	1
Waffle Cone	140	2

(See Fast Foods for other nutrient data.)

BORDEN

Per ½ Cup (4 fl.oz)		
Buttered Pecan (Lady Borden)	180	12
Chocolate Swirl; Strawberry	130	6
Dutch Choc. (Olde Fashioned)	130	6
Strawberries 'n Cream	130	5
Vanilla (Eagle Brand)	150	9
Vanilla (Olde Fashioned)	130	7
Ice Milk: Chocolate, ½ cup	100	2
Strawberry/Vanilla, ½ cup	90	2
Orange Sherbet, ½ cup	110	1

DAIRY QUEEN

See Fast Foods Section (Page 115).

DREYER'S OR EDY'S

GRAND ICE CREAM Per ½ Cup (4 fl.oz)	CALS	FAT (g)
Almond Praline	150	7
Black Cherry Vanilla	140	7
Butter Pecan; Candy Bar	160	9
California Crunch	170	9
Chocolate; Mint Choc. Chip	160	9
Chocolate Chip	150	9
Chocolate Chocolate Chip	160	10
Coffee	140	8
Cookies 'n Cr; Caramel Nut	160	9
Double Trouble	170	13
French Vanilla	160	10
Malt Ball 'n/Marble Fudge	150	8
Mocha Almond Fudge	160	9
Mom's Lemon Cream Pie	160	8
Rocky Road	170	10
Strawberry	130	6
Toasted Almond	150	9
Vanilla; Van. Choc. Strawb.	160	10
GRAND LIGHT — Per 4 fl.oz		
Almond Praline	140	5
Banana-Politan	110	4
Butter Pecan; Candy Bar	140	4
Cafe Au Lait	110	4
Chocolate Chip	120	4
Chocolate Fudge Mousse	130	4
Cookies 'n Cream	120	5
Dreamy Caramel Cream	140	4
Malt Ball 'n Fudge	140	5
Marble Fudge	120	4
Mocha Almond Fudge	140	5
Peanut Butter & Chocolate	130	5
Raspberry Truffle	110	5
Rocky Road	130	5
Strawberry; Van.Choc.Strawb.	110	4
Vanilla	100	4
AMERICAN DREAM - Per 4 fl.oz		
Chocolate	120	1
Choc. Chip; Cookies 'n Cr.	135	1
Mocha Almond Fudge	145	1
Rocky Road; Toasted Almond	145	1
Strawberry	95	<1
Vanilla	105	<1
Vanilla-Chocolate-Strawberry	105	<1

(Continued Next Page.)

25

ICECREAMS & ICES (CONT)

DREYER'S OR EDY'S (CONT)

FROZEN DESSERTS

	CALS	FAT
Dietary Dairy Dessert: Per 3 fl.oz		
Chocolate, 1 scoop, 3 fl.oz	110	3
Marble Fudge	120	3
Vanilla	100	3
Nonfat Frozen Dairy Dessert:		
Strawberry, 1 scoop, 3 fl.oz	70	<1
Chocolate Chip	100	1

DOLE BARS

Fruit 'n Juice: Pina Colada	90	3
Other types	70	0
Fruit & Cream: Choc./Banana	175	9
Chocolate/Strawberry	140	8
Other types	90	1
Fruit & Yogurt: All types	75	<1
Fresh Lites: All types	25	<1
Sun Tops: All types	40	<1

ESKIMO PIE

Bars: Dark Choc., 3 fl.oz	180	12
5 fl.oz size	280	21
Sugar Free, 2½ fl.oz	140	11
w/Crisped Rice, 2½ fl.oz	150	11
Choc. Fudge Bar, 2½ fl.oz	90	0
Kreme Kooler	80	2
Sandwiches: Ice Cream	180	6
Sugar Free	170	6
Fat Freedom	130	0
Sugar Free Cone, 3.4 fl.oz	210	12

"Of course we want you to eat properly, but you're practising too much!"

FLAV·O·RICH

Per ½ Cup (4 fl.oz)	CALS	FAT (g)
Butter Almond/Pecan	150	9
Chocolate/Choc. Chip	150	7
Coffee; Peach	130	7
Cookies 'N Cr.; Heavenly Hash	160	8
Fudge Ripple; Neopolitan	140	7
Strawberry	130	6
Swiss Choc. Almond	170	10
Vanilla; Spumoni	140	7
Vanilla (Old Fashioned)	150	8

FRUSEN GLADJE

Butter Pecan (Per ½ cup)	280	16
Chocolate	240	15
Chocolate Chip, Choc/Vanilla	270	17
Mocha Chip; Praline & Cream	280	17
Strawberry	250	16
Swiss Almond Chocolate	270	17
Vanilla: Reg./Raspb. Swirl	230	14
Swiss Almond	270	18
Toffee Chunk	270	17

HAAGEN·DAZS

Per ½ Cup (4 fl.oz)		
Blueberry & Cream	190	8
Butter Pecan	290	17
Chocolate; Coffee	270	17
Choc Choc Chip/Mint	290	18
Deep Choc Fudge	300	15
Deep Choc Peanut	330	19
Honey	250	16
Lime & Cream	190	8
Macadamia Nut	330	24
Macadamia Brittle	290	18
Maple Walnut	310	25
Mocha Double Nut	290	20
Orange & Cream	200	8
Raspberry & Cream	180	7
Rum Raisin; Strawberry	250	17
Vanilla; Vanilla Fudge	260	17
Vanilla Swiss Almond	290	19
Vanilla Peanut Butter Swirl	280	20
BARS: Deep Choc: All flavors	320	21
Vanilla: w. Milk Chocolate	290	20
with Semi-Sweet Choc.	310	22

ICECREAMS & ICES (CONT)

NESTLE (BARS)

	CALS	FAT
Alpine White Candytops	250	18
Crunch: Chocolate; Vanilla	190	12
Lite	150	10
Milk Choc. with Almonds	350	23
Quik; 100 Grand Candytops	210	14
Oh Henry!	320	20

SIMPLE PLEASURES

Frozen Dairy Dessert
(with Simplesse fat substitute)

Coffee; Strawberry, ½ cup	120	<1
Rum Raisin; Toffee Crunch	130	<1
Peach, ½ cup, 4 fl.oz	135	<1
Chocolate, ½ cup	140	<1

WEIGHT WATCHERS

Per ½ Cup (4 fl.oz)

Choc., Vanilla, Neopolitan	100	3
Pecan, Choc. Chip Swirl	120	3
Fudge Marble; Strawb./Creme	120	3
Choc. Fudge; Swiss Vanilla	105	3
BARS: Chocolate Dip	110	7
Chocolate Treat	100	1
Choc. Mousse; Fruit Juice	35	<1
Peanut Butter Fudge	60	<1
Double Fudge; Choc. Mint Tr.	60	1
Sugar Free Orange Vanilla	30	<1
Vanilla Sandwich	150	3

TOFUTTI

Non-Dairy Frozen Desserts
(Nil cholesterol, nil lactose.)

Tofutti (Hard) — Per ½ Cup, 4 fl.oz

Better Pecan, ½ cup, 4 fl.oz	240	17
Chocolate; Wildberry	210	13
Chocolate Cookies Supreme	230	13
Deep Choc. Fudge; Vanilla	200	10
Vanilla Almond Bark	230	14
Tofutti (Soft Serve): Vanilla	160	8
Lite Lite Tofutti: Choc. Fdge	100	<1
All other flavors	90	<1
Tofutti Cuties: All flav., each	130	5
Better Than Cheesecake:		
Blueb; P/apple, 1 sl., 3½ oz	210	10
Choc; Choc. Brownie, 3½ oz	280	18
Better Than Yogurt, 4 fl.oz	70	<1

MISCELLANEOUS ICECREAMS, ICES, BARS

	CALS	FAT
Believe: Chocolate, 4 fl.oz	260	17
Raspberry, ½ cup, 4 fl.oz	190	1
Vanilla, ½ cup, 4 fl.oz	240	12
Borden: Light Dream Pops	30	0
Ice Pop, regular	40	0
Carnation: Bon Bons, 5 pce	170	12
Heaven, average	225	13
Crystal Light: All flavors	14	0
Cool N' Crmy: Orange; Van.	30	1
Other flavors, average	55	2
Drumstick	185	10
Fudgesicle	90	0
Fla-Vor-Ice: Regular size	30	0
Fudge Sundae (Bak.Fudgetastic)	220	15
Jell-O: Pops Bars	35	0
Pudding Bars	80	2
Snowburst	45	0
Klondike, Lite w/choc coating	140	10
Kool-Aid Pops	40	0
Cream Pops	50	2
Light N' Lively: Choc., ½ cup	110	3
Oreo: Cookies 'n Cream Bar	220	15
Sandwich	240	11
Popsicles: Big Stick	80	0
Regular Ice Pop	50	0
Sugar-free: Ice Pop	18	0
Creamsicle	25	1
Fudge Pops	35	1
Rice Dream: Vanilla, ½ cup	130	5
Sealtest (Kraft/Knudsen):		
Chocolate, ½ cup, 4 fl.oz	140	6
Fat Free, Choc., ½ cup	100	0
Fat Free Bars, 1 bar	90	0
Sherbet: Borden/Dryers, ½ cup	110	1
Land O'Lakes, all flav., ½ c	130	2
Sorbet: Fruit (no fat), ½ cup	110	0
Shamitoff, Choc/Cocon, ½ c	280	15
Haagen-Dazs: Oran./Vanilla	210	9
Raspb./Vanilla, ½ cup	180	9
3 Musketeers, Van/Choc Bars	170	10
Vitari, soft serve, 4 fl.oz	80	0
Welch's Fruit Juice Bars:		
All flavors, 1¾ fl.oz bar	45	0
3 fl.oz bar	80	0
No Sugar Added, 1 bar	25	0
Fruit & Cream, 1 bar	45	0

FATS, SPREADS, OILS

BUTTER & MARGARINE

	CALS	FAT (g)
Butter, Margarine, Blends		
Regular: 1 tsp, 5g	35	4
1 Pat, 5g	35	4
1 Tbsp, approx. ½ oz	100	11
2 Tbsp, 1 oz	205	23
1 Stick/½ cup, 4 oz	810	92
1 Pound, 2 cups, 16 oz	3240	368
Whipped: 1 tsp, 4g	25	3
1 Tbsp, 11g	80	9
1 Stick, ½ cup, 2⅔ oz	540	61
Unsalted: Same as Salted		

REDUCED FAT MARGARINE & SPREADS

Per Tbsp

	CALS	FAT (g)
Blue Bonnet: Light Tasty	60	7
Diet/Soft, whipped	70	7
Chiffon Whipped, 1 Tbsp	70	8
Fleischmann's Light	80	8
'I Can't Believe It's Not Butter!'	90	10
Imperial Light, 1 Tbsp	60	6
Kraft: 'Touch of Butter'		
40% fat (bowl)	50	6
50% fat (stick)	60	7
Land O'Lakes: Country Morn. Blend,		
Light Soy Oil Sprd. (64%)	75	9
Mother's Spread, 1 Tbsp	70	8
Mrs Filbert's Spread 25	80	8
Miracle: Whipped bowl	60	7
Stick	70	7
Nucoa, HeartBeat Margarine	25	3
Parkay: Margarine, whipped	60	7
Soft Diet, reduced cal.	50	5
Spreads: 50% Veg. Oil	60	7
Light Corn Oil	70	8
Squeeze Spread	90	10
Promise, 1 Tbsp	90	10
Shedd's Spread, Squeezable	80	9
Weight Watchers, Light	50	6

FOR COMPARISON

	CALS	FAT (g)
Mayonnaise: Regular, 1 Tbsp	100	11
Light, average, 1 Tbsp	50	5
(See Salad Dressings for extra listings.)		
Peanut Butter, 1 Tbsp	100	8
Avocado, mashed, 1 Tbsp	25	2.5

COOKING FATS & OILS

ANIMAL FATS	CALS	FAT (g)
Average all types:		
(Beef Tallow/Drippings, Lard (Pork),		
Chicken, Duck, Goose, Turkey)		
1 Tbsp, 13g	115	13
2¼ Tbsp, 1 oz	255	28
1 Cup, 7¼ oz	1850	205
½ Pound, 8 oz	2040	227
Ghee/Butter Oil: 1 Tbsp, 13g	110	13
2¼ Tbsp, 1 oz	250	28

VEGETABLE SHORTENING

Average all types (e.g. Crisco):	CALS	FAT (g)
1 Tbsp	113	13
2¼ Tbsp, 1 oz	250	28
1 Cup, 7¼ oz	1810	205

VEGETABLE OILS

All types: Includes almond, canola, corn, coconut, grapeseed, linseed, palm, peanut, rice-bran, safflower, sesame, sunflower, soybean, wheatgerm.

	CALS	FAT (g)
1 tsp	45	5
1 Tbsp	120	14
2 Tbsp, 1 oz	250	28
1 Cup, 7¾ oz	1930	218

SPRAYS, SPRINKLES

	CALS	FAT (g)
No-Stick Sprays (Pam, Mazola):		
Negl. cals/fat per serving	2	<1
2-3 second spray	8	1
Butter Buds, 1 serving, ½ tsp	4	<1
Molly McButter, ½ tsp	4	<1

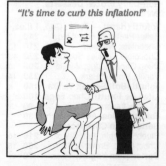

"It's time to curb this inflation!"

CREAM

CREAM

	CALS	FAT
Half & Half Cream: 1 Tbsp	20	2
1 Cup	315	28
Light, coffee/table (20% fat),		
1 Tbsp	30	3
1 Cup	470	46
Medium (25% fat), 1 Tbsp	40	4
Sour Cream: Regular, 1 Tbsp	30	3
1 Cup	490	48
Light, 1 Tbsp	20	1
Half & Half, 1 Tbsp	20	2
Whipping Cream:		
Heavy (37% fat):		
1 Tbsp fluid/2 Tbsp whipped	50	6
¼ cup whipped	100	12
½ cup fluid/1 cup whipped	410	44
Light (30% fat):		
1 Tbsp fluid/2 Tbsp whipped	45	5
½ cup fluid/1 cup whipped	350	37

WHIPPED TOPPINGS

	CALS	FAT
Cream:		
Pressurized, aver., 1 Tbsp	10	1
¼ cup (Kraft Real Cr.)	30	2
Frozen, ¼ cup	25	2
Imitation Cream: Per ¼ Cup (4 Tbsp)		
Birds Eye Cool Whip: Lite	30	2
Extra Creamy, ¼ cup	55	4
Non-Dairy	50	4
Dream Whip, prep. w/milk	40	4
D-Zerta, reduced cal.	30	4
Featherweight, 2 Tbsp	8	0
Kraft Whipped Topping, ¼ c.	35	3
La Creme, ¼ cup	50	4
Reddi-wip Lite, 1 Tbsp	6	<1
¼ cup/4 Tbsp	24	2

COFFEE CREAMERS

	CALS	FAT
Powder: Per Rounded tsp (3g)		
Coffee-Mate, Cremora: Reg.	16	1
Light	12	<1
Liquid: Coffee-Mate, 1 Tbsp	16	1
Mocha Mix, 1 Tbsp	19	1
Farm Rich, 1 Tbsp	18	2
Non-Dairy Imitation Cream:		
Powdered, 1 Tbsp	35	2
Frozen, 1 fl.oz	40	3
1 Cup	325	24
Sour, 1 Tbsp	30	3

EGGS

	CALS	FAT (g)
Chicken Egg:		
Raw, weight with shell		
Jumbo, 2½ oz	100	7
Extra Large, 2¼ oz	90	6
Large, 2 oz (USDA, 1989 fig.)	75	5
Medium, 1¾ oz	70	5
Small, 1½ oz	65	4
Egg Yolk, 1 large	60	5
Egg White, 1 large	15	0
Dried: Whole, ¼ cup, 1 oz	170	12
Eggwhite, 1 oz	105	0
Fried: 2 large with 1 tsp fat	100	8
Dry-fried, non-stick pan	75	5
Scrambled: 1 large egg		
w. 1 Tbsp milk & 1 tsp fat	120	9
with skim milk, no fat	80	5
1 Egg + 2 whites, no fat	110	5
Omelette: Plain, 2 lge eggs	230	19
+ ½ oz cheese	280	23
Spanish, 3 eggs	425	32
(w. cheese, butter, tomato)		
Eggnog, ½ cup, 4 fl.oz	160	8
Other Eggs: Duck, Turkey	130	10
Goose egg	275	19

EGG SUBSTITUTES

Equivalent to 1 Egg

	CALS	FAT
Egg Beaters (Fleischm.), ¼ cup	25	0
Egg Magic (F/weight), ½ pkg	60	2
Egg Watchers (Tofutti), 2 oz	55	2
Eggstra, ½ envelope	50	2
Scramblers (M/St. Farms) ¼ c	60	2

Note: Above products contain no cholesterol.

EGG DISHES

	CALS	FAT
Devilled Eggs: Reg. 2 halves	140	13
Lowfat (½ yolk), 2 halves	70	4
Quiche: Regular, 5 oz	350	26
Lowfat (cott. chse., skim milk)	160	7
Souffle, cheese, 1 cup, 3½ oz	210	16

FAST FOOD OUTLETS

	CALS	FAT
Burger King: Scr. Egg Platter	550	34
Carls: Scrambled Eggs	120	9
Jack In The Box: Scr. Eggs	430	21
McDonalds: Egg McMuffin	290	11
Scrambled Eggs	140	10
Roy Rogers: Egg & Bisc. Plat.	395	27

Extra Listings — See Fast Foods Section.

Note: Cooking reduces weight of meat by 20-45% due to water and fat losses. Average weight loss is 30%. Actual loss depends on cooking method and cooking time. Examples:

4 oz raw wt. = approx. 3 oz cooked wt.
4 oz cooked wt. = approx. 5½ oz raw wt.

WHAT 3 oz COOKED MEAT LOOKS LIKE

● Half the size of this book (4¼" x 3" x ⅜" thick)
● Rectangular piece (4" x 2½" x ½" thick)
● Pack of cards (3½" x 2½" x ⅝" thick)

STEAK READY RECKONER

SIRLOIN (Choice Grade) External fat trimmed to ¼"	CALS	FAT (g)
BROILED, Edible Portion (no bone)		
Small Serving, 3 oz		
(3 oz cooked, from 4-4½ oz raw)		
Lean + fat (¼"), 3 oz	**230**	14
Lean + marbling, 3 oz	**195**	10
(External fat trimmed **before** cooking)		
Lean only, 3 oz	**170**	7
(No external fat or marbling)		
Medium/Regular Serving, 5 oz		
(from approx. 7 oz raw)		
Lean + fat (¼"), 5 oz	**470**	29
Lean + marbling, 5 oz	**400**	20
Lean only, 5 oz	**350**	14
Large Serving, 8 oz		
(from 11-12 oz raw)		
Lean + fat, 8 oz	**610**	38
Lean + marbling, 8 oz	**520**	26
Lean only, 8 oz	**454**	18
Extra Large Serving, 12 oz		
(from approx. 16-17 oz raw)		
Lean + fat (¼"), 12 oz	**915**	57
Lean + marbling, 12 oz	**780**	39
Lean only, 12 oz	**680**	27
PAN-FRIED		
Sirloin (choice), medium serving:		
Lean + fat (¼"), 5 oz	**450**	32
Lean only, 5 oz	**330**	15

HINT TO SAVE FAT & CALORIES

Save extra calories with broiled steak by trimming off the external fat **before** cooking. This prevents external fat liquefying and migrating into the lean meat.

OTHER STEAKS

Filet Mignon (Tenderloin):	CALS	FAT (g)
1 medium steak, 6 oz raw wt.		
Broiled, with ¼" fat trim		
Lean + fat (¼"), 4 oz	**340**	24
Lean only, 3½ oz	**210**	10
Broiled, (¼" fat removed before cooking)		
Lean + marbling, 3¼ oz	**220**	12
Lean only, 3 oz	**180**	8

New York/Club Steak:		
Top Loin/Short Loin		
1 steak, regular (9¼ oz raw, ¼" fat)		
Broiled:		
Lean + fat (¼"), 6¼ oz	**510**	35
Lean + marbling, 5½ oz	**330**	16
Lean only, 5¼ oz	**310**	14

Porterhouse Steak:		
1 medium, 6 oz raw wt. (no bone)		
Broiled: Lean + fat (¼"), 4¼ oz	**370**	27
Lean only, 3½ oz	**220**	11

T-Bone Steak:		
1 medium, 8 oz raw wt.		
Broiled: Lean + fat	**380**	27
Lean only	**220**	10

AVERAGE ALL CUTS

Average all Retail Cuts
Edible weight (no bone)

RAW		
(1 lb raw yields approx. 11-12 oz cooked)		
Lean + fat (¼" trim), 1 oz	**70**	5.5
½ Pound, 8 oz	**560**	44
Lean only, 1 oz	**40**	2
½ Pound, 8 oz	**320**	16
Fat only, 1 oz	**190**	20

COOKED (No Added Fat)		
Lean + fat (¼"), 1 oz	**86**	6
Small serving, 3 oz	**260**	18
Lean + marbling, (no ext. fat), 1 oz	**78**	5
Small serving, 3 oz	**235**	15
Lean only, 1 oz	**60**	3
Small serving, 3 oz	**180**	9
Fat only, 1 oz	**193**	20

BEEF — INDIVIDUAL CUTS

Average All Grades Edible Weight (no bone)	CALS	FAT (g)
Brisket, whole, braised:		
Lean + fat (¼"), 3 oz	330	27
Lean + marbling, 3 oz	250	17
Lean only, 3 oz	205	11
Chuck, blade, braised:		
Lean + fat (¼"), 3 oz	290	22
Lean + marbling, 3 oz	285	20
Lean only, 3 oz	210	11
Flank: Raw, 4 oz	200	12
Braised, 3 oz	225	14
Broiled, 3 oz	190	11
Ribs, whole (ribs 6-12):		
Average all grades, roasted		
(1lb raw yields 10¼ oz roasted)		
Lean + fat (¼")		
(3.6 oz w/bone, 3 oz no bone)	300	25
Lean only, 3 oz (no bone)	200	11
Round, bottom, braised:		
Lean + fat (¼"), 3 oz	235	14
Lean only, 3 oz	180	7
Round, eye/tip, roasted:		
Lean + fat (¼"), 3 oz	200	11
Lean, 3 oz	145	4
Round, top, Per 3 oz:		
Braised, Lean + fat	210	10
Lean only	175	5
Broiled, Lean + fat	185	8
Lean only	155	4
Pan-fried, Lean + fat	235	13
Lean only	190	7

GROUND BEEF

	CALS	FAT
Raw: Reg. (73% lean), 4 oz	350	30
Lean (80% lean), 4 oz	300	24
Extra lean (85% lean)	250	17
Baked/Broiled: Reg., 3 oz	250	18
Lean, 3 oz	230	16
Extra lean, 3 oz	200	12
Pan-fried: Regular, 3 oz	260	19
Lean, 3 oz	230	16
Extra lean, 3 oz	200	12
Ground Beef Patties: Average		
Frozen, raw, 4 oz	320	26
Broiled, 3 oz	240	17

LAMB

CHOICE GRADE	CALS	FAT (g)
Leg (Whole), roasted:		
Lean + fat, 3 oz	220	14
Lean only, 3 oz	160	7
Leg (Sirloin Half), roasted:		
Lean + fat, 3 oz	250	18
Lean only, 3 oz	175	8
Leg (Shank Half), roasted:		
Lean + fat, 3 oz	190	11
Lean only, 3 oz	155	6
Loin Chop, broiled:		
1 chop (raw wt., 4¼ oz):		
Lean + fat (2¼ oz edible)	200	15
Lean only (1.6 oz edible)	100	5
Rib Chop, broiled/roasted:		
1 chop (raw wt., 3½ oz)		
Lean + fat (2½ oz edible)	255	21
Lean only (1¾ oz edible)	120	7
Shoulder (Arm/Blade):		
Braised: Lean + fat, 3 oz	290	21
Lean only, 3 oz	240	14
Broiled: Lean + fat, 3 oz	240	16
Lean only, 3 oz	180	9
Roasted: Similar to Broiled		
Cubed Lamb (Leg/Shoulder):		
For stew or kabob		
Raw, lean only, 8 oz	310	12
Braised, lean only, 3 oz	190	8
Broiled, lean only, 3 oz	160	6
New Zealand Lamb (Imported):		
Similar calories and fat to domestic.		

VEAL

Edible weights	CALS	FAT
Leg (Top Round):		
Braised: Lean + fat, 3 oz	180	6
Lean only, 3 oz	170	5
Pan-fried, breaded:		
Lean + fat, 3 oz	195	8
Lean only, 3 oz	175	6
Pan-fried, not breaded:		
Lean + fat, 3 oz	180	7
Lean only, 3 oz	155	4
Roasted: Lean + fat, 3 oz	135	4
Lean only, 3 oz	130	3

Continued Next Page.

VEAL (CONT)

	CALS	FAT
Loin Chop: 1 chop, 7 oz raw wt.		
Braised: Lean + fat	**230**	14
Lean only	**155**	6
Roasted: Lean + fat	**175**	10
Lean only	**125**	5
Rib, roasted: Lean + fat, 3 oz	**195**	12
Lean only, 3 oz	**150**	7
Shoulder, Arm/Blade, roasted:		
Lean + fat, 3 oz	**155**	7
Lean only, 3 oz	**145**	6
Sirloin, roasted:		
Lean + fat, 3 oz	**170**	9
Lean only, 3 oz	**145**	6
Cubed for Stew, braised:		
Leg/Shoulder, lean only, 3 oz	**160**	4
(1 lb raw wt. yields 9¼ oz cooked)		

PORK

Figures based on NLMB data (1990)

FRESH PORK (Cooked Wt., no bone)
(4 oz raw wt. = approx. 3 oz cooked wt.)

	CALS	FAT
Blade Steak, broiled:		
Lean + fat, 3 oz	**220**	15
Lean only, 3 oz	**190**	11
Country Style Ribs, broiled:		
Lean + fat, 3 oz	**270**	22
Lean only, 3 oz	**205**	13
Leg (Ham), roasted:		
Lean + fat, 3 oz	**250**	18
Lean only, 3 oz	**180**	9
(Ham, cured — See Cold Meats)		
Loin Chops, broiled: Average		
(From 1 chop: 5 oz raw wt. w/bone or 4 oz raw wt., no bone)		
Lean + fat, 3 oz	**200**	11
Lean only, 3 oz	**165**	7
Rib Chops, broiled:		
Lean + fat, 3 oz	**215**	13
Lean only, 3 oz	**180**	7
Rib Roast, roasted:		
Lean + fat, 3 oz	**210**	13
Lean only, 3 oz	**175**	9
Loin Roast, roasted:		
Lean + fat, 3 oz	**190**	10
Lean only, 3 oz	**160**	7
Back Ribs, broiled:		
Lean + fat	**310**	25

PORK (CONT)

	CALS	FAT
Sirloin Chop, broiled:		
Lean + fat, 3 oz	**175**	8
Lean only, 3 oz	**155**	6
Sirloin Roast, roasted:		
Lean + fat, 3 oz	**215**	14
Lean only, 3 oz	**180**	9
Tenderloin, roasted:		
Lean + fat, 3 oz	**140**	4
Lean only, 3 oz	**135**	4
GROUND PORK		
Raw: Average, ¼ lb, 4 oz	**300**	24
Broiled, 3 oz	**245**	18
Pan-fried, drained, 3 oz	**250**	19

BACON, HAMS

BACON

	CALS	FAT
Raw: 1 med. slice (20/lb), ¾ oz	**125**	13
1 thick slice (12/lb), 1⅓ oz	**210**	22
(1 lb raw yields approx. 5 oz cooked)		
Broiled/Pan-fried: 1 md. sl., 6g	**36**	3
3 medium slices	**110**	9
1 thick slice, 12g	**70**	6
Canadian-style Bacon:		
As purchased, 1 sl., 1 oz	**45**	4
Cooked, 1 slice	**43**	4
Bacon Bits, 1 Tbsp, ¼ oz	**20**	1
Breakfast Strips:		
Broiled, 1 slice, 12g	**50**	4

HAM

	CALS	FAT
Boneless Ham, cooked:		
Regular, (approx. 11% fat):		
Unheat. (as purch.), 1 oz	**52**	3
Roasted, 3 oz	**150**	8
Extra Lean (5% fat):		
Unheated, 1 oz	**37**	2
Roasted, 3 oz	**125**	5
Whole Ham, cooked:		
Lean + fat (as purchased)		
Unheated, 1 oz	**70**	5
Roasted, 3 oz	**345**	26
Lean only, unheated, 1 oz	**40**	2
Roasted, 3 oz	**135**	5
Canned Ham: Similar to boneless ham		
Chopped, canned, 3 oz	**260**	21
Ham Patties, ckd, 1 pty, 2¼ oz	**205**	18
Ham Steak, extra lean, 2 oz	**70**	2
Ham Slices: See Cold Processed Meats.		

MEATS (CONT)

GAME MEATS

	CALS	FAT
Antelope, roasted, 3 oz	130	3
Buffalo, roasted, 3 oz	160	6
Boar (wild), roasted, 3 oz	140	4
Caribou, roasted, 3 oz	140	4
Deer/Venison, roasted, 3 oz	135	3
Rabbit: Roasted, 3 oz	130	6
Stewed, 1 cup, diced, 5 oz	300	14

VARIETY & ORGAN MEATS

Per 3 oz, Edible Weight

	CALS	FAT
Brains: Braised, 3 oz	130	9
Pan-fried, 3 oz	200	14
Chitterlings, pork, simmered	260	25
Ears, pork, simmered, 1 ear	180	12
Feet, pork: Simmered, 3 oz	165	11
Cured, pickled	170	14
Heart: Aver., braised, 3 oz	140	5
Jowl, pork, raw, 4 oz	750	80
Kidneys, simmered, 3 oz	130	4
Liver: Raw, 4 oz	160	5
Braised, 3 oz	140	4
Pan-fried, 3 oz	200	9
Chicken, 4 livers, ckd, 3 oz	195	
Pancreas, braised, 3 oz	200	13
Spleen, braised, 3 oz	130	4
Stomach, pork, raw, 4 oz	180	11
Sweetbreads: Beef, ckd., 3 oz	270	20
Lamb, cooked, 3 oz	150	5
Tail, pork, simmered, 3 oz	340	31
Tongue, braised, 3 oz:		
Beef/Lamb/Pork, aver.	240	17
Veal	170	9
Tripe, beef, raw, 4 oz	110	5
Tallow, Lard — See Fats.		

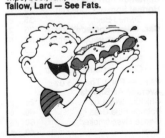

SAUSAGES

FRESH SAUSAGES

Pork/Beef: Aver. all types	CALS	FAT
Medium size, 2 oz: Raw	235	23
Broiled/Pan-fried	100	8
Small, 1 oz: Raw	120	12
Broiled/Pan-fried	50	4

(Note: Fat is lost in broiling/pan-frying.
Cooked wt. = approx. 60-70% raw wt.)

Turkey, Shelton's Brand:		
Breakfast Saus., 1.7 oz: Raw	115	10
Broiled/Pan-fried	70	6
Italian Sausage: Raw, 2 oz	135	12
Broiled/Pan-fried	90	7

FRANKS & WEINERS

Average All Brands
Regular/Smoked: Per Frank

	CALS	FAT
2 oz link (8/16 oz pkg)	180	16
1.6 oz link (10/16 oz pkg)	140	13
1½ oz link (8/12 oz pkg)	135	12
1.2 oz link (10/12 oz pkg)	110	10
1 oz link (16/16 oz pkg)	90	8
Small/Little (50/lb), each	30	3

Light/Fat-reduced (Osc. Mayer):

2 oz link (8/16 oz pkg)	130	11
1 oz link (16/16 oz pkg)	70	6

Pork: Eckrich, reg., 2 oz | 260 | 26
Brown 'n Serve (Swift)	95	9
Jimmy Dean, cooked	140	13
Little Friers (Osc. Mayer)	80	8

Turkey Franks:

Louis Rich: Reg. (8/16 oz), 2 oz	130	11
(8/12 oz pkg), 1½ oz	100	9
Cheese (10/16 oz pkg), 1.6 oz	110	7
Shelton's: 1 frank, 1.2 oz	80	6
Chicken Franks (Shelt.), 1.2 oz	95	8

HOT DOGS, CORN DOGS

HOT DOGS, Ready-To-Go
(Includes Ketchup/Relish)

	CALS	FAT
Small (1 oz furter/1 oz roll)	200	8
Regular (1½ oz furter/2 oz roll)	280	16
Large (2 oz furter/2 oz roll)	330	24
Super/Giant (3 oz furter/3 oz roll)	520	27
Extras: Chili Sce — Add 40 calories/3g fat		
Cheese — Add 50 calories/5g fat		
Mustard — Add 15 calories/nil fat		

CORN DOGS

Beef/Pork frank, average	250	17
Turkey: *Gobblers!* (Shelton's)	220	11

COLD MEATS (PROCESSED)

HAM, LUNCHEON, SAUSAGE

Abbrev. (O.M.) = Oscar Mayer

Average All Brands	CALS	FAT
Bar-B-Q Loaf (O.M.), 1 oz	45	2
Beef, chopped, smoked, 1 oz	40	2
Beef Jerky, 6" stick, 0.2 oz	25	1
Berliner (pork/beef), 1 sl., ¾ oz	50	4
Blood Sausage, 1 slice, 1 oz	100	9
Bologna: Regular, aver., 1 oz	90	8
Light, average, 1 oz	70	6
Bratwurst, 1 oz	90	8
Braunschweiger: Hormel, 1 oz	80	7
Eckrich, 1 oz	70	6
Oscar Mayer, 1 oz	100	9
Chicken Breast: Smoked (O.M.)	25	<1
Oven-roasted (O.M.), 1 oz	30	<1
Louis Rich, 1 oz	40	2
Chicken Roll, 1 slice, 1 oz	45	2
Corned Beef, jellied, 1 oz	30	1
1 thin slice (O.M.), 0.6 oz	16	<1
Ham, deviled, 1 Tbsp	35	3
Ham, luncheon:		
Regular (11% fat), 1 oz	52	3
Lean (5% fat), 1 oz	37	1.5
Oscar Mayer, Jubilee:		
Boneless, 1 oz	45	3
Chopped (Light), 1 oz	40	2
Canned, 1 oz	30	1
Smoked, sliced, ¾ oz	20	<1
Armour: Chopped, 1 oz	80	6
Boneless, lower salt	35	2
Canned (star), 1 oz	40	2
Hormel: Chopped, 1 oz	55	3
Light & Lean, 1 oz	35	2
Eckrich: Chopped, ¾ oz	35	2
Ham Loaf, 1 oz	70	6
Ham & Chse. Loaf (O.M.), 1 oz	70	5
Head Cheese (O.M.), 1 oz	60	4
Italian Sausage, 1 oz	90	7
Kielbasa (Polish Saus.), 1 oz	85	7
Knockwurst, 1 oz	90	8
Livercheese, 1 slice, 1⅓ oz	115	10
Liver Pate, aver., 2 Tbsp, 1 oz	100	9
Liverwurst, 1 oz	95	8
Luncheon Meat, average, 1 oz	90	8
Mortadella, 1 oz	95	8
New Engl. Brand Saus., 1 oz	40	2
Old Fash./Olive Lf. (O.M.), 1 oz	60	4

	CALS	FAT
Pastrami, Beef, 1 oz	100	8
Osc. Mayer, 2 sl., 1 oz	32	<1
Pepperoni, average, 3 sl., 1 oz	140	13
Salami: (Approx. 3 thin slices/1 oz)		
Beef/Pork, ckd (moist), 1 oz	70	6
Dry/Hard, 1 oz	130	10
Turkey Salami, 1 oz	55	4
Armour, lower salt	80	7
Osc. Mayer: Cotto, 1 sl., ¾ oz	45	4
Genoa, 3 slices, 1 oz	105	9
Salami for Beer, ¾ oz	50	4
for Beer, beef, ¾ oz	70	6
Eckrich: Beer; Cotto, 1 sl.	70	6
Best's (Kosher), 1 sl., ¾ oz	50	4
Hormel: Beef, 1 slice	40	3
Genoa, 1 oz	110	10
Hard, sliced, 3 sl., 1 oz	105	9
Sausage Sticks: Tombstone	130	12
Smoked, average, ½ oz	80	7
Spam: All flavors, 1 oz	85	8
Deviled, 1 Tbsp, 1½ oz	35	34
Summer Sausage (Thuringer/Cervelat)		
Reg./Beef (O.M.), ¾ oz	70	6
Turkey, Louis Rich products:		
Bologna, 1 oz	60	5
Breast, average, 1 oz	35	1
Ham (round), 1 oz	35	1
Luncheon loaf, 1 oz	45	3
Pastrami (round), 1 oz	30	1
Salami, reg./Cotto, 1 oz	55	4
Summer Sausage, 1 oz	55	4

SPREADS, PATE

Per 1 Tbsp (½ oz)		
Carnation Spreads: Average	25	2
Hormel Spreads: Chicken	30	2
Corned Beef	35	3
Osc. Mayer Spreads: S/wich	35	2
Braunschweiger (German)	50	5
Ham & Cheese	35	3
Ham Salad	30	2
Chili con Carne Concentr.	40	3

PATE — Per 1 Tbsp, ½ oz		
Average All Brands		
Chicken liver, 1 oz	25	2
Pate de Foie Gras	60	6
Goose Liver, smoked	60	6
Liver	40	4

CHICKEN

QUICK GUIDE

From 3 lb ready-to-cook chicken

	CALS	FAT
BREAST/WING QUARTER		
Roasted: With skin	300	15
Without skin	190	5
Fried, batter dipped	480	26
LEG QUARTER		
Thigh & Drumstick		
Roasted: With skin	265	15
Without skin	180	8
Fried, batter dipped	430	26
Kentucky Fried Chicken — See Fast-Foods		

AVERAGE — ALL MEATS

Average of Light & Dark Meats
Per 4 oz Serving (no bone)

	CALS	FAT
Roasted: With skin	270	15
Without skin	215	8
Stewed: With skin	250	14
Without skin	200	8
Fried: Batter-dipped	330	20
Flour-coated	305	17

CHICKEN PARTS

BROILERS OR FRYERS
Edible Weights (No Bone)

Breast: Per ½ Breast

	CALS	FAT
Raw: With skin, 5 oz	245	13
Without skin, 4¼ oz	130	2
Roasted: With skin, 3½ oz	195	8
Without skin, 3 oz	140	3
Stewed: With skin, 4 oz	210	8
Without skin, 3¼ oz	140	3
Fried: Batter-dipped, 5 oz	370	19
Flour-coated, w/skin,3½ oz	220	9

Drumstick: Per Drumstick

	CALS	FAT
Roasted: With skin, 2 oz	125	6
Without skin, 1½ oz	75	2
Fried: Batter-dipped, 2½ oz	195	11
Flour-coated, 1¾ oz	120	7
Stewed: With skin, 2 oz	115	6
Without skin, 1½ oz	80	3

Thigh Portion: Edible Wt. (no bone)

	CALS	FAT
Raw: With skin, 3.3 oz		
(4¼ oz with bone)	200	14
Without skin, 2.4 oz	80	3
Roasted: With skin, 2¼ oz	155	10
Without skin, 2 oz	110	6

Thigh Portion (Cont.)	CALS	FAT (g)
Stewed: With skin, 2½ oz	160	10
Without skin, 2 oz	105	5
Fried: Batter-dipped, 3 oz	240	14
Flour-coated, 2¼ oz	165	9

Wing: Per Wing
Raw Weight 3.2 oz (with bone)

	CALS	FAT
Raw: With skin	110	8
Without skin	35	1
Roasted: With skin	105	7
Without skin	45	2
Fried: Batter-dipped	160	11
Flour-coated	105	7
Stewed: With skin	100	7
Neck: Simmered, with skin	95	7
Without skin	30	2

Skin Only: Skin From ½ Chicken

	CALS	FAT
Raw, 2¾ oz	275	26
Roasted, 2 oz	255	22
Stewed, 2½ oz	260	24
Fried, flour-coated, 2 oz	280	24
Fried, batter-dipped, 6¾ oz	750	55

ROASTERS
Average of Light & Dark Meat:

	CALS	FAT
Roasted: With skin, 4 oz	250	15
Without skin, 4 oz	190	8
Light Meat: Without, skin, rst.	175	5
Dark Meat: Without skin, rst.	206	10

STEWING CHICKEN
Stewed: Per 4 oz Serving
Average of Light & Dark Meat:

	CALS	FAT
With skin	325	21
Without skin	270	14
Light Meat: Without skin	240	9
Dark Meat: Without skin	295	17

CAPON CHICKEN

	CALS	FAT
Roasted: With skin, 4 oz	260	13
½ Chicken, with skin	1460	74

MISCELLANEOUS

	CALS	FAT
Giblets, simmered, 1 cup	230	7
Fried, flour-coated, 1 cup	400	20
Gizzard, simmered, 1 cup	220	5
Heart, simmered, 1 cup	270	12
Liver: Raw, 4 oz	140	5
Simmered, 1 cup	220	8
Liver Pate, 1 Tbsp, ½ oz	60	8

35

TURKEY

FRYER-ROASTERS

	CALS	FAT
Roasted: Per 3 oz Serving		
Light Meat: With skin	140	4
Without skin	120	1
Dark Meat: With skin	155	6
Without skin	140	4

½ of Whole Turkey:
(Approx. 3¼ lbs raw wt. w/out neck
and giblets; 2 lb 6 oz cooked wt.)

	CALS	FAT
Roasted: With skin	1400	46
Without skin	1030	18

Ground Turkey, Raw:	CALS	FAT
Regular (85% lean), 4 oz	180	10
Lean (90% lean), 4 oz	160	4
Breast, no skin, 4 oz	115	1
(4 oz raw wt. = 3 oz cooked wt.)		

TURKEY PARTS

Roasted, Edible Weights (no bone)

	CALS	FAT
Breast (½): (from 17¼ oz raw wt. w/bone)		
With skin, 12 oz (no bone)	525	11
Without skin, 10¾ oz	415	2
Back (½): With skin, 4½ oz	265	13
Without skin, 3½ oz	165	5
Leg (Thigh & Drumstick):		
(from 1 lb raw wt. w/bone)		
With skin, 8½ oz (no bone)	420	13
Without skin, 7¾ oz	355	8
Wing: (from 7¼ oz raw wt. w/bone)		
With skin, 3 oz (no bone)	185	9
Without skin, 2 oz	100	2
Neck: Simmered, 1 neck		
(9 oz w/bone)	275	11
Giblets, simm., 1 c, 5 oz	240	7

YOUNG HENS (ROASTED)

	CALS	FAT
Light Meat: With skin, 3 oz	175	8
Without skin, 3 oz	135	3
Dark Meat: With skin, 3 oz	200	11
Without skin, 3 oz	165	7
Young Toms — Similar to Young Hens		

DUCK, GOOSE, QUAIL

	CALS	FAT
Duck, roasted, with skin, 3oz	285	24
Without skin, 3 oz	170	10
½ whole duck, with skin	1300	108
Goose, roast, with skin, 3 oz	260	19
Without skin, 3 oz	200	11
Pheasant, ½ bird, raw	720	37
Quail, 1 whole, raw	210	13

36

POULTRY PRODUCTS

	CALS	FAT
Armour, Turkey: Patt., 2¼ oz	170	11
Breast Fillets w/cheese, 5 oz	300	16
Turkey Sticks, 2 oz	150	10
Banquet/Country Pride: Pages 40-42		
Crystal Springs (Natural/Lite):		
Chicken; Turkey, 5 oz can	130	<1
Louis Rich:		
Breast of Turkey, fully cooked:		
BBQ'd/Smoked/Rstd, 3 oz	105	3
Fresh Turkey Cust, cooked:		
Breast Cuts, 3 oz	120	3
Drumsticks/Wings, 3 oz	105	8
Luncheon Slices — See Cold Meats (p. 34)		
Franks: Medium, 1½ oz	100	79
Large, 2 oz	130	11
Smoked Saus./Kielbasa, 1 oz	40	2
Turkey Nuggets, cooked, each	60	4
Turkey Patties, cooked, each	210	13
Turkey Sticks, cooked, each	80	5
Shelton's: Gobblers! Corn Dog	220	11
Turkey Sausage Patty, each	180	17
Pot Pies (whole wheat): Turkey	350	12
Chicken Pot Pie	430	20
Turkey Jerky, ½ oz packet	45	<1
Franks & Sausages — Page 33		
Swanson — See Page 44		
Turkey Store:		
Breast Slices, 1 slice, 2½ oz	70	1
Breast Sirloins, each, 10 oz	285	3
Drumstick Steaks, 3½ oz	110	4
Ground Turkey, lean, ¼ lb	160	8
Ground Turkey Breast, ¼ lb	115	1
Breakfast Sausage Links, 1 oz	70	6
Tyson, Chicken Products:		
Breast Chunks, 3 oz serving	240	17
Breast Fillets: Regular, 3 oz	190	9
Marinated, butter/garlic, 3½ oz	160	7
Other flavors, aver., 3½ oz	125	2
Breast Patties, each, 2½ oz	220	15
Brst. Tenders, Sthn. fried, 3 oz	220	15
Chick'n Chunks/Chedd., 2½ oz	220	15
Chicken Pie, 6 oz	230	11
Microwave Tenders, 3½ oz	230	11
Microwave Chunks, 3½ oz	220	15
M/wave S/wiches: Breast	275	12
BBQ Chicken	210	4
Wings: All flavors, 3½ oz	220	14
Tyson Frozen Dinners — See Page 46		

FISH

FRESH FISH (READY RECKONER)

LOW OIL (Less than 2.5% fat)
White/pale colored flesh. Examples:
Cod, Flounder, Haddock, Halibut, Monkfish, Perch, Pike, Pollock, Snapper, Sole, Whiting

Per 4 oz Edible Portion	CALS	FAT
Raw, 4 oz (no bones)	90	1
Steamed, Broiled, Baked	130	1
Fried: Lightly Floured	210	8
Breaded	260	12
In Batter	320	16

MEDIUM OIL (2.5-5% fat)
Pale colored flesh. Examples:
Bluefin Tuna, Catfish, Kingfish, Salmon (Pink), Swordfish, Rainbow Trout, Yellowtail

Raw, 4 oz (no bones)	140	5
Baked, Broiled, 4oz	175	6
Fried, 4 oz	230	11

HIGH OIL (Over 5% fat)
Darker colored flesh. Examples:
Albacore Tuna, Bluefish, Herring, Mackerel, Orange Roughy, Salmon (Atl./Chinook/Sockeye), Sardines, Trout, Whitefish

Raw, 4 oz (no bones)	230	16
Baked, Broiled, 4 oz	275	17
Fried, 4 oz	340	23

Cooking Yields (Fin fish):
4 oz Raw wt. = 3½ oz Cooked wt.
4 oz Cooked wt. = 5 oz Raw wt.

Calorie & Fat Variations
The amount of fat/oil in fish varies with the species, season and locality. Within the same fish, fat/oil content is generally higher towards the head.

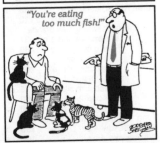

"You're eating too much fish!"

FISH & SHELLFISH

Edible Wts. (no bones/shell)	CALS	FAT
Abalone: Raw, 4 oz	120	1
Anchovy: Paste, 1 Tbsp, ¼ oz	15	1
Cnd. in oil, drnd., 5 only, ¾ oz	40	2
Pickled, 1 oz	50	3
Barracuda (Pacific), raw, 4 oz	130	3
Bass: Black, raw, 4 oz	105	1
Striped, raw, 1 fillet, 5½ oz	150	4
Blue Fish, raw, 1 fillet, 5¼ oz	185	6
Butterfish, raw, 4 oz	165	9
Carp, raw, 4 oz	145	6
Catfish: Raw, 4 oz	130	5
Fried, bread., 1 fillet, 3 oz	200	12
Caviar: black/red, 1 Tbsp	40	3
Clams: Raw, 3 oz (4 lge/9 sm)	65	1
Fried, breaded, 3 oz	170	10
Canned, 3 oz	125	2
Cod, Atl./Pacific: Raw, 4 oz	95	1
Baked/Broil., 1 fill., 6¼ oz	135	2
Canned, 3 oz	90	1
Crab: Alaska King, raw, 4 oz	95	1
1 leg, cooked, 4¾ oz	130	2
Blue, raw, 1 crab (⅓ lb whole crab, ¾ oz flesh)	18	<1
Canned, ½ cup, 2½ oz	65	<1
Dungeness, 1 crab, 5¾ oz edible (from 1½ lb whole crab)	140	2
Imitation Crab Legs/Stix, 3 oz	80	1
Crayfish, raw, 4 oz (edible)	100	1
Croaker, raw, 4 oz	120	3
Cuttlefish, raw, 4 oz	90	1
Dolphinfish, raw, 4 oz	95	1
Eel: Raw, 4 oz	210	13
Smoked, 2 oz	190	16
Fish Fillets/Sticks/Nuggets — See Fish Products, Page 39.		
Flounder/Sole, raw, 4 oz	80	<1
Gefilte Fish: See Jewish Foods, p.103		
Grouper, raw, 4 oz	105	1
Haddock: Raw, 4 oz	100	<1
Broiled, 1 fillet, 5¼ oz	170	1
Smoked, 2 oz	22	<1
Halibut, Raw, 4 oz	125	3
Herring: Atlantic, raw, 4 oz	180	10
Pickled, 2 pieces, 1 oz	60	4
In Sour Cream, 1 oz	50	5
Rollmops, 1½ oz	110	8

Herring, canned — Next Page.

37

FISH & SHELLFISH (CONT)

	CALS	FAT
Herring, Can: Plain w/liq., 4 oz	235	15
in Tomato Sauce, 4 oz	200	12
Smoked, kippered, 4 oz	245	14
Jellyfish: Raw, 4 oz	30	<1
Salted, 4 oz	40	<1
Kingfish, raw, 4 oz	120	3.5
Ling, raw, 4 oz	100	<1
Lobster, Northern: Raw, 4 oz	105	1
1 Lobster, 6¼ oz		
(from 1½ lb whole lobster)	135	1.3
Cooked, 1 cup, 5 oz	140	1
Lobster Newberg, ¾ cup	360	22
Lobster Thermidor, 1 serv.	370	20
Lobster Salads, 1 cup	220	13
Lox, Regular/Nova, 2 oz	65	2
Mackerel: Atlantic, raw, 4 oz	235	16
Jack, can., ½ cup, 3⅓ oz	150	6
King, raw, 4 oz	120	2
Pacific/Jack, raw, 4 oz	180	9
Spanish, raw, 4 oz	160	7
Mahi-Mahi, raw, 4 oz	140	5
Monkfish, raw, 4 oz	75	1
Mullet, striped, raw	135	4
Mussels: Raw, 4 oz (edible)	100	2
1 cup, 5¼ oz (edible)	130	3
Cooked, moist heat, 3 oz	150	4
Ocean Perch, raw, 4 oz	90	1.5
Octopus, common, raw, 4 oz	95	1
Orange Roughy, raw, 4 oz	145	9
(Cals may be much lower. Over 90% of total fat is waxester which may not be metabolized)		
Oysters: Common, raw, 3 oz	70	1
Eastern, raw:		
6 medium, 3 oz	60	2
1 cup, 8¾ oz	170	6
Fried/brd., 6 medium, 3 oz	170	11
Pacific, raw, 1 med., 1¾ oz	40	1
Oysters Rockefeller, 6 oyst.	220	13
Perch, average, raw, 4 oz	105	2
Pollock, raw, 4 oz	100	1
Pompano, Florida, raw, 4 oz	190	10
Porgy/Scup, raw, 4 oz	130	4
Rockfish, Pacific, raw, 4 oz	110	2
Roe, raw, 1 oz	40	2
Sablefish, raw, 4 oz	220	18
Salmon, Raw: Chinook, 4 oz	205	7
Atlantic; Coho/Silver, 4 oz	160	7
Chum; Pink, 4 oz	135	4
Red/Sockeye, 4 oz	190	10

	CALS	FAT
Salmon, Canned: Average all brands		
Pink/Humpback, 1 oz	40	2
½ Cup, 3½ oz	140	6
3¾ oz Can, whole	155	6
7¾ oz Can, whole	320	12
Red/Sockeye, 1 oz	48	2.5
3¾ oz Can, whole	200	8
Atlantic, ½ cup, 3½ oz	230	14
Chinook/King, ½ cup	210	14
Chum, ½ cup, 3½ oz	140	5
Coho/Silver, ½ cup	155	5
Sardines, Canned: Aver. All Brands		
In Oil, undrained, 1 oz	85	7
Drained of oil, 1 oz	60	3
3¾ oz can, drain. (3¼ oz)	190	11
1 lg./2 md. 3"/5 sm., 0.8 oz	50	3
In Tom./Mustard Sce, 1 oz	45	3
3¾ oz can (8 sardines)	170	11
Scallop: Raw, 6 lg./14 sm., 3 oz	75	<1
Breaded/fried, 6 lge, 3 oz	200	10
Shark: Raw, 4 oz	150	6
Batter-dipped, fried, 4 oz	260	16
Shrimps: Raw, in shell, ½ lb	140	2
Raw, shelled, 3 oz (12 lge)	90	1.5
Bread./fried, 3 oz (11 lge)	210	11
Canned, 2 oz	60	1
Smelt, Rainbow, raw, 4 oz	115	3
Snapper, raw, 4 oz	115	1
Sole, Lemon, raw, 4 oz	90	1
Squid, raw, 4 oz	105	1
Surimi: See Japanese Dishes (p. 102).		
Surimi, Imit. Crablegs/Shrmp., 4 oz	110	1
Swordfish, raw, 4 oz	140	5
Trout, Rainbow, raw, 4 oz	135	4
Crystal Springs, 5 oz can	150	7
Tuna: Raw, Bluefin, 4 oz	165	6
Skipjack; Yellowfin	120	1
Canned: Average all brands		
In Water: Drained, 1 oz	37	<1
Flaked w/liq., 1 oz	30	<1
¼ cup, 2 oz	60	1
6½ oz can, whole	205	1
In Oil: Drained, 1 oz	53	2.3
Flaked with oil, 1 oz	75	6.5
¼ cup, 2 oz	150	13
6½ oz can, whole	490	42
Tuna Salad, ½ cup, 3½ oz	200	10
Whitefish, raw, 4 oz	155	7
Whiting, raw, 4 oz	100	1.5

FISH — FROZEN PRODUCTS

GORTON'S

	CALS	FAT
Crispy Batter: Fish Sticks, 4	260	18
Fish Fillets, 2	290	19
Crunchy: Fish Sticks, 4	210	13
Fish Fillets, 2	230	13
Microwave Sticks	225	15
Microwave Fillets, 2	340	26
Value Pack: Fish Sticks, 4	190	11
Fish Portions, 1	180	11
Fishmarket Fresh: Perch, 5 oz	140	3
Cod/Hadd./Flounder/Sole	110	1
Light Recipe: Tempura Fillet	200	14
Lightly breaded fillets, 1	180	8
Microwave Entrees:		
Baked Scrod	320	18
Fillets in Herb Sauce	190	8
Haddock in Lemon Butter	360	21
Shrimp Scampi	390	30
Sole in Lemon Butter	380	24
Sole in Wine Sauce	180	8
Stuffed Flounder	350	18

MRS PAUL'S

	CALS	FAT
Battered: Fish Sticks, 4	210	12
Fish Portions, 2	300	19
Batter Dipped: Fish Fillets, 2	330	17
Crispy Crunchy: Fish Sticks, 4	190	8
Fish Fillets, 2	220	9
Breaded Fish Portions, 2	230	15
Breaded Minced Sticks, 4	140	6
Crunchy Batter: Fish Fillets, 2	280	14
Flounder Fillets, 2	220	9
Haddock Fillets, 2	190	5
Light Breaded Fillets:		
Average, ½ pkg, 4½ oz	240	10
Light Fillets 'N Sauce, 1 fillet	140	6
Deviled Crabs, 1 cake, 3 oz	180	9
Fish Cakes, 2 cakes, 4 oz	190	7
Fish Scallops, ½ pkg, 3 oz	160	7
Fried Clams, ½ pkg, 2½ oz	200	9
Fried Shrimp, ½ pkg, 3 oz	200	11

(Light Seafood Entrees: Page 43)

VAN DE KAMP'S

	CALS	FAT (g)
Battered: Fish Sticks, 4	170	9
Fish Fillets, 1	170	9
Haddock Fillets, 2	250	13
Halibut Fillets, 2	180	9
Perch Fillets, 2	280	14
Breaded: Fish Sticks, 4	190	10
Fish Fillets, 2	280	15
Haddock Fillets, 2	260	15
Crispy Microwave:		
Fish Sticks, 4	200	11
Fish Fillets, 1	130	7
Light Fillets: Average, 1	250	12
Natural Fillets: Per 4 oz		
Cod/Flounder/Hadd./Sole	90	1
Ocean Perch	110	2

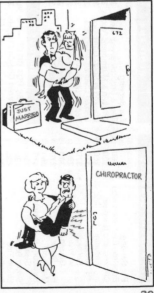

OTHER FISH DISHES

- Frozen Entrees/Dinners — Pp. 40-47.
- Ethnic Restaurant Foods — Pp. 101-104.
- Long John Silver — p. 124.
- Red Lobster — p. 134.

ARMOUR CLASSICS

Per Serving	CALS	FAT (g)
Boneless Beef Short Ribs	380	16
Chicken: and Noodles	230	7
Fettucini	260	9
Mesquite	370	16
Parmigiana	370	19
w. Wine & Mushroom Sce	280	11
Glazed	300	16
Ham Steak	270	7
Meat Loaf	360	17
Salisbury: Parmigiana	410	21
Steak	350	17
Sirloin Roast	190	4
Sirloin Tips	230	7
Swedish Meatballs	330	18
Turkey w. Dressing & Gravy	320	12
Veal Parmigiana	400	22
Yankee Pot Roast	310	12

ARMOUR CLASSICS LITE

Per Serving	CALS	FAT (g)
Baby Bay Shrimp	220	6
Beef Pepper Steak	220	4
Beef Stroganoff	250	6
Chicken: a la King	290	7
Burgundy	210	2
Marsala	250	7
Oriental	180	1
Sweet & Sour	240	2
Salisbury Steak	300	11
Seafood w. Natural Herbs	190	2
Shrimp Creole	290	9
Steak Diane	290	9

BENIHANA

Per Serving	CALS	FAT
Beef & Broccoli w/veg/rice	300	6
Chicken & Mushrooms/Veges	350	5
Chicken in Spicy Garlic Sce	300	4
Glazed Chicken w/veg/rice	270	1
Pepper Steak w/Rice	340	5
Shrimp & Cashews w/Rice	270	4
Shrimp & Oriental Veges	260	2
Sweet & Sour Chicken	390	3

BANQUET

CHEESE HOT BITES — Per Nugget	CALS	FAT
Mozzarella Cheese Nuggets	240	13
BONELESS CHICKEN HOT BITES		
Breast Patties, each	210	13
Breast Tenders, each	150	6
Chicken: Drum-Snackers	220	15
Nuggets, each	210	14
Nuggets with Cheddar	250	18
Hot 'n Spicy Nuggets	250	19
Sticks, each	220	15
Southern Fried: Per Portion		
Breast Patties	210	12
Breast Tenders	160	7
Chicken Nuggets	220	14
MICROWAVE CHICKEN HOT BITES		
Breast Patty & Bun	310	14
South'n Fried Brst Patty/Bisc.	320	14
Breast Tenders	260	10
Chicken Nuggets:		
with Sweet & Sour Sauce	360	21
Hot 'n Spicy with BBQ Sce	360	21
South'n Fried Chicken Breast		
Nuggets w. BBQ Sauce	370	23

BANQUET (CONT)

CHICKEN PRODUCTS	CALS	FAT (g)
Fried Chicken	330	19
Breast Portions	220	11
Thighs & Drumsticks	250	14
Hot 'n Spicy: Fried Chicken	330	19
Snack 'n Chicken	140	9
COOKIN' BAGS		
BBQ Sauce & Sliced Beef	100	2
Breaded Veal Parmigiana	230	11
Chicken: & Veg. Primavera	100	2
a la King	110	5
Creamed Chipped Beef	100	4
Gravy: & Salisbury Steak	190	14
with Sliced Beef/Turkey	100	5
Meat Loaf	200	14
Mushr. Grvy/Chbrld Beef Patty	210	15
CASSEROLES		
Macaroni & Cheese	350	17
Spaghetti with Meat Sauce	270	8
DINNERS		
Beans & Frankfurters	520	25
Beef Enchilada	500	15
Cheese Enchilada	550	19
Chicken & Dumplings	430	24
Chopped Beef	420	32
Fried Chicken	400	22
Macaroni & Cheese	420	20
Meat Loaf	440	27
Mexican Style	490	18
Combination	520	17
Noodles & Chicken	350	15
Salisbury Steak	500	34
Spaghetti & Meatballs	290	10
Turkey	390	20
Western	630	41

BANQUET, BUDGET GOURMET

BANQUET (CONT)

	CALS	FAT
EXTRA HELPING DINNERS		
Beef	870	61
Chicken Nuggets: w. BBQ Sce	640	36
Fried Chicken,	570	28
Salisbury Steak	910	60
Turkey	750	42
PLATTERS		
Chicken: average all varieties	430	21
Beef	460	34
Fish	450	22
Ham	400	17
FAMILY ENTREES		
Per 1/4 Package Serving		
Beef Stew	140	5
Chicken: with Dumplings	280	14
w. Vegetables Primavera	140	3
Chili Gravy & Beef Enchiladas	270	13
Gravy: with Salisbury Steak	300	22
with Sliced Beef	160	5
with Sliced Turkey	150	8
Lasagne with Meat Sauce	270	10
Macaroni & Cheese	290	13
Mostaccioli & Meat Sauce	170	3
Mushr. Gravy & Beef Patties	290	21
Noodles & Beef with Gravy	200	7
Onion Gravy & Beef Patties	300	21
Veal Parmigianan Patties	370	18
MEAT PIES		
Beef Pie; Turkey Pie	510	33
Chicken Pie	550	36
Tuna Pie	540	33
SUPREME MICROWAVE MEAT PIES		
Beef Pie	440	29
Chicken Pie; Turkey Pie	430	28

BUDGET GOURMET

	CALS	FAT
ENTREES		
Beef Cantonese	260	9
Cheese Macaroni	430	25
Chicken: w. Egg Noodles	440	25
Sweet & Sour	340	5
with Fettucini	400	21
Marsala	270	8
Italian Sausage Lasagne	430	23
Linguini w. Shrimp & Clams	270	10
Pepper Steak with Rice	330	10
Roast Sirloin Supreme	320	15
Seafood Newburg	350	13
Shrimp with Fettucini	370	22
Sirloin: Cheddar Melt	390	22
Tips & Country Vegetables	300	17
Swedish Meatballs w. Noodles	580	37
Three Cheese Lasagne	390	18
Turkey a la King with Rice	390	16
THREE DISH DINNERS		
Beef Mexicana	520	18
Chicken: Cacciatore	470	27
Mexicana	560	20
Scallops & Shrimp Marinara	330	9
Sirloin: Salisbury Steak	450	24
Tips in Burgundy Sauce	340	14
Swiss Steak	410	22
Veal Parmigiana	490	25
Yankee Pot Roast	360	18
SIDE DISHES		
Cauli. w/Cheddar Cheese Sce	130	9
Cheddared: Potatoes	260	16
Potatoes with Broccoli	150	8
Cheese Tortellini	210	8
Macaroni & Cheese	240	35
Mandarin Vegetables	160	11
Nacho Potatoes	200	12

BUDGET GOURMET (CONT)

	CALS	FAT
SIDE DISHES (CONT)		
New England Recipe Veg.	230	14
Oriental Rice w. Veg.	290	12
Pasta Alfredo w. Broccoli	230	11
Peas & Califlower/Cream Sce	150	8
Peas & Waterchestnuts Orient.	110	4
Rice Mexicana	240	9
Rice Pilaf w. Greenbeans	240	11
Spinach Au Gratin	160	12
Three Cheese Potatoes	230	11
Ziti in Marinara Sauce	200	9

BUDGET GOURMET LIGHT

	CALS	FAT
ENTREES: Beef Stroganoff	290	12
Cheese: Ravioli; Lasagne	290	10
Chicken: Au Gratin	250	11
Enchilada Suiza	290	12
French Recipe	240	9
Mandarin	300	7
Orange Glazed	250	3
Glazed Turkey	270	5
Ham & Asparagus Au Gratin	290	12
Lasagne with Meat Sauce	290	12
Linguini with Scallops & Clams	290	11
Mandarin Vegetables	160	11
Oriental Beef	290	9
Sirloin: Beef in Herb Sauce	270	10
Beef Enchilada Ranchero	280	10
Salisbury Steak	260	13
DINNERS		
Chicken: Breastin Wine Sauce	250	5
Roast with Herb Gravy	270	9
Teriyaki	290	9
Sliced Turkey Brst/Herb Gravy	290	8
Special Recipe Sirloin of Beef	260	10

FROZEN ENTREES & MEALS (CONT)
CHUN KING, DINING LITE, KRAFT, HEALTHY CHOICE, LA CHOY

CHUN KING

EGG ROLLS — Each	CALS	FAT
Chicken, Meat & Shrimp	220	8
Shrimp	200	6
ENTREES		
Beef: Pepper Oriental	310	3
Teriyaki	380	2
Chicken: Chow Mein	370	6
Crunchy Walnut	310	5
Imperial	300	1
Sweet & Sour Pork	400	5
Szechuan Beef	340	3
PEA PODS		
Chinese Pea Pods, ¼ package	20	0
SIDE DISHES		
Fried Rice: with Chicken	260	4
with Pork	270	6

COUNTRY PRIDE

Per ¼ Package Serving	CALS	FAT
Chicken: Chunks, Sticks	240	15
Nuggets, Patties	250	16
Southern Fried Chunks	280	20

DINING LITE

	CALS	FAT
Beef Teriyaki	270	5
Cheese Cannelloni	310	9
Cheese Lasagne	260	6
Chicken: a la King/Noodle	240	7
Chow Mein	180	2
Glazed	220	4
Fettucini with Broccoli	290	12
Lasagne with Meat Sauce	240	6
Oriental Pepper Steak	260	6
Salisbury Steak	200	8
Spaghetti with Beef	220	8
Sauce & Swedish Meatballs	280	10

DINNER SUPREME (STOUFFER)

DINNER SUPREME	CALS	FAT
Baked Chicken Brst. w. Gravy	300	11
Barbeque-Style Chicken	390	23
Cheese Stuffed Shells	310	14
Chicken Florentine	430	18
Chicken Parmigiana	360	15
Chicken with Supreme Sauce	360	12
Fried Chicken	450	23
Glazed Ham Steak	380	15
Roast Turkey Breast	330	10
Salisb. Stk.; Homest. Meatlf.	400	23
Veal Parmigiana	350	13

KRAFT

	CALS	FAT
Barbeque Beef with Corn	340	12
Beef Stew, 10 oz	250	12
Chicken a la King	350	14
Chicken & Egg Noodles	420	20
Chili w/Beef & Beans	380	22
Lasagne w/Meat Sauce	390	16
Macaroni & Beef in Sauce	370	16
Ravioli, 10 oz	320	11
Spaghetti & Meatballs	340	15
Salisb. Steak; Tuna Noodle	370	20
Turkey & Dressing, 9 oz	300	10

KID CUISINE

	CALS	FAT
Cheese Beef Patty Sandwich	400	19
Cheese Pizza	240	4
Pepper Steak	400	19
Chicken Nuggets	320	15
Fish Nuggets	420	22
Fried Chicken	380	14
Macar/Cheese w. Mini Franks	380	14
Mini-Cheese Ravioli	250	2
Spaghetti with Meat Sauce	310	12

HEALTHY CHOICE

DINNERS	CALS	FAT
Breast of Turkey	290	5
Beef Pepper Steak	290	6
Chicken: Oriental	220	2
Parmigiana	280	3
and Pasta Divan	310	4
Herb Roasted	260	3
Mesquite	310	2
Sweet & Sour	280	2
Salisbury Steak	300	7
Shrimp: Creole	210	1
Marinara	220	1
Sirloin Tips	290	6
Sole Au Gratin	270	5
Yankee Pot Roast	260	4
ENTREES		
Beef Pepper Steak	250	4
Chicken: a l'Orange	260	2
Chow Mein	220	3
Glazed	220	3
Fettucini Alfredo	240	7
Lasagne with Meat Sauce	260	5
Linguini with Shrimp	230	2
Seafood Newburg	200	3
Sole with Lemon Butter Sauce	230	4
Spaghetti with Meat Sauce	310	6

LA CHOY

	CALS	FAT
Sweet & Sour Chicken	280	4
Beef Teriyaki	280	5
Pepper Steak	290	9
Spicy Chicken Oriental	290	5
Egg Rolls: Chicken, 3 rolls	90	3
Lobster, 3 rolls	80	2
Meat & Shrimp, 3 rolls	80	2
6 rolls	100	3

LE MENU, LEAN CUISINE, LOONEY TUNES, MRS PAUL'S

LE MENU

	CALS	FAT (g)
ENTREES		
Beef Burgundy	330	23
Chicken Kiev	530	39
Manicotti, Cheese filled	410	20
Oriental Chicken	330	9
LIGHT STYLE DINNERS		
Chicken Cacciatore	270	8
Chicken Cannelloni	270	5
Chicken Chow Mein	260	4
Chicken Empress	210	4
Glazed Chicken Breast	270	6
Herb Roasted Chicken	220	6
Salisbury Steak	220	7
3-Cheese Stuffed Shells	280	8
Turkey Divan	280	9
Veal Marsala	260	6
DINNERS		
Beef Sirloin Tips	400	19
Beef Stroganoff	450	25
Chicken a la King	330	14
Chicken Cordon Bleu	470	20
Chicken Florentine	340	10
Chicken Parmigiana	400	20
Chopped Sirloin Beef	440	25
Ham Steak	300	10
Pepper Steak	370	13
Sliced Breast of Turkey with Mushroom Gravy	270	6
Sole, fillet of	360	14
Sweet & Sour Chicken	450	22
Yankee Pot Roast	370	15

MRS T'S PIEROGIES

	CALS	FAT (g)
Potato & Cheese Pierogies, 1	60	<1

LEAN CUISINE

	CALS	FAT (g)
ENTREES — Per Package		
Beef & Bean Enchiladas	280	10
Beef/Pork Cannell. w/Mornay	260	10
Beefsteak Ranchero	270	9
Breast of Chicken:		
in Herb Cream Sauce	260	10
Marsala with Vegetables	190	5
Parmesan	260	8
Cheese Cannelloni/Tom. Sce	260	10
Chicken: a l'Orange/Alm. Rice	260	5
and Veg. w. Vermicelli	250	7
Cacciatore w. Vermicelli	250	5
Chow Mein w. Rice	250	5
Enchanadas	270	9
Fiesta	250	8
Oriental	230	9
Filet of Fish: Divan	260	7
Florentine	230	8
Jardiniere w/Souffl'd Pot.	290	10
Glazed Chicken w. Veg. Rice	270	8
Lasagne with Meat & Sauce	270	8
Linguini with Clam Sauce	270	8
Meatball Stew	250	10
Oriental Beef w. Veg. & Rice	250	7
Rigatoni Bake/Meat Sce/Ch.	260	10
Salisbury Steak/Ital. Sce/Veg	280	15
Shrimp & Chicken Cantonese	270	9
Sliced Turkey Brst/Mushr. Sce	240	7
Spaghetti w. Beef/Mushr. Sce	280	7
Stuffed Cabb./Meat/Tom. Sce	220	10
Szechwan Beef/Noodles/Veg	260	10
Tuna Lasagne	270	10
Turkey Dijon	270	10
Veg & Pasta Mornay w. Ham	280	11
Zucchini Lasagne	260	7

LEAN CUISINE (CONT)

	CALS	FAT (g)
PASTA SALADS — Per Package		
Country Mustard/Swiss Ch.	290	10
Creamy Dill with Tuna	250	8
Creamy Tarragon w. Chicken	240	7
Oriental with Chicken	230	4
Salsa Mexicana w. Turkey	240	6
Zesty Ital. w. Cheese & Salami	280	9

LEGUME & NASOYA

See Vegetarian Section — Page 50.

LOONEY TUNES

	CALS	FAT (g)
Bugs Bunny Chicken Chunks	370	20
Daffy Duck Spagh/Meatballs	300	15
Road Runner Chick. S/wich	320	11
Speedy Gonzales Beef Ench.	400	16
Sylvester Fish Sticks	300	15
Tweety Macaroni & Cheese	280	8
Wile E. Coyote H/burg. Pizza	300	12
Yosemite Sam BBQ Chicken	420	21

MRS PAUL'S

	CALS	FAT (g)
LIGHT SEAFOOD ENTREES		
Fish Dijon	200	5
Fish Florentine	220	8
Fish Mornay	230	10
Seafood Lasagne	290	8
Seafood Rotini	240	6
Shrimp and Clams w. Linguini	240	5
Other Fish Products — See Page 39.		

43

MORTON, PATIO, RIGHT COURSE, STOUFFER'S

MORTON

	CALS	FAT (g)
DINNERS		
Beans & Frankfurters	350	13
Fish	370	13
Ham	290	4
Meat Loaf	310	17
Mexican Style	300	10
Salisbury Steak	300	17
Sliced Beef	220	5
Spaghetti & Meatball	200	3
Turkey	200	6
Veal Parmigian	260	8
Western	290	14
MEAT PIES		
Beef Pie	430	31
Chicken, Turkey Pie	420	28

PATIO

	CALS	FAT (g)
BRITOS — Per Brito		
Beef & Bean, Green Chili	250	10
Nacho Beef	270	13
Nacho Chse, Spicy Chicken	250	10
Red Chili	240	10
BURRITOS		
Beef & Bean	370	16
Green Chili	330	12
Red Chili	340	13
Red Hot	360	15
MEXICAN DINNERS		
Beef Enchilada	520	24
Cheese Enchilada	380	10
Tamale	470	21
Fiesta	470	20
Mexican Style	540	25

RIGHT COURSE

RIGHT COURSE ENTREES	CALS	FAT (g)
Per Package		
Beef: Dijon w. Pasta & Veg.	290	9
Ragout with Rice Pilaf	300	8
Chicken Tenderloins:		
in Barbeque Sauce	270	6
in Peanut Sauce	280	8
Chicken Italiano/Fettucini/Veg.	280	8
Fiesta Beef with Corn Pasta	280	7
Homestyle Pot Roast	220	7
Sesame Chicken	320	9
Sliced Turkey in a Mild Curry Sauce with Rice Pilaf	320	8
Shrimp Primavera	240	7
Vegetarian Chili	280	7

STOUFFER'S

MEALS/ENTREES — Per Package	CALS	FAT (g)
Beef: Chop Suey w. Rice	300	9
Pie	500	32
Short Rib in Gravy	350	20
Stroganoff with Noodles	390	20
Teriyaki w. Rice & Veg.	290	8
Cashew Chicken w. Rice	380	16
Cheese Enchiladas	590	40
Chicken: a la King with Rice	290	9
Chow Mein w/out Noodles	130	4
Divan	320	20
Enchiladas	490	29
Pie	530	33
Chili con Carne with Beans	260	10
Creamed: Chicken	300	21
Chipped Beef	230	16
Escalloped Chicken & Noodles	420	25
Fiesta Lasagne	430	22
Green Pepper Steak w. Rice	330	11

STOUFFER'S (CONT)

MEALS/ENTREES (CONT)	CALS	FAT (g)
Ham & Asparagus Bake	510	35
Homestyle Chicken & Noodles	310	15
Lasagna, single serving	360	13
Lobster Newburg	380	32
Macaroni: & Beef w. Tomatoes	170	7
& Cheese, 12 oz	250	13
Pasta Shells Chse/Tom. Sce.	330	15
Salisbury Steak in Gravy	250	14
Spaghetti: with Meatballs	380	15
with Meat Sauce	370	11
Stuffed Green Peppers w/ Beef	200	9
Swedish Meatballs w/ Noodles	480	26
Tortellini: Beef/Marinara Sce.	360	12
Cheese Alfredo	600	40
Cheese with Tomato Sce	360	16
Tortilla Grande	530	33
Tuna Noodle Casserole	310	13
Turkey: Cass. w/ Gravy/Dress.	360	17
Pie	540	36
Vegetable Lasagna, 1 serve	420	24
Welsh Rarebit	350	30
SIDE DISHES — Per Package		
New England Clam Chowder	180	9
Corn Souffle	160	7
Creamed Spinach	170	14
Fettucini Alfredo	270	19
Green Bean Mushroom Cass.	160	11
Noodles Romanoff	170	9
Pasta: Carbonara	620	45
Oriental	300	14
Primavera	270	21
Potatoes au Gratin	110	6
Scalloped Potatoes	90	4
Spinach Souffle	140	9

SWANSON ENTREES & DINNERS

SWANSON

GREAT STARTS BRKFAST
Per Whole Package

	CALS	FAT (g)
French Toast (Cinnamon Swirl) with Sausages	470	26
French Toast w. Sausages	450	25
Omelet w.Cheese Sauce/Ham	380	29
Pancakes & Blueberries/Sce	410	10
Pancakes & Sausages	470	22
Pancakes & Strawberries/Sce	430	11
Scrambled Eggs & Sausage with Hashbrowns	430	35
Scrambled Eggs, Home Fries	280	21
Scr. Eggs & Bacon w/Fries	360	28
Spanish Style Omelet	240	16

GREAT STARTS BREAKFASTS ON A BISCUIT

	CALS	FAT (g)
Egg, Canadian Bac/Cheese	420	22
Egg, Sausage & Cheese	460	29
Sausage	410	22

BREAKFASTS ON A MUFFIN

	CALS	FAT (g)
Egg, Beefsteak & Cheese	380	22
Egg, Canadian Bac/Cheese	300	16

CHICK. DUET GOURMET NUGGETS

	CALS	FAT (g)
All varieties, average	200	12

CHICKEN DUET ENTREES

	CALS	FAT (g)
All varieties, average	330	19

PLUMP & JUICY CHICKEN

	CALS	FAT (g)
Chicken Dipsters/Drumlets	220	14
Chicken Nibbles	300	20
Fried Chicken, breast portions	360	22
1 lb T/Out Pre-Fried Chicken	270	17
Take-Out Fried Chicken	270	17
Thighs & Drumsticks	280	19

SWANSON (CONT)

HOMESTYLE RECIPE ENTREES

	CALS	FAT (g)
Chicken Cacciatore	260	8
Chicken Nibbles	340	24
Chicken Pie	380	19
Chili Con Carne	270	10
Fish 'n' Fries	350	17
Fried Chicken	380	21
Lasagne with Meat Sauce	400	16
Macaroni & Cheese	400	21
Salisbury Steak	480	34
Scalloped Potatoes & Ham	340	16
Seafood Creole with Rice	240	6
Sirloin Tips in Burgundy Sce	270	10
Spag. w. Ital/Style Meatballs	460	19
Swedish Meatballs	350	22
Turkey w. Dressing/Potatoes	290	13
Veal Parmigiana	330	13

HUNGRY MAN DINNERS

	CALS	FAT (g)
Boneless Chicken	700	28
Chopped Beef Steak	640	37
Fried Chicken, white meat	870	46
Fried Chicken, dark meat	860	45
Mexican	820	41
Salisbury Steak	680	41
Sliced Beef	450	12
Turkey	550	18
Veal Parmigiana	560	23

3-COMPARTMENT DINNERS

	CALS	FAT (g)
Beans & Franks	440	20
Fried Chicken Platter	340	16
Macaroni & Beef	370	15
Macaroni & Cheese	380	15
Noodles & Chicken	260	9
Spaghetti & Meatballs	370	16

SWANSON (CONT)

4-COMPARTMENT DINNERS

	CALS	FAT
Beef	340	8
Beef in Barbeque Sauce	460	15
Beef Enchiladas	480	22
Chicken in Barbeque Sauce	460	13
Chicken Nuggets	460	25
Chopped Sirloin Beef	370	19
Fish 'n Chips	500	20
Fish Nuggets	410	19
Fried Chicken, BBQ flavoured	520	21
Fried Chicken, white meat	560	25
Fried Chicken, dark meat	560	28
Loin of Pork	310	12
Meatloaf	430	22
Mexican Style Combination	520	24
Salisbury Steak	410	18
Sweet 'n Sour Chicken	380	11
Swiss Steak	340	11
Turkey	350	11
Veal Parmigiana	450	22
Western Style	450	21

POT PIES

	CALS	FAT
7 oz Pie: Beef	380	20
Chicken	370	22
Macaroni & Cheese	220	9
Turkey	390	22
16 oz Pie: Beef	700	36
Chicken	740	41
Turkey	750	42

TYSON, VAN DE KAMP'S, WEIGHT WATCHERS

TYSON

GOURMET DINNERS	CALS	FAT (g)
A L'Orange, whole pkg.	300	8
Beef Champignon	370	10
Chicken & Beef Luau	330	10
Dijon	310	17
Francais	280	14
Kiev	520	33
Lasagne; Parmigiana	380	14
Marsala	300	13
Mesquite	320	10
Oriental	270	7
Peking	390	20
Pepper Steak	330	11
Picatta	450	17
Pasta Trio	240	10
Salisbury Supreme	380	11
Sweet & Sour	430	26
Turkey	420	15
	380	11
Other Chicken Products – See p.36		

VAN DE KAMP'S

MEXICAN HOLIDAY CLASSIC	CALS	FAT (g)
Beef Enchilada, 7½ oz	250	15
Beef & Bean Burrito, 5 oz	320	9
Beef Enchilada Dinner, 12 oz	390	15
Beef Tostada Supreme, 8½ oz	530	30
4 Cheese Enchiladas, 8½ oz	370	20
Cheese Enchilada, 7½ oz	270	15
Cheese Ench. Dinner, 12 oz	450	20
Cheese Ench. w/Rice & Beans	620	30
Chicken Enchilada, 7½ oz	250	10
Chick. Suiza w/Rice & Beans	550	20
Grande Burrito w/Rice & Beans	530	20
Mexican Style Dinner	420	20
Shrd. Beef Enchil. w/Rice/Corn	490	15
Sirloin Burrito Grande	440	15

WEIGHT WATCHERS

BREAKFAST ITEMS	CALS	FAT (g)
Pancakes: Per Pancake		
Buttermilk, 2 pancakes	150	3
w. Strawberry Topping	230	4
w. Blueberry Topping	260	4
with Links	240	10
French Toast:		
with Links, 1 pkg	260	12
with Cinnamon, ½ pkg	170	2
Breakfast Sandwiches: Per Package		
Egg, Canadian Style Bacon & Cheese Muffin	230	8
Sausage Biscuit	220	11
Sweet Rolls: Per ½ Package		
Cheese	180	5
Strawberry	170	5
Coffee Cakes/Muffins: Per ½ Pkg		
Blueberry Muffins	170	5
Banana Nut Muffins	170	5
Coffee Cake w. Cinn. Streusel	190	7

FROZEN ENTREES — Per Pkg.	CALS	FAT (g)
Poultry:		
Chicken: Fettucini	290	10
a la King	220	8
Breaded Cordon Bleu	230	11
Imperial	220	4
Nuggets	270	12
Southern Fried Patty	340	16
Sweet 'n Sour Tenders	240	1
Stuffed Turkey Breast	260	10

Continued Next Column.

WEIGHT WATCHERS (CONT)

FROZEN ENTREES (CONT)	CALS	FAT (g)
Beef/Veal:		
Beef: Stroganoff	320	13
Salisbury Steak Romana	310	13
Sirloin Tips & Mushr. in Wine Sauce	250	8
London Broil in Mushroom Sce	140	3
Veal Patty Parmigiana	220	10
Fish: Oven Fried	300	13
Fillet of Fish Au Gratin	200	6
Seafood Linguini	210	7
Stuffed Sole w. Newburg Sce	310	9
Baked Potato:		
Broccoli & Cheese	250	7
Chicken Divan	270	4
Italian:		
Baked Cheese Ravioli	290	12
Cheese Manicotti	300	13
Garden Lasagne	380	14
Italian Cheese Lasagne	380	14
Lasagne with Meat Sauce	330	11
Pasta Primavera	260	11
Pasta Rigati	290	9
Spaghetti with Meat Sauce	280	7
Mexican:		
Burritos: Beefsteak	310	12
Chicken	310	13
Enchiladas: Beef Ranchero	300	13
Cheese Ranchero	360	18
Chicken Suiza	330	15
Fajitas: Beef	250	7
Chicken	230	5

WORTHINGTON

See Vegetarian Section — Page 51.

FROZEN PIZZAS

FAST-FOODS RESTAURANTS
Pizza Hut, Domino's, Shakey's, Godfather's:
See Fast-Foods Section.

BANQUET
	CALS	FAT
Zap French Bread: Cheese	310	10
Pepperoni	350	16
Deluxe	330	13

CELESTE
	CALS	FAT
Per 6 oz (1/4 Large or 1/2 Small)		
Cheese, Vegetable	320	17
Deluxe, Sausage, Pepperoni	380	22
Supreme	380	24
Pizza For One: Cheese	500	25
Pepperoni	545	30
Sausage, Deluxe	570	32
Suprema	680	39
Vegetable	490	26

FOX, MR P'S
	CALS	FAT
DELUXE — Per 1/2 Pizza		
Golden Topping	240	11
Other varieties, average	260	13

JENO'S
	CALS	FAT
CRISP 'N TASTY — Per 1/2 Pizza		
Canadian Style Bacon	250	11
Cheese	270	14
Comb. Sausage & Pepperoni	300	16
Hamburger, Pepperoni	290	15
Sausage	300	16
PIZZA ROLLS — Per 6 Rolls (3 oz)		
Microwave varieties	250	13
Other varieties	240	13
4-PACK PIZZA — Per Pizza		
Cheese	160	8
Other Flavors	180	9

LEAN CUISINE
	CALS	FAT
Cheese, 1 whole pizza	310	10
Other Pizzas, average	350	12

PAPPALO'S
	CALS	FAT
PAN PIZZA — Per 1/6 Pizza		
Combination, Pepperoni	340	15
Hamburger	310	12
Sausage	360	18
THIN CRUST — Per 1/6 Pizza		
Hamburger	240	8
Pepp./Saus./Combin., average	260	10
FRENCH BREAD PIZZA — Whole		
Combination	430	21
Cheese	360	15
Pepperoni, Sausage	410	20

PEPPERIDGE FARM
	CALS	FAT
CROISSANT PASTRY PIZZA		
Cheese, Pepperoni	490	26
Deluxe, Hamburger	520	27
Sausage	540	29

PILLSBURY
	CALS	FAT
MICROWAVE — Per 1/2 Pizza		
Cheese	240	10
Pepperoni, Combination	310	15
Sausage	280	13
FRENCH BREAD PIZZA		
Cheese, 1 pizza	370	15
Pepperoni, 1 pizza	430	19
Sausage, 1 pizza	410	16
& Pepperoni Combination	450	21
ALL READY PIZZA CRUST		
Pizza Crust, 1/4 whole	180	2

STOUFFER'S
	CALS	FAT
TRADITIONAL PIZZAS		
Cheese, 1/2 pkg	320	15
Other types, average, 1/2 pkg	370	19
FRENCH BREAD PIZZAS — 1/2 Pkg		
Canadian Style Bacon	360	14
Cheese	340	13
Deluxe; Vegetable Deluxe	430	21
Double Cheese; Sausage	410	18
Hamburger, Pepperoni	410	20
Pepperoni & Mushroom	430	22
Sausage & Pepperoni	450	23

TOTINO'S
	CALS	FAT
PARTY PIZZA — Per 1/2 Pizza		
Cheese	340	17
Canadian Bacon; Vegetable	310	14
Combination, Sausage, Bacon	385	21
Hamburger, Pepperoni	370	19
PAN PIZZA — Per 1/6 Pizza		
Three Cheese	290	10
Sausage, Pepperoni	330	14
MY CLASSIC DELUXE — Per 1/6 Pizza		
Deluxe Cheese	210	9
Combination, Pepperoni	270	14
MICROWAVE (Small) — 1 Pizza		
Cheese	250	8
Sausage, Saus./Pepp. Comb.	320	16
Pepperoni	280	12
Pizza Slices: Cheese	170	7
Sausage/Pepp./Combination	200	10

WEIGHT WATCHERS
	CALS	FAT
Cheese; Sausage, 1 pizza	310	8
Combination, 1 pizza	300	9
Pepperoni, 1 pizza	320	9
French Bread Pizzas, average	310	13

CANNED & PACKAGED (NON-FROZEN) ENTREES, MEALS & FOOD PRODUCTS

CAMPBELL'S

	CALS	FAT
Barbecue Beans (Per 8 oz)	210	4
Home Style Beans	230	4
Old Fash. Beans in Molasses	230	3
Pork & Beans in Tomato Sce	190	2
Ranchero Beans	180	4

CHEF BOYARDEE

Microwave Meals (7½ oz):

	CALS	FAT
ABC's & 123's; Tic Tac Toes	260	11
Beef Ravioli	220	5
Beefaroni	220	7
Cheese Ravioli	200	3
Dinosaurs: Pasta w/Cheese	160	1
with Meatballs	230	8
Elbows Macaroni & Beef	210	7
Lasagne: with Beef	230	9
w/Garden Veges	230	7
Rigatoni; Shells (Tom./Meat Sce)	210	6
Spaghetti & Meatballs	240	10

ESTEE

	CALS	FAT
Beef Ravioli; Beef Stew	210	8
Spaghetti & Meatballs	240	15
Chili with Beans	390	28

FEATHERWEIGHT

	CALS	FAT
Chicken/Dumplings (Per Pkg)	160	5
Beef Ravioli	220	4
Chili with Beans	280	10
Spagh./Meatballs; Beef Stew	160	3
Chicken Stew; Spanish Rice	140	1

FRANCO-AMERICAN

Pasta — Per Serving, 7½ oz

	CALS	FAT
Beef RaviolO's in Meat Sce	250	8
Hearty Pasta: Beef Ravioli	280	11
Macaroni w/Beef in Tom. Sce	200	5
Macaroni & Cheese	170	2
Spaghetti: in Tom. Sce/Cheese	190	2
w. Meatballs in Tom. Sce	220	8
Circus O's/Spaghetti O's, reg.	170	2
w. Meatballs/Beef Franks	210	8

HAIN

3-Grain Side Dishes — Per ½ Cup

	CALS	FAT
Rice Almondine/Oriental	130	5
Chicken Meatless Style	100	1
Herb Side Dish	80	1

HAIN (CONT)

Canned Chili — Per 7½ oz

	CALS	FAT
Spicy Chili with Chicken	130	2
Spicy Tempeh	160	4
Spicy Vegetarian	160	1

HAMBURGER HELPER

Made as directed — ⅕ Pkg (1 Cup)

	CALS	FAT
Cheeseburger Macaroni	370	19
Creamy Stroganoff	390	20
Meatloaf	360	22
Beef Noodle; Hamburger Stew	320	15
Potatoes Au Gratin; Stroganoff	320	15
Pizzabake; Sloppy Joe, ⅙ pkg	320	14
Tamale Pie	380	16
Other flavors, average ⅕ pkg	350	14

HEALTH VALLEY — P. 50

HEINZ

	CALS	FAT
Pork 'N' Beans/Tom. Sce, 4 oz	125	1
Veget. Beans/Tom. Sce, 4 oz	115	<1

HORMEL MICRO CUP

Per Cup (7½ oz)

	CALS	FAT
Chili with Beans	250	11
Chili, no Beans	380	28
Chili Mac	200	10
Dinty Moore Beef Stew	190	9
Lasagne	250	13
Macaroni & Cheese	190	6
Noodles & Chicken	180	7
Pork & Beans	250	5
Ravioli in Tomato Sauce	250	11
Spaghetti & Meatballs	205	7
Scalloped Potatoes & Ham	260	16

KRAFT

SIDE DISHES
Made as directed — Per ½ Cup

	CALS	FAT
Velveeta Shells & Cheese	210	8
Pasta & Cheese: All types	180	8
Pasta Salad: with Creamy Dill	190	11
Homestyle; Rancher's	240	16
Garden Primavera	170	7
Vegetable with Parmesan	210	11
Potatoes & Cheese: All types	140	5
Rice & Ch.: Cheddar/Broccoli	180	8
Other varieties	150	4

CANNED & PACKAGED (NON-FROZEN) ENTREES, MEALS & FOOD PRODUCTS

LA CHOY

	CALS	FAT
Entrees, Canned — Per ¾ Cup		
Oriental: Beef Pepper	90	2
Sweet & Sour w/Chicken	240	2
Sweet & Sour w/Pork	250	4
Bi-packs — Per Serving		
Chicken/Pork Chow Mein	80	3
Beef Pepper Oriental	100	3
Beef/Shrimp Chow Mein	70	1
Sukiyaki	70	1
Vegetable Chow Mein	50	2

LITTLE BEAR

	CALS	FAT
Baked Beans, 7½ oz	240	1
Chili, Vegetarian, 7½ oz	160	1
Refried Beans, 4 oz	90	3

LUNCH BUCKET

	CALS	FAT
Beef Ravioli (Per Serving)	260	4
Beef Stew	190	6
Chicken Noodle; Hearty Chick.	110	3
Chili (Reg./Hot) w/Beans	330	16
Country Vegetable Soup	90	3
Lasagne; Spagh. N' Meat Sce	260	5
Pasta N' Chicken	220	8
Macaroni & Beef	250	4

NASOYA — See Page 50

SWANSON

	CALS	FAT
Canned — Per Serving		
Chicken a la King, 5¼ oz	180	12
Chicken & Dumplings, 7½ oz	220	12
Chicken Stew, 7½ oz	170	7
Chunk Mixin' Chicken, 2½ oz	130	8
Chunky Chicken Spread, 1 oz	60	4
Premium Chunk Poultry		
White & Dark Chicken, 2½ oz	100	4
White Turkey, 2½ oz	90	2
White & Dark Turkey, 2½ oz	90	3

TOP SHELF (HORMEL)

	CALS	FAT
Beef Oriental/Stroganoff	300	10
Boneless Beef Ribs	400	19
Italian Style Lasagne	350	16
Spaghettini w/Meat Sauce	260	6
Tender Beef Roast	250	7

ROSARITA

	CALS	FAT (g)
Refried Beans:		
Reg./Spicy, ½ cup, 4½ oz	140	4
Vegetarian, ½ cup, 4½ oz	120	2

TUNA HELPER

	CALS	FAT
Made as directed — Per ⅕ Pkg		
Tuna Au Gratin; Buttery Rice	280	11
Cheesy Ndls; Tuna Tetrazzini	250	9
Creamy: Mushroom	220	6
Noodles; Fettucini Alfredo	300	13
Tuna Salad; Pot Pie (5oz)	420	27

VAN CAMP'S

	CALS	FAT
Per 1 Cup (8 oz)		
Pork & Beans	220	2
Baked Beans	260	2
Deluxe Baked Beans	320	4
Brown Sugar Beans	290	5
Butter Beans	160	1
Chili with Beans	350	23
Chili without Beans	410	34
Kidney Beans		
Dark/Light/New Orleans	180	1
Mexican Style Chili Beans	210	2
Red Beans	190	1
Vegetarian Style Beans	210	1
Spanish Rice	160	4
Tamales with Sauce	290	16
Beanee Weenee	330	15
Chili Weenee	310	16
Noodlee Weenee	240	8
Spaghetti Weenee	240	7

WOLF BRAND

	CALS	FAT
Per 1 Cup (8 oz)		
Beef Stew	180	8
Chili with Beans	350	22
Chili without Beans	390	27
Extra Spicy Chili with Beans	330	21
Extra Spicy Chili w/out Beans	360	25
Chili-Mac	320	20
Chili Hot Dog Sauce, ⅙ cup	40	2
Tamales	350	24

WORTHINGTON — Page 51

VEGETARIAN MEALS & PRODUCTS

FANTASTIC FOODS

Mixes - Made-up, cooked:	CALS	FAT (g)
Fantastic Falafil, fried, 6 small balls, 3 oz	240	14
Nature's Burger (Original) + fat, 1 burger, 3 oz	200	9
Tofu Burger, 1 burger	135	5
Tofu Scrambler (+ fat), ½ cup	160	12
Tofu Classics (+ fat/oil), average, ½ cup, 4 oz	140	8
Veg. Chili (+ beans), ½ c.	105	1

HEALTH VALLEY

FAST MENU — Per ½ Can (7½ oz)		
Amaranth with Garden Veg.	140	3
Hearty Lentil & Vegetables	150	4
Honey Baked Org. Beans Tofu	140	4
Oat Bran Pilaf w. Vegetables	210	7
Organic Black Beans w. Tofu	150	4
Organic Lentils with Tofu	170	5
Western Black Bean w. Veg.	160	5
Chili Beans & Sauce:		
Boston Baked Beans, 7½ oz	190	<1
Mild Veg. Chili/Beans, 5 oz	160	3
Mild Veg. Chili/Lentils, 5 oz	140	4
Tomato Sauce, 1 cup	70	<1
Veg. Beans w/Miso, 7½ oz	180	<1

Other Products: See separate sections for cereals, cookies, snacks, soups, muffins.

LEGUME

FROZEN ENTREES — Per Serving		
Classic Manicotti	220	11
Classic Lasagne, ½ pkg	210	8
Hearty Vegetarian Stew	350	8
Manicotti Florentine	260	7
Mexican Enchiladas	270	8
Pasta Primavera	180	5
Stuffed Shells Provencale	240	11
Vegetable Bean Ragout	190	4
Vegetable Lasagne/Ravioli	240	8
Vegetarian Chili	245	8
Vegetarian Franks & Beans	280	7
Vegetable Tortellini	240	5

MANDARIN SOYFOODS

Garden Patties w. Cheese, (1)	147	2
Tofu Patties w. Cheese, (1)	150	3
Plain w. Herbs/Veg., (1)	145	1

MORNINGSTAR FARMS

FROZEN PRODUCTS	CALS	FAT (g)
Country Breakfast: Per Serving		
with Hashbrowns	360	23
with Pancakes	380	19
French Toast & Patties	380	15
Country Crisp Patties, each	220	15
H/style Country Crisps, 3 oz	250	16
Breakfast: Strips, 3 strips	80	6
Links, 3 links	190	14
Patties, 2 patties	190	12
Grillers, 1 patty	180	12
Scramblers, ¼ cup	60	3

MUDPIE

Vegie Burgers, 1 patty, 3 oz	200	11

NASOYA

FROZEN PRODUCTS — Per Serving		
Classic Lasagne, ½ package	210	8
Classic Manicotti, ½ package	220	11
Manicotti, 2 manicotti	320	14
Manicotti Florentine, 1 pkg	260	7
Mexican Enchiladas, 1 pkg	270	8
Ravioli, ¼ pkg, 7-8 ravioli	255	7
Stuffed Shells: 2 shells	315	15
Provencale, 1 pkg	240	12
Tortellini, ½ package	275	4
Vegetable Lasagne, 1 package	240	8
TOFU PRODUCTS		
Tofu: Soft, 4 oz	70	6
Premium Soft, 4 oz	80	4
Silken, 4 oz	50	5
Firm, 4 oz	100	5
Extra Firm, 4 oz	140	8
Chinese 5 Spice Tofu, 5 oz	150	8
French Cntry. Herb Tofu, 5 oz	150	8
Vegi-Dressings, 1 Tbsp, ½ oz	40	3
Wonton Skins, 1 skin	22	0
Egg Roll Wrappers, each	22	0

NILE SPICE

Per ½ Cup		
Rozdali: Spicy Currant	161	4
Vegetable Curry	154	4
Couscous Salad, ½ cup	103	5
Couscous Whole Wheat	153	4

VEGETARIAN MEALS & PRODUCTS

WORTHINGTON

FROZEN PRODUCTS	CALS	FAT (g)
Beef Pie, Vegetarian, 1 pie	360	16
Bolono, 2 slices	60	2
Chicken Pie, Vegetarian, 1 pie	380	20
Chicken, Meatless, ½ cup, 3 oz	190	13
Chic-Ketts, ½ cup, 3 oz	160	7
Chik Stiks, 1 stik	110	7
Crispy Chik, 3 oz	280	19
Crispy Chik Patties, 1 patty	220	15
Dinner Roast, 4 oz	240	16
Dixie Dogs, 1 dog	200	10
Egg Rolls, Vegetarian, 1 roll	160	6
Fillets, Vegetarian, 2 fillets	180	9
Fripats, 1 piece, 2¼ oz	180	12
Golden Croquettes, each	280	14
Harvest Bake, Lentil Rice Loaf, 2½ slices, 4 oz	190	9
Leanies, 1 link	100	6
Meatless: Beef Style, 3 sl., 2 oz	100	5
Chicken, 2 slices, 2 oz	130	9
Corned Beef, 4 sl., 2 oz	120	6
Salami, 2 slices, 1½ oz	90	5
Smoked Beef, 3 sl., 2 oz	120	6
Smoked Turkey, 3 sl., 2 oz	135	9
Okara Patties, 1 patty	160	10
Prosage Roll, 2 slices (³/₈")	180	12
Prosage Links, 3 links	190	14
Prosage Patties, 2 patties	210	14
Stakelets, 1 piece, 2½ oz	150	8
Stripples, 4 strips	120	9
Tofu Garden Patties, 1 patty	90	4
Tuno, ¼ cup, 2 oz	100	7
Veelets, 1 piece	230	14
Wham, 3 slices, 2½ oz	120	7

CANNED & DRY PRODUCTS		
Chik: Diced, ¼ cup, 2 oz	90	8
Sliced, 2 slices, 2 oz	90	8
Chili, ²/₃ cup, 5 oz	190	10
Choplets, 2 slices, 3¼ oz	100	2
Country Stew, 1¼ cup, ½ can	220	10
Fri-Chik, 2 pieces, 3 oz	180	13
Gran Burger, dry, 6 Tbsp	110	1
Multi-grain Cutlets, 2 sl., 3¼ oz	90	2
Non-Meatballs, 3 balls, 2 oz	100	6
Numete, ½" slice, 2½ oz	160	11
Prime Stakes, each, 3¼ oz	160	10

WORTHINGTON (CONT)

CANNED & DRY PRODUCTS (CONT)	CALS	FAT
Protose, ½" slice, 2½ oz	180	8
Saucettes, 2 links	140	9
Savory Slices, 2 slices, 2 oz	100	6
Super Links, 1 link	100	7
Turkee Slices, 2 slices	130	9
Vege Steaks, 2½ pieces	110	2
Vegetarian Burger: ½ cup, 4 oz	150	4
No Salt added, ½ cup	160	6
Veget. Skallops, ½ cup, 3 oz	90	2
No Salt, ½ cup, 3 oz	80	1
Veja-Links, 2 links	140	10

NATURAL TOUCH		
Taco Mix, 2 Tbsp (made up)	90	2
Loaf Mix, ¼ package	180	7
Vegetarian Chili, ²/₃ cup	230	12
Dinner Entree, 1 patty. 3 oz	230	14
Stroganoff Mix, ¼ package	90	3
Caroby, Milk Bar, 4 sections	150	9

VEGGIE POCKETS

Ken & Robert's (Imagine Foods):		
Greek Style	360	15
Pizza Style; Tex-Mex	390	18

SOYBEAN PRODUCTS

	CALS	FAT
Curd Cheese, 1 oz	30	2
Miso, ½ cup, 5 oz	280	8
Natto, ½ cup, 3 oz	190	10
Tempeh, 1 piece, 3 oz	170	6
Fried, 3 oz	250	14
Tofu: Mori-Nu Tofu, Silken:		
Soft, 4 oz	60	3
Firm, 4 oz	70	3
Extra Firm, 4 oz	70	2
Hinoichu Tofu: Soft, 4 oz	60	3
Reg. (Japanese), 4 oz	80	4
Firm (Chinese), 4 oz	90	5
Nasoya Tofu: See opposite page		
Tofu, stir-fried, 4 oz	120	8
Soybean Protein (T.V.P.), 1 oz	90	0
Soy Drinks: See Page 20		

WHOLEFOOD PRODUCTS

Beans/Lentils — Pp. 92-95.
Cereals/Flours/Grains — Pp. 62-67.
Nuts/Seeds — Pp. 86-87.

51

CANNED, CONDENSED — Made as Directed

RED & WHITE LABEL Per 8 oz Serving	CALS	FAT (g)
Bean with Bacon	120	4
Beef	80	2
Beef Broth (Bouillon)	16	0
Beef Noodle	70	3
Beefy Mushroom	60	3
Black Bean	110	2
Cheddar Cheese	130	8
Chicken Alphabet/Barley	70	2
Chicken Broth	35	2
Chicken Broth & Noodles	60	2
Chicken Broth & Rice	50	1
Chicken 'n Dumplings	80	3
Chicken Gumbo	60	2
Chicken Noodle/Noodle'O's	70	2
Chicken with Rice	60	2
Chicken & Stars	60	2
Chicken Vegetable	70	3
Chili Beef	140	5
Clam Chowder, Manhattan	70	2
Clam Chowder, New England	80	3
made with Milk (whole)	150	7
Consomme (Beef) with Gelatin	25	0
Cream of Asparagus	90	4
Cream of Celery	100	7
Cream of Chicken	110	7
Cream of Mushroom	100	7
Cream of Potato	70	3
made w. Water & Milk	110	4
Cream of Shrimp	90	6
made with Milk (whole)	160	10
Creamy Chicken Mushroom	120	8
Curly Noodle with Chicken	80	3
French Onion	60	2
Golden Mushroom	80	3
Green Pea	160	3
Homestyle Beef Noodle	80	3
Homestyle Chicken Noodle	70	3
Homestyle Cream of Tomato	110	3
made with Milk (whole)	180	7
Homestyle Vegetable	60	2
Meatball Alphabet	100	4
Minestrone	80	2
Nacho Cheese	110	8
Noodles & Ground Beef	90	4
Old Fashioned Tomato Rice	110	2

RED & WHITE LABEL (CONT)	CALS	FAT (g)
Old Fashioned Vegetable	60	2
Oyster Stew	80	5
made with Milk (whole)	150	9
Pepper Pot	90	4
Scotch Broth	80	3
Split Pea with Ham & Bacon	150	4
Tomato	90	2
made with Milk (whole)	160	6
Tomato Bisque	120	3
Turkey Noodle	70	3
Turkey Vegetable	70	3
Vegetable	80	2
Vegetable Beef	70	2
Vegetarian Vegetable	80	2
Won Ton Soup	45	1
Zesty Tomato	90	1

CREAMY NAT. GOLD LABEL — 8 oz	CALS	FAT (g)
Asparagus, with water	100	5
made with Milk (whole)	170	9
Broccoli, with water	70	3
made with Milk (whole)	140	7
Cauliflower, with water	130	9
made with Milk (whole)	200	13
Potato, with water	120	7
made with Milk (whole)	190	11

GOLDEN CLASSIC — 8 oz	CALS	FAT (g)
Chicken Veg. w. Wild Rice	80	3
Sirloin Beef	70	3
Tortellini & Vegetable	80	3

SPEC. REQUEST 1/3 LESS SALT - 8 oz	CALS	FAT (g)
Bean with Bacon	120	4
Chicken Noodle	70	2
Chicken with Rice	60	2
Cream of Chicken	110	7
Cream of Mushroom	100	7
Tomato	90	2
Vegetable	80	2
Vegetable Beef	70	2

LOW SODIUM — Per Can, 10½ oz	CALS	FAT (g)
Chicken Broth	40	2
Chicken with Noodles	160	5
Chunky Chicken Vegetable	240	11
Cream of Mushroom	190	13
Split Pea	240	5
Tomato with Tomato Pieces	180	5

SOUPS (CONT)

CAMPBELL'S (CONT)

	CALS	FAT (g)
MICROWAVE CHUNKY		
Beef with Country Veges.	170	4
Chicken Noodle w. Mushr.	180	7
New Engl. Clam Chowder	250	15
Old Fash. Chick./Country Veg.	150	4
Sirloin Burger w/Country Veg.	200	8
HOME COOKIN' 19 oz — Per ½ Can		
Chicken with Noodles	120	3
Country Vegetable	110	2
Hearty Beef; Minestrone	130	3
Hearty Lentil	150	1
Split Pea with Ham	190	4
Tomato Garden; Veget. Beef	130	3
CHUNKY, 19 oz SIZE — Per ½ Can		
Beef	170	4
Chicken Noodle; Chicken Veg.	180	6
Clam Chowder, Manhattan	150	4
Clam Chowder, New England	250	15
Minestrone; Steak & Potato	170	5
Old Fashioned Bean with Ham	250	8
Old Fashioned Chicken	150	4
Old Fashioned Vegetable Beef	160	5
Split Pea with Ham	210	5
SOUP-FOR-ONE — Per Can, 7¾ oz		
Clam Chowder, New England	130	4
Golden Chicken and Noodles	120	4
Old Fashioned Bean with Ham	220	7
Old World Vegetable	130	4
Savory Cream of Mushroom	180	13
Tomato Royale	180	3
CAMPBELL'S CUP 2 MIN. SOUP MIX		
Chicken Noodle/Vegetable	90	2
Creamy Chicken w.White Meat	120	5
Noodle with Chicken Broth	100	2
Vegetable Beef w. Sirloin Beef	110	2
QUALITY SOUP & RECIPE MIX		
Chicken Noodle, Noodle	100	2
Chicken Rice with White Meat	90	2
Onion, Onion Mushroom	50	<1
INSTANT SOUP CUPS		
Chicken Flavor Noodle	140	3
Noodle w/Chicken Broth	130	2
INSTANT SOUP (PACKETS)		
Noodle w/Chicken Broth	110	2
Onion	30	0

CUP-A-SOUP (LIPTON)

	CALS	FAT
Chicken Broth, 6 fl.oz	20	<1
Chicken Noodle	50	1
Chicken Vegetable	45	1
Cream of Chicken	80	4
Creamy Chicken w/Veges.	90	4
Creamy Broccoli	60	2
Creamy Broccoli & Cheese	70	3
Cream of Mushroom	70	3
Country Style: Chicken Supr.	110	6
Harvest Vegetable	100	1
Hearty Chicken	70	1
Green Pea	110	4
Onion	25	<1
Tomato	100	1
Lite: Chicken Florentine	40	1
Creamy Tomato & Herb	70	<1
Golden Broccoli; Spr. Veg.	40	1
Lemon Chicken	45	<1
Oriental Cup	45	2

CUP O' NOODLES (NISSIN)

	CALS	FAT
Cup O' Noodles:		
Aver. all varieties, ½ pkg	145	7
Twin Pack: Average, 1 cup	150	7
Oodles of Noodles (Top Ramen):		
Beef/Chicken, aver. ½ pkg	200	9
Hearty Cup O' Noodles:		
Aver. all varieties, ½ pkg	150	7

Note: Cholesterol in above range: < 5 mg

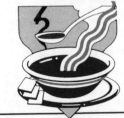

Lower calorie soups are useful fillers for dieters. Avoid high-fat rich soups. Nutritious soups can also aid health recovery.

SOUPS (CONT)

CROSSE & BLACKWELL

Per ½ Can, 6½ oz	CALS	FAT
Black Bean w. Sherry	80	3
Clam Chowder: Manhattan	50	1
New England	90	4
Consomme; Gazpacho	25	<1
Crab a la Maryland	50	1
Minestrone	90	3
Mushr. Bisque; Crm Shrimp	90	5
Vichyssoise, Cream of	70	3

ESTEE

	CALS	FAT
Chunky Chicken Veg., 7½ oz	120	6
Chunky Minestrone, 7½ oz	160	5
Chunky Vegetable Beef, 7½ oz	140	7
Dry Mixes: Per 6 oz Serving		
Mushroom; Tomato	40	1
Chicken/Beef Noodle; Onion	25	<1

FANTASTIC NOODLES

	CALS	FAT
Creamy Cheddar (Per ½ pkg)	180	8
Miso Vegetable, Curry Veg.	150	7
Tomato Vegetable	160	7

FEATHERWEIGHT

	CALS	FAT
Chicken Noodle (Per 7½ oz)	70	1
Mushroom	60	1
Tomato	80	1
Vegetable Beef	100	2

HAIN

CANNED — Per Serving		
Chicken Broth	70	6
Chicken Noodle Soup	120	4
Creamy Mushroom Soup	110	4
Italian Vege-Pasta Soup	160	5
Minestrone Soup; Split Pea	170	2
New England Clam Chowder	180	4
Vegetarian Lentil Soup	160	3
Vegetarian Vegetable Soup	140	4
SOUP MIXES — Per 6 oz Serving		
Cheese & Broccoli	310	22
Minestrone Savory	110	1
Potato Leek Savory	260	18
Split Pea Savory	310	10
Tomato Savory; Mushr. Sav.	220	14
Vegetable Savory	80	1

HEALTH VALLEY

Per ½ Can (7½ oz)	CALS	FAT
Beef Broth	10	<1
Black Bean	150	2
Chicken Broth	35	2
Chunky 5 Bean Vegetable	110	2
Chunky Vegetable Chicken	125	2
Green Split Pea	180	<1
Lentil	220	4
Minestrone; Tomato	130	3
Manhattan Clam Chowder	110	2
Mushroom Barley	100	2
Vegetable	110	1
Fat Free Range: ½ can	60-80	<1

HORMEL

Micro Cup Hearty Soup, 7½ oz		
Bean & Ham	190	3
Beef Vegetable	80	1
Chicken Noodle	110	3
Chicken w/Rice Veg; Minestrone	110	2
Country Vegetable	90	2
New Engl. Clam Chowder	120	5

LIPTON

INSTANT SOUPS — Per 8 fl.oz		
Beef Oriental Noodle	180	<1
Chicken Oriental Noodle	180	2
Garden Veg; Oriental Noodle	200	1
COUNTRY STYLE — Per 8 fl.oz		
Creamy Chicken Vegetable	145	9
Vegetable w/Meatballs	135	3
Virginia Pea	200	8
LOTS-A-NOODLES		
Beef, 9 oz	170	<1
Chicken; Other flavors	180	2
HEARTY ONES		
Homestyle Chicken Noodle	230	4
Classic Italian Pasta Soup	330	2
Old Fash. Beef Noodle	230	3

NILE SPICE

Per 8 oz Serving		
Golden Couscous: Lentil	175	<1
Vegetable Chicken	175	4
Vegetable Parmesan	160	3
Tomato Minestrone	160	0
Potato: All flavors	130	5

MANISCHEWITZ

Per 8 oz Serving	CALS	FAT (g)
Beef Cabbage	60	<1
Borscht with Beets	80	0
Low Calorie Borscht	20	0
Chicken (Clear)/Rice	45	<1
Chicken Barley	83	<1
Chicken Vegetable	55	<1
Mushroom Barley	70	<1
Schav	11	0
Split Pea	135	<1
Tomato/Vegetable	60	<1
Soup Mixes: Average, 6 fl.oz	50	<1

PROGRESSO

Per 9½ oz (½ of 19 oz Can)		
Beef; Hearty Beef, average	160	5
Beef Barley/Vegetable	150	4
Beef Minestrone	170	5
Chicken Broth, 8 oz	16	0
Chicken Noodle	120	4
Chicken Rice/Vegetable	130	3
Corn Chowder	200	10
Cream of Chicken	180	11
Cream of Mushroom	160	10
Hearty Chicken; Chickarina	130	4
Clam Chowder: Manhattan	120	2
New England Style	220	12
Green Split Pea	160	3
Ham & Bean	180	2
Homestyle Chicken	110	3
Hearty Chicken	130	4
Lentil	140	4
Lentil with Sausage	180	7
Minestrone	130	4
Split Pea with Ham	170	4
Tomato	120	3
Tomato Beef w/Rotini	170	4
Tortellini	90	3
Vegetable	80	2
Zesty Minestrone	150	8

SNOW'S

Made as Directed: Per 7½ oz		
Clam Chwdr, New Eng/Manhat	140	6
Corn Chowder	150	6
Fish/Seafood Chowder	130	6

PRITIKIN

Per ½ Can	CALS	FAT (g)
Beef Broth	20	<1
Chicken Broth	15	0
Chicken w. Pasta; Mushroom	60	<1
Chicken Veg.; Manhat. Clam	70	<1
Tomato; Vegetable	70	0
Minestrone	110	<1
Split Pea; Navy Bean	130	0

ROKEACH

Made Up: Per 8 oz Serving		
Borscht	120	<1
Celery, Cream of	90	4
Mushroom, Cream of	135	7
Tomato	90	1
Tomato with Rice	170	5
(Add extra if made with milk)		

STOUFFER'S

Cream of Spinach, 8 oz	210	15
New Eng. Clam Chowder, 8 oz	180	9

WEIGHT WATCHERS

Per 10½ oz Serving		
Chicken Noodle	80	2
Vegetable with Beef Stock	90	2
Turkey Vegetable	70	2
Chunky Vegetarian	100	2
Cream of Mushroom	90	2
Instant Broth	8	0

BOUILLON CUBES & POWDERS		
Bouillon Cubes: Aver. all types		
Regular, 1 cube	8	0
Low Sodium (LiteLine)	12	<1
Powders: Average, 1 tsp	8	0
Herb-Ox:		
Instant Broth & Seasoning:		
Beef, 1 envelope	8	0
Chicken, Vegetarian	12	<1
Onion	14	<1
Herbs, Spices: 1 tsp	5	0
SOUP OYSTER CRACKERS		
40 small/20 large, ½ oz	60	2

SAUCES & CONDIMENTS

SAUCES & CONDIMENTS

	CALS	FAT
Average of Brands & Homemade:		
Apple Sce: Swtnd., ¼ c, 2¼ oz	45	0
Unsweetened., ¼ cup, 2 oz	27	0
Barbecue, average, 1 Tbsp	20	0
Bearnaise Sce, ¼ cup, 2½ oz	190	19
Catsup (Ketchup): Reg., 1 Tbsp	16	0
Heinz Lite, 1 Tbsp	8	0
Cheese, h/made, ¼ c, 2½ oz	150	10
Chili Sauce: Heinz, 1 Tbsp	17	0
Del Monte, 1 Tbsp	35	0
Wolf Hot Dog, 1 Tbsp	15	<1
Cranberry Sce, jelled, ¼ c, 2½ oz	105	0
Escoffier Sauces, 1 Tbsp	20	<1
Horseradish: Kraft, 1 Tbsp	10	1
Heinz, 1 Tbsp	70	7
Sauceworks, 1 Tbsp	50	5
Mushroom Sauce, ¼ cup, 2 oz	50	2
Mustard, average, 1 tsp	5	0
Hot Must. (Sceworks), 1 tsp	12	<1
Pizza Sauce, cnd, ¼ cup, 2 oz	40	2
Salsa (La Victoria), aver., 1 T	5	0
Seafood Cocktail Sce, 1 Tbsp	20	1
Soy Sce, all types, av., 1 Tbsp	10	0
Spaghetti Sce: ½ cup, 4½ oz	135	6
(Also see Prego/Ragu — Next Page)		
Steak Sauce: A.1., 1 Tbsp	12	<1
Lea & Perrins, 1 Tbsp	20	<1
Heinz — See next column.		
Strawberry Puree Sauce,		
unsweet., 2 Tbsp, 1 oz	9	0
Sweet & Sour Sauce:		
Contadina, ¼ cup, 2 oz	75	<1
Kikkoman, 2 Tbsp, 1 oz	35	<1
La Choy, 2 Tbsp, 1 oz	60	<1
Tabasco Sauce, 1 Tbsp	2	0
Taco Sauce, average, ¼ cup	20	0
Tartar Sauce, 1 Tbsp	75	7
Teriyaki Sauce, 1 Tbsp	15	0
Tomato Ketchup (Heinz), 1 Tbsp	16	0
Weight Watchers, 1 Tbsp	12	0
Tomato Paste, 6 oz pkg/¾ cup	150	0
Tomato Puree, ½ cup	50	0
Tomato Sauce, ½ cup, 4¼ oz	40	0
Vinegar: White or wine, 1 fl.oz	4	0
Great Impressions, 1 fl.oz	14	0
White Sauce, ½ cup, 5 oz	130	7
Worcestershire Sce, 1 Tbsp	10	0

HEINZ

Per 1 Tbsp — Approx. ½ oz	CALS	FAT (g)
Barbecue Sauces: All flavors	18	0
Chili Sauce; 57 Sauce	15	0
Horseradish Sauce	70	7
Mustard: Pourable/Mild	8	<1
Spicy Brown	13	1
Seafood Cocktail Sauce	16	0
Steak Sauce (Traditional)	11	0
Tartar Sauce	66	7
Tomato Ketchup	16	0
Worcestershire Sauce	8	0

KRAFT

All Natural Sauces: 2 Tbsp, (⅒ Pkg)		
Alfredo, 1 oz	50	4
Bearnaise Herb Butter, 1 oz	70	7
Cheese: Ched./Nacho/Triple	60	4
Hollandaise, 1 oz	80	7
Barbecue Sauces:		
Average all types, 2 Tbsp	50	1
Other Sauces: Per 1 Tbsp		
Horseradish: Reg./Cream Style	10	0
Mustard	10	0

ESTEE

Barbecue Sauce, 1 Tbsp	18	<1
Spaghetti Sauce, ½ cup, 4 oz	60	2
Steak Sauce, 1 Tbsp	14	<1

FEATHERWEIGHT

Barbecue Sauce, 1 Tbsp	14	0
Catsup, Chili Sauce, 1 Tbsp	8	0
Mustard, 1 tsp	5	0
Spaghetti Sce w. Mushr., 4 oz	60	2

NEWMAN'S OWN

Spaghetti Sauce, ½ cup, 4 oz	70	2
Bandito Diavalo Spicy, ½ cup	70	2

PRITIKIN

Mexican Sauce, ¼ can, 4 oz	50	1
Spaghetti/Mushrooms, ¼ can	60	0

ROSARITA

Enchilada Sauce, ¼ cup, 2 oz	12	0
Nacho Cheese, ¼ cup, 2¼ oz	105	8
Taco Sauce, ¼ cup, 2 oz	20	0

SAUCES, GRAVIES, PICKLES

SPAGHETTI SAUCES

Per ½ Cup, 4 oz	CALS	FAT (g)
Prego: Al Fresco, all flavors	100	5
Extra Chunky: Saus./Pepp.	170	9
Other flavors	110	6
Marinara	100	5
Meat Flavored	150	6
Mushroom	140	5
No Salt Added	100	6
Regular	140	6
Ragu: Chunky Garden Style	70	3
Fresh Italian	90	3
Pizza Quick	35	2
Spaghetti	80	4
Thick & Hearty	100	3
Weight Watchers: With Meat	75	2
With Mushrooms	60	<1

(Also See Estee/F'therwt/Newman's/Pritikin.)

SAUCE MIXES

BORDEN (Made up)		
El Molino: Hot Enchilada, ¼ c.	32	2
Mild Gr. Chili; Red Taco, ¼ c.	20	0
Snow's: Newburg, ⅓ cup	120	8
Welsh Rarebit Ch., ½ cup	170	11
HAIN — Pasta & Sauce		
Creamy Parmesan, ¼ pkg	150	3
Fettucini Alfredo, ¼ pkg	180	4
Italian Herb, ⅕ pkg	110	2
Marinara, ¼ pkg	120	1
Primavera, ¼ pkg	140	4
McCORMICK — Per ½ Package		
Beef Stew; Beef Stroganoff	65	<1
Cheese Sauce	70	3
Chili Season.; Meat Marinade	55	1
Hamburger	65	2
Hollandaise	100	8
Nacho Cheese	85	3
Sour Cream	90	6
Spaghetti Sce; Taco Seasoning	65	<1
Pasta Prima (McCormick):		
Alfredo, ½ cup (made up)	255	13
Herb & Garlic, ½ cup	325	12
Marinara, ½ cup	330	8
Pesto, ½ cup	195	6
Pasta Salad, ½ cup	390	23

GRAVIES

Homemade Gravy:	CALS	FAT
Thin, little fat, 2 Tbsp, 1 oz	20	1
Thick, 2 Tbsp, 1¼ oz	50	2
¼ cup, 2½ oz	100	4
Franco-American (Canned)		
Au Jus Gravy, ¼ cup, 2 oz	10	0
Beef Gravy w. Onions, 2 oz	25	1
Chicken Gravy, 2 oz	50	4
Mushroom Gravy, 2 oz	25	1
Pork Gravy, 2 oz	40	3
Turkey Gravy, 2 oz	30	2
Estee (Gravy Mixes) — Made Up		
Brown Gravy, ¼ cup, 2 oz	14	0
Chicken & Herb, ¼ cup, 2 oz	20	<1
Pillsbury (Gravy Mixes)		
Brown; Homestyle, ¼ cup	15	0
Chicken, as prep., ¼ cup	25	1

PICKLES & RELISHES

Average of Brands		
Bread & Butt. Pickles, 4 sl., 1 oz	20	0
Chutney, 2 Tbsp, 1¼ oz	40	0
Dill: 1 md., (3¾"x1¼" diam.), 2¼ oz	7	0
1 large (4"x1¾" diameter), 5 oz	15	0
Halves: Small, 1 oz	3	0
Large, 2½ oz	8	0
Slices, 4 slices, 1 oz	3	0
Sweet, small, ½ oz	22	0
Gherkins, sweet, 1 med., 1 oz	15	0
Horseradish, 1 Tbsp	10	0
Lemon Juice, 1 Tbsp	4	0
Mustard, aver. all brands, 1 tsp	5	0
Olives — See Page 89.		
Peppers: Hot/Mild, 1 oz	8	0
Pickled: Beets, ½ cup, 4 oz	75	0
Onions, 1 medium, ¾ oz	10	0
Cocktail Onion, 1 onion	2	0
Red Cabbage, ½ cup, 3 oz	60	0
Pickles, sweet, 2 Tbsp, 1 oz	35	0
Relishes: S/wich Spread, 1 tsp	20	1
Cranberry-Orange, 1 Tbsp	30	0
Hot Dog (Heinz), 1 Tbsp	17	0
Sweet Pickle, 1 Tbsp	20	0
Sauerkraut, ½ cup, 3½ oz	25	0
Sweet Cauliflower	35	0
Salsa: Average all types		
Regular, no oil, 2 Tbsp	15	0
w/Oil, homemade, 2 Tbsp	40	3

SALAD DRESSINGS

Per Tablespoon, Approx. ½ oz (14g)

BERNSTEIN

	CALS	FAT
Blue Cheese, Caesar, French	50	5
Herb & Garlic Italian	60	6
Italian: Low Calorie	4	<1
Restaurant	65	7
with Cheese	45	3
with Cheese, Low Calorie	12	1
with Cheese & Garlic	50	5
Roquefort; Thousand Island	65	7
Vinaigrette Low Calorie	2	<1

COOK'S CLASSICS

	CALS	FAT
Apple/Honey Mustard	50	6
Cook's Caesar	50	5
Country French/Dijon	10	0
Dill; Italian Garlic	5	0
Tarragon, Garlic Lover's	50	5

ESTEE

	CALS	FAT
Blue Cheese	8	<1
Creamy: Dijon	8	<1
Garlic	2	0
Italian	4	0
French	4	0
Red Wine Vinegar	2	0
Thousand Island	8	0
Mayonnaise: 1 Tbsp	50	5

FEATHERWEIGHT

	CALS	FAT
Creamy: Cucumber	4	0
Dijon	20	2
French	14	0
Garden Herb	25	2
Italian	4	0
Italian Cheese; Oriental Spice	20	2
Russian; Red Wine Vinegar	6	0
Mayonnaise: 1 Tbsp	30	2
Soyamaise: 1 Tbsp	100	11

HOLLYWOOD

	CALS	FAT
Caesar; Crmy French, 1 Tbsp	70	7
Dijon Vinaigrette	60	6
Italian/Creamy Italian	90	9
Italian Cheese	80	8
Old Fashion Buttermilk	75	8
Poppy Seed Rancher's	75	8
Thousand Island	60	6

GOOD SEASONS (MIX)

	CALS	FAT (g)
Made as Directed		
Bleu Cheese & Herbs	70	8
Buttermilk Farm Style	60	6
Cheese: Garlic/Italian	70	8
Classic Herb, Garlic & Herbs	70	8
Italian: Regular	70	8
Lite, Lite Cheese	25	3
Lite Zesty	25	3
Mild/Zesty	70	8
No Oil	6	0
Lemon & Herbs	70	8
Ranch: Regular	60	6
Lite	30	2

HAIN

	CALS	FAT
Creamy: Caesar/Low-Salt	60	6
French	60	6
Italian/No Salt Added	80	8
Cucumber Dill	80	8
Dijon Vinaigrette	50	5
Garlic & Sour Cream	70	7
Honey & Sesame	60	5
Italian Cheese Vinaigrette	55	6
Old Fashioned Buttermilk	70	7
Poppyseed Rancher's	60	7
Savory Herb — No Salt Added	90	10
Swiss Cheese Vinaigrette	60	7
Thousand Island	50	5
Traditional Italian	80	8
No Salt Added	60	6
Mayonnaise: Light	60	6
All other varieties	110	12

HERB MAGIC

	CALS	FAT
Reduced Calorie: Herb Basket	6	0
Sweet & Sour	14	0
1000 Island; Crmy Cucumber	8	0
Zesty Tomato	18	0

HIDDEN VALLEY RANCH

	CALS	FAT
Take Heart: Bleu Cheese	12	0
French	20	0
Italian	16	0
Original Ranch	20	0
Thousand Island	20	0

58

SALAD DRESSINGS (CONT)

KRAFT

Per Tbsp, ½ oz	CALS	FAT (g)
Bacon & Tomato	70	7
But/milk Crmy; Bacon B/milk	80	8
Chunky Blue Cheese	60	6
Cole Slaw	70	6
Creamy: Garlic; Italian	50	5
Cucumber; On. & Chives	70	7
Russian	60	5
French; Italian	60	6
Miracle French; Gold. Caesar	70	6
Miracle Whip/Cholesterol Free	70	7
Oil & Vinegar; Presto Italian	70	8
Oil-Free Italian	4	0
Russian; 1000 Island & Bac.	60	5
Reduced Calorie:		
Bacon & Tomato/Buttermilk	30	2
Blue Cheese; Crmy Bacon	30	2
Crmy Cucumber; Crmy Italian	25	2
French	25	1
Italian, House	30	3
Italian, Zesty	20	2
Miracle Whip Light	45	4
Russian; 1000 Island	30	1
Kraft Free (No Fat): Italian	6	0
Catalina; Ranch	16	0
French; Thousand Island	20	0
Mayonnaise: Real	100	12
Light Reduced Calorie	50	5
Cholesterol Free	90	10
Cholesterol Free Light	45	5
Catalina: French	60	5
Reduced Calorie Dressing	18	1
Ranchers Choice: Creamy	90	10
Reduced Calorie Creamy	30	3
Roka: Blue Cheese	60	6
Reduced Cal. Blue Ch.	16	1

MARZETTI

	CALS	FAT
Buttermilk & Herb	90	10
Caesar	75	8
French: Regular	55	6
Light French	18	1
Honey Dijon; Red Wine Vin.	65	6
Italian: Reg./Gusto	55	6
Light Italian	30	3
Sweet & Saucy Red French	60	5
Thousand Island	70	7

NASOYA (TOFU-BASE)

	CALS	FAT
Creamy Dill; Garden Herb	40	3
Italian Vegi; Sesame Garlic	40	3
Nayonaise	40	4

NEWMAN'S OWN

	CALS	FAT
Olive Oil & Vinegar, 1 Tbsp	80	9

PRITIKIN

	CALS	FAT
Italian: Regular	0	0
Italian Creamy; Russian	12	0
French; Vinaigrette	10	0
Ranch Salad; Zesty Tomato	18	0

SEVEN SEAS

	CALS	FAT
Buttermilk Recipe	80	8
Creamy: French	60	6
Italian	70	7
LIGHT		
Buttermilk Recipe; Ranch	50	5
French	35	3
Thousand Island	30	2

VIVA

	CALS	FAT
Herb & Spice	60	6
Italian; Red Wine Vinegar & Oil	70	8
Ranch	80	8
LIGHT		
Italian	40	4
Creamy Italian; Red Wine	45	4
Herbs & Spices	30	3

SUDDENLY SALAD (MIX)

Made as directed: Per Tbsp	CALS	FAT
Caesar; Classic Pasta	20	1
Creamy Macaroni; Pasta Prim.	25	1
Italian Pasta; Tortellini Italian	20	<1
Ranch & Bacon	26	2

WALDEN FARMS

	CALS	FAT
Bleu Cheese	27	2
Creamy Italian with Parmesan	35	3
French	33	2
Italian: Regular/Sodium Free	9	<1
No Sugar Added	6	<1
Ranch	35	2
Thousand Island	24	2

Continued Next Page

SALAD DRESSINGS
(CONT)

WEIGHT WATCHERS

Per Tablespoon, ½ oz	CALS	FAT
Caesar	4	0
Creamy: Italian	50	5
Ranch	25	0
French Style	10	0
Italian Style	6	0
Russian; Thousand Island	50	5
Tomato Vinaigrette	8	0
Whipped	45	4
Single Serve: Caesar	6	0
Creamy Ranch	35	0
Italian Style	9	0
Mayonnaise: All types	50	5

WESTBRAE NATURAL

	CALS	FAT
Oriental Style; Lemon & Spice	40	3
Oriental Orange; Sesame	40	3

WISHBONE

Per Tablespoon (approx. ½ oz)	CALS	FAT
Caesar with Olive Oil	50	5
French, Deluxe/Sweet Spicy	60	6
Italian: Reg/Blend/Robusto	45	4
Creamy with cheese	60	6
Ranch	80	8
Red Wine Olive Oil Vinaigrette	35	3
Russian	45	2
Thousand Island	60	6
Lite: Chunky Blue Cheese	40	4
Classic Dijon Vinaigrette	30	3
Creamy Italian	25	2
French Style	30	<1
Italian	6	0
Olive Oil Vinaigrette	16	2
Olive Oil Caesar	30	3
Olive Oil Italian	20	2
Ranch	45	4
Red Wine Vinaigrette	20	2
Russian	20	<1
Sweet 'n Spicy French	16	0
Thousand Island	35	3

OTHER MAYONNAISES

	CALS	FAT
Heart Beat Reduced Calorie	40	4
Hellmann's Chol.Free Red.Cal.	50	5
Bestfoods Light/Chol. Free	50	5
Nalley Reduced Calorie	45	5
Vons	100	11

HERBS & SPICES

Per 1 teaspoon	CALS	FAT (g)
Average all types: 1 tsp	5	0
Allspice, ground	5	0
Chili powder	8	<1
Cinnamon, ground	6	0
Curry Powder	6	<1
Garlic Powder	9	0
Nutmeg, ground	12	1
Onion Powder	7	0
Parsley, dried	4	0
Pepper, black/red/white, aver.	6	0
Saffron	2	0
Tumeric, ground	8	0
Seeds: Fenugreek	12	<1
Mustard, yellow	15	1
Poppyseed	15	1
Other types, average	7	<1
Parsley Patch,		
salt-free blends, average	10	0
All-purpose, 1 tsp	6	0
Sesame, 1 tsp	16	<1
Perc Salt-free Seasoning, 1 tsp	8	0
Vegit seasoning mix, 1 tsp	5	0

SEASONINGS & FLAVORINGS

	CALS	FAT
Accent Flavor Enhancer, 1 tsp	10	0
Angostura Bitters, 1 tsp	12	0
Bacon Bits, average, 1 Tbsp	30	1
Bacon Chips (Durkee), 1 Tbsp	45	2
Bac 'N Pieces Chips, 1 Tbsp	25	<1
Best O'Butter, 1 tsp	10	<1
Butter Buds, 1 tsp	8	<1
Garlic Bread Sprinkle, 1 tsp	8	<1
Garlic Salt, 1 tsp	2	0
Italian Seasoning, 1 tsp	4	0
Lemon Pepper Season., 1 tsp	7	0
Meat Tenderizer, aver., 1 tsp	3	0
Molly McButter, 1 tsp	8	<1
Parsley Patch (see Herbs/Spices)		
Perc Salt-free Seasoning, 1 tsp	8	0
Salad Sprinkles (Lawry's), 1 tsp	16	<1
Salad Supreme (McCormick), 1 tsp	11	<1
Salt: Regular, Sea Salt	0	0
Morton Lite Salt	0	0
Seasoned Salts	2	0
Salt Substitutes (Potass. Chloride)	0	0
Seasoning Mixes, aver., ¼ pkg	25	<1
Taco Seasoning, aver., ¼ pkg	30	<1

BABY FOODS

- Do not overly restrict calories or fat in baby's food. Adequate calories and nutrients are required for normal growth. Seek professional advice if in doubt.
- When stopping breast-feeding or formula milk, use whole milk for babies less than 2 years. Fat-reduced milks may not have sufficient calories.
- High-fiber diets are too low in calories for babies, and are unsuitable.

BABY CEREALS (Dry):	CALS	FAT
Average all brands, ½ oz	60	1
with 2½ fl.oz milk	100	4
INFANT FORMULAS		
Average, made-up, 5 fl.oz	100	5.5

BEECH-NUT

STAGE 2 — Per 4½ oz Jar

Dinners: Beef; Turkey	120	6
Beef & Egg Noodle; Macar.	90	4
Chicken Noodle	90	3
Chicken & Rice; Veget. Ham	80	3
Veget. Beef/Lamb/Chicken	90	4
Desserts & Yogurts:		
Yogurts: Banan./Peach/Frt.	120	2
Cottage Chse. w/Pineapple	130	7
Vanilla Custard Pudding	130	4
Guava/Mango/Papaya	100	0

STAGE 3 — Per 6 oz Jar

Dinners: Beef & Egg Noodle	110	5
Chicken Noodle	100	3
Macaroni & Beef	130	6
Spagh. & Beef; Veg. Beef	120	5
Turkey Rice	90	3
Vegetable Chicken	110	4
Vegetables: Carrots	60	0
Green Beans	45	0
Sweet Potatoes	110	0
Fruits & Desserts: Peaches	90	0
Apple Sce & Banan./Cherries	100	0
Bananas w/Pears; Frt Dess.	130	0
Cottage Cheese w/Yogurt	170	2
Mixed Fruit w/Yogurt	160	2
Vanilla Custard Pudding	180	5
Fruit Juices: Average, 4 fl.oz	60	0

GERBER

STRAINED: Cereals w/Frt, aver.	100	1
Juices: Average all types	70	0
Fruits: Average all types	80	1
Banan./Prunes w/Tapioca	110	1
Desserts: Average all types	100	1
Vegetables: Carrots; Squash	35	0
Creamed Corn	80	1
Other varieties, average	60	1
Dinners (4½ oz): Average	90	3

GERBER (CONT)

JUNIOR — Per 6 oz Jar

	CALS	FAT
Cereals with Fruit, average	140	2
Fruits: Apple; Blueberry	80	1
Banan/Plums w/Tapioca, av.	130	1
Pears/Peaches/Banana, av.	100	1
Desserts: Hawaiian; Van. Custard	150	2
Peach; Fruit Dess; Apple	130	1
Dinners: Vegetable Bacon	140	6
Other varieties, average	110	3
Meats/Lean Meats: Average	100	5
Vegetables: Brocc./Carr./Chse.	50	1
Mixed Vegetables	70	1
Carrots; Green Beans; Peas	80	1
Sweet Potatoes	110	1

CHUNKY PRODUCTS — Per 6 oz Jar

Noodles & Beef	150	6
Noodles & Chicken	110	3
Rice w/Chick; Veg. & Turkey	120	3
Rice w/Beef; Macar. Alphab.	140	4
Spaghetti Tom. Sce & Beef	160	5
Vegetables & Beef/Ham	130	5
Vegetables & Chicken	140	5

HEINZ

STRAINED DINNERS — Per 4½ oz Jar

Beef/Egg Noodles; Chick. Noodle	70	2
Vegetables & Bacon/Beef	75	3
Vegetables & Ham/Lamb	55	1
Veg., Egg Noodles & Chick./Tky	75	2

JUNIOR FOODS — Per 6 oz Jar

Dinners: Chicken Noodle	95	3
Bf. & Egg Ndls; Macar. Beef	90	2
Spagh. w/Tom. Sce & Meat	100	3
Turkey Rice w/Vegetables	75	2
Vegetables & Bacon/Beef	95	3
Veg. & Ham/Dumpl. & Beef	95	3
Veg./Egg Noodles/Chicken	100	3
Veg., Egg Noodles & Turkey	80	3
Vegetables: Carrots	45	1
Creamed Green Beans	90	3
Cr. Corn; Sweet Potatoes	140	2
Desserts: Custard Pudding	160	2
Other varieties, average	150	0
Fruits: Apples & Apricots/Pears	120	0
Other varieties, average	150	0

BREAKFAST CEREALS

COOKED CEREALS

	CALS	FAT (g)
Buckwheat Groats, roasted:		
Dry, ½ cup, 3 oz	**280**	2
Cooked, 7 oz	**180**	1
Bulgur: Dry, ½ cup, 2½ oz	**240**	1
Cooked, 1 cup, 6½ oz	**150**	<1
Corn/Hominy Grits:		
Dry, ¼ cup, 1.4 oz	**145**	<1
3 Tbsp, 1 oz	**110**	<1
Cooked, ¾ cup, 6½ oz	**110**	<1
Instant, 1 pkt, 0.8 oz	**80**	<1
w/Imit. Bacon Bits, 1 oz	**100**	<1
Cream of Rice, ckd, ¾ c, 6 oz	**90**	0
Cream of Wheat:		
Regular, ckd, ¾ cup, 6 oz	**180**	<1
Quick, ckd, ¾ cup, 6 oz	**95**	<1
Instant, ckd, ¾ cup, 6 oz	**110**	<1
Farina: Cooked, ¾ cup, 6 oz	**85**	0
Millet, dry, ¼ cup, 1 oz	**100**	1
Oat Bran, raw, ⅓ cup, 1 oz	**75**	2
Cooked, ½ cup	**45**	<1
Oatmeal: Dry, ⅓ cup, 1 oz	**110**	0
Regular, ckd, ¾ cup, 6 oz	**110**	2
1 cup, 8 oz	**145**	3
Instant: Regular aver., 1 oz	**100**	2
Flavored, average	**150**	2
Quaker — See p.65		
Total: Regular, 1.2 oz	**110**	2
Flavored, average	**160**	2
Under Cover Bears, aver.	**170**	3
Roman Meal, ckd, ¾ cup, 6½ oz	**110**	<1
Wheat Hearts, 1 oz dry/¾ c. ckd	**110**	1

COLD CEREALS

Average All Brands

	CALS	FAT
Bran (processed), ⅓ cup, 1 oz	**70**	<1
Bran Flakes, ¾ cup, 1 oz	**90**	<1
Corn Flakes, 1 cup, 1 oz	**110**	<1
Granola, ¼ cup, 1 oz	**130**	4
Oat Bran Cereal, ⅓ cup, 1 oz	**110**	1
Puffed Rice, 1 cup, ½ oz	**55**	0
Puffed Wheat, 1 cup, ½ oz	**55**	0
Raisin Bran, ½ cup, 1 oz	**85**	<1
Rice Crisps, 1 cup, 1 oz	**110**	<1
Shredded Wheat, 1 bisc., ¾ oz	**80**	<1
Sugar-frosted Flakes, ¾ c, 1 oz	**110**	<1
Wheat Flakes, 1 cup, 1 oz	**105**	<1

BRANS & WHEATGERM

	CALS	FAT (g)
Bran: Wheat, unprocessed,		
1 Tbsp, 3g	**10**	0
Rice Bran, raw, 1 Tbsp, 5g	**16**	1
⅓ cup, 1 oz	**90**	6
Oat Bran, 1 Tbsp, 5g	**15**	<1
⅓ cup, 1 oz	**75**	2
Wheat Germ, 1 Tbsp, ¼ oz	**27**	1
¼ cup, 1 oz	**108**	3

CEREAL ADD-ONS

	CALS	FAT
Milk: Per ½ Cup, 4 fl.oz		
Whole, ½ cup	**80**	4.5
2% Fat, ½ cup	**60**	2.3
Skim, ½ cup	**43**	0
Yogurt: Per ½ Cup, 4 fl.oz		
Plain: Whole	**90**	4
Skim	**60**	0
Fruit: Whole	**125**	2.6
Lowfat	**120**	2
Non-fat	**60**	0
Fibresonic (Matol), 1 pkt	**40**	2
with 8oz skim milk	**120**	2
Fruit: Dried, average, 1 oz	**80**	0
Banana, ½ medium	**50**	0
Prunes, in Syrup, 5 (3 oz)	**90**	0
Lecithin Granules, 1 Tbsp, 8g	**40**	5
Nuts: Almonds, 6 (¼ oz)	**40**	4
Pollen (Bee) Granules, 1 T., 8 g	**25**	1
Seeds: Sunflower, 1 Tbsp	**65**	6
Sugar: 1 heaping tsp	**22**	0
1 Tbsp, ½ oz	**55**	0
Honey: 1 Tbsp, ¾ oz	**65**	0

MAXIMUM DESIRABLE DAILY FAT INTAKE
(for various calorie levels)

1200 Calories — 30 grams
1500 Calories — 40 grams
2000 Calories — 60 grams
2500 Calories — 80 grams
3000 Calories — 100 grams

1 teaspoon fat has 4g fat
1 teaspoon oil has 5g fat

BREAKFAST CEREALS (CONT)

ARROWHEAD MILLS

HOT CEREALS
Per 1 oz Serving (Dry)	CALS	FAT (g)
Bear Mush	100	0
Cracked Wheat Cereal	90	<1
Four Grain Cereal	95	<1
Oatmeal (Instant): Regular	100	2
Fruit/Nut types, average	130	3
Oats — Steel Cut	110	2
Rice & Shine, ¼ oz	160	1
Seven Grain Cereal	100	1

COLD CEREALS — Per 1 oz
	CALS	FAT
Apple/Maple Corns	100	1
Arrowhead Crunch	120	3
Bran Flakes	100	1
Corn Flakes	110	1
Maple-Nut Granola	125	5
Nature O's	110	1
Oat Bran Flakes	110	2
Puffed Corn/Millet	100	0
Puffed Rice/Wheat	100	0
Wheat Bran	25	1
Wheat Flakes	110	1
Wheat Germ, raw	108	3

BARBARA'S BAKERY

	CALS	FAT
Breakfast O's, ¾ cup, 1 oz	120	2
Brown Rice Crisps, 1 cup, 1 oz	120	1
Corn Flakes, 1 cup, 1 oz	110	0
14 Grains Hot Cereal, 1¼ oz	105	1
Raisin Bran, 1 oz	110	<1
Breakfast Biscuits, 2 biscuits	120	1
Crunchy Oat Bran, 1 oz	120	4

BREADSHOP

	CALS	FAT
Granola: Breadshop, aver., 1 oz	125	5
Nectar-Sweet, aver., 1 oz	110	4
Muesli, Rye Date/Oat Bran, 1 oz	100	2
Triple Bran/Oat Bran, 1 oz	100	2

EREWHON

Per 1 oz Serving	CALS	FAT
Aztec Corn & Amaranth	100	0
Crispy Brown Rice Cereal	110	1
Raisin Bran	100	0
Wheat Flakes	100	0

GENERAL MILLS

Per Serving, 1 oz	CALS	FAT (g)
Body Buddies, Nat. Fruit, 1 cup	110	1
Booberry, 1 cup	110	1
Cheerios: Regular, 1¼ cup	110	2
Apple Cinnamon, ¾ cup	110	2
Honey Nut, ¾ cup	110	1
Cinnamon Toast Crunch, ¾ cup	120	3
Clusters, ½ cup	110	3
Cocoa Puffs, 1 cup	110	1
Count Chocula, 1 cup	110	1
Country Corn Flakes, 1 cup	110	<1
Crispy Wheats 'n Raisins, ¾ cup	100	1
Fiber One, ½ cup	60	1
Frankenberry, 1 cup	110	1
Fruity Yummy Mummy, 1 cup	110	1
Golden Grahams, ¾ cup	110	1
Kaboom, 1 cup	110	1
Kix, 1½ cups	110	1
Lucky Charms, 1 cup	110	1
Oatmeal: Crisp, 1 cup	110	2
Raisin Crisp, ½ cup	110	2
Raisin: Nut Bran, ½ cup	110	3
Oat Bran, ¾ cup, 1½ oz	150	2
Total: Regular, 1 cup	100	1
Corn Flakes, 1 cup	110	1
Raisin Bran, 1 cup, 1½ oz	140	1
Trix, 1 cup	110	1
Wheaties, 1 cup	100	1

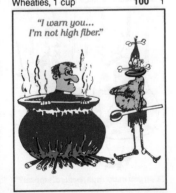

"I warn you... I'm not high fiber."

HEALTH VALLEY

Per 1 oz Serving	CALS	FAT (g)
Amaranth: w/Bananas, ½ cup	110	2
Crunch w/Raisins, ¼ cup	110	3
10 Bran Cereal (Fat Free) ¾ cup	90	<1
Bran Cereal (w/Fruit), ¼ cup	100	1
Corn Flakes: Reg (¾ c.); Blue (½ c)	90	<1
Crisp Brown Rice, ¾ cup	90	<1
Fiber 7 Flakes (100% Org.), ½ c.	90	<1
Fruit & Fitness, 1 cup, 2 oz	220	4
Fruit Lites, all types, ½ cup, ½ oz	45	0
Granola (Fat Free), ¼ cup	90	<1
Healthy Crunch (no fat ad) ¼ c.	90	1
Healthy O's (100% Org.), ¾ cup	90	1
Lites Puffed Cereals, ½ cup	50	1
Oat Bran Flakes, all types, ½ c.	100	<1
Orangeola: (No fat added), ¼ c.	90	1
Real Oat Bran Cereal: (No Fat Added)		
Almond Crunch, ¼ cup	90	1
Hawaiian Fruit; Raisin Nut	100	1
Rice Bran Cereal, ½ cup	110	3
Rice Bran O's, ½ cup	110	1
Sprouts 7: Banan./Hawn. Frt., ¼ c.	90	1

KASHI

Kashi, Puffed, 1 cup, ¾ oz	75	<1
7 Grains (Bkfst Pilaf):		
cooked, ⅔ cup, 5 oz	175	1
5 Bran Kashi, ½ pkt, 2½ oz	280	6

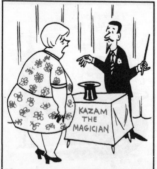

"Can you make my appetite disappear?"

KAZAM THE MAGICIAN

KELLOGGS

Per 1 oz Serving	CALS	FAT (g)
All-Bran, ⅓ cup	70	1
with Extra Fiber, ½ cup	50	0
Apple Jacks, 1 cup	110	0
Apple Raisin Crisp, ⅔ cup	130	0
Bigg Mixx, ½ cup	110	2
with Raisins, ½ cup	140	2
Bran Buds (w/Psyllium), ⅓ c.	70	1
Branflakes (40% Bran), ⅔ cup	90	0
Cocoa Krispies, ¾ cup	110	0
Common Sense O/Bran, ½ cup	100	1
with Raisins, ½ cup	120	1
Corn Flakes, 1 cup	100	0
Corn Pops, 1 cup	110	0
Cracklin Oat Bran, ½ cup	110	4
Crispix, 1 cup	110	0
Froot Loops, 1 cup	110	1
Frosted Flakes/Krispies, ¾ cup	110	0
Frosted Mini-Wheats, 4 bisc.	100	1
Bite Size, ½ cup	100	0
Fruitful Bran, ⅔ cup, 1½ oz	120	1
Heartwise, ⅔ cup	90	1
Honey Smacks, ¾ cup	110	1
Just Right (w/Fiber Nug.), ⅔ c.	100	1
w/Fruit & Nuts, ⅔ cup	140	1
Kenmei Rice Bran, ¾ cup	110	1
Almond & Raisin, ¾ cup	150	2
Mueslix: Crispy Blend, ⅔ cup	160	2
Golden Crunch, ½ cup	120	2
Nut & Honey Crunch, ⅔ cup	110	1
Crunch O's, ⅔ cup	110	2
Nutra-Grain:		
Almond Raisin, ⅖ cup	140	2
Wheat, ⅔ cup	100	0
Raisin Bran, 1 cup	130	0
Oatbake: Honey Bran, ⅓ cup	110	3
Raisin Bran, ⅓ cup	110	3
Product 19, 1 cup	100	0
Raisin Bran, ¾ cup	120	1
Rice Krispies, 1 cup	110	0
Shredded Wheat Squares:		
All types, ½ cup	90	0
Special K, 1 cup	110	0

NECTAR SWEET

Granola: All types, aver., 1 oz	110	4

NABISCO

Per 1 oz Serving	CALS	FAT
100% Bran	110	2
Cream of Wheat, 1 oz	100	0
Fruit Wheats; Raisin/Strawb.	100	0
Oat Bran, instant: Reg., 1 oz	80	2
Apple Cinnamon, 1⅜ oz	130	2
Shredded Wheat, 1 biscuit	84	<1
Bite-size, ⅔ cup	110	1
Shredded Wheat w/Oat Bran	100	1
Team Flakes, ¾ cup	110	1
Toasted Wheat & Raisins, 1.4 oz	140	2

NATURE VALLEY

Per Serving, 1 oz		
Cinnamon & Raisin, ⅓ cup	120	4
Fruit & Nut, ⅓ cup	130	5
Toasted Oat, ⅓ cup	130	5
Wheat Hearts, 1 oz	110	1

POST

Per 1 oz Serving		
Branflakes, ¾ cup	90	0
Cocoa/Fruity Pebbles, 1 cup	110	1
Fruit & Fibre, ½ cup	85	1
Grape Nut Flakes, 1 cup	100	1
Grape Nuts, ¼ cup	110	0
Honey Bunches with Almonds	120	3
Honey Roasted	110	2
Honeycomb, 1⅓ cup	110	0
Oat Flakes (fortified), ⅔ cup	110	1
Raisin Bran, ½ cup	85	0
Raisin Grape Nuts, ½ cup	100	0
Smurf — Magic Berries, 1 cup	120	1
Toasties Corn Flakes, 1¼ cups	110	0

RALSTON

Per 1 oz Serving		
Almond Delight, ¾ cup	110	2
Corn/Rice Chex, 1 cup	110	0
Fruit Muesli, ½ cup, 1½ oz	150	3
Honey Graham Chex, ⅔ cup	110	1
Multi Bran Chex, ⅔ cup	90	0
Oat Chex, ½ cup	100	1
Batman/Barbie Swtn'd, 1 cup	110	1
Teen. Mut. Ninja Turtles, 1 cup	110	0

STONE — BUHR

Apple Granola, 1 oz	100	2

QUAKER

(Ready-To-Eat): Per 1 oz	CALS	FAT
Crunchy Bran, ⅔ cup	90	1
Oat Squares, ½ cup	100	2
100% Natural, ¼ cup	130	6
Apple & Cinn., ¼ cup	130	5
Raisin & Date, ¼ cup	120	5
Puffed Rice; Wht., 1 cup, ½ oz	50	0
Shredded Wheat, 2 bisc.	130	1
Unproc. Bran, 2 Tbsp, ¼ oz	8	0
Instant Grits: Per Pouch		
White Hominy	80	0
w/Imitation Bacon Bits	100	<1
w/Cheddar Cheese Flavor	105	<1
Oat Bran, High Oat Fiber:		
Regular, 1 pouch, 1 oz	100	2
Apple/Raisin, 1¼ oz	120	2
Instant Quaker Oatmeal: Per Pouch		
Oatmeal: Regular, 1 oz	90	2
Apples & Cinn., 1¼ oz	120	1
Blueberries, 1¼ oz	130	2
Cinnamon & Spice, 1½ oz	160	2
Maple/Br. Sug; Rais./Spice	150	2
Strawb./Peaches & Cream	130	2
Raisin/Date/W'lnut, 1¼ oz	140	4
Extra Fortified Oatmeal: Per Pouch		
Regular, 1 oz	100	2
Apples & Spice, 1¼ oz	130	2
Raisins & Cinn., 1¼ oz	130	2
Quaker/Mother's: Cooked, ⅔ cup,		
Oat Bran	90	2
Whole Wheat Hot Natural	90	1
Oats Quick & Old Fash.	100	2

OTHER QUAKER BRANDS

Cap'n Crunch: Reg./berries, ¾ c.	120	2
Peanut Butter Crunch, ¾ c.	120	3
Crunchy Nut Oh!s, 1 cup	130	4
Honey Graham Oh!s, 1 cup	120	3
King Vitaman, 1½ cups	110	1
Kretschmer Wh/Germ, ¼ cup	100	3
Honey Crunch Wh/Germ, ¼ c.	110	3
Toasted Wheat Bran, ⅓ cup	60	2
Life, ⅔ cup, 1 oz	100	2
Popeye Sweet Crunch, 1 cup	120	2
Sun Country Granola with		
Raisins, ¼ cup	120	5
100% Nat. Granola w/alm., ¼ c.	130	5

CEREAL GRAINS & FLOURS

Per ½ Cup (8 level Tbsp)	CALS	FAT
Amaranth, ½ cup, 3½ oz	**365**	6
Arrowroot, ½ cup, 2¼ oz	**230**	0
Barley: Regular, ½ cup, 3¼ oz	**325**	2
Pearled, raw, 3½ oz	**350**	1
cooked, 2¾ oz	**100**	<1
Flakes, ½ cup, 1½ oz	**150**	<1
Buckwheat: Regular, ½ cup, 3 oz	**290**	3
Groats, roasted, dry, 3 oz	**285**	2
roasted, cooked, 3½ oz	**90**	<1
Flour, whole-groat	**200**	2
Bulgur, dry, ½ cup, 2½ oz	**240**	1
cooked, ½ cup, 3¼ oz	**75**	<1
Carob Flour, ½ cup, 1.8 oz	**95**	<1
Corn, kernels (blue/yellow), 3 oz	**300**	4
Corn Bran, ½ cup, 1.4 oz	**85**	<1
Corn Flour/Masa, 2 oz	**210**	2
Corn Grits, dry, ½ cup, 2¾ oz	**290**	1
cooked, ½ cup, 4¼ oz	**75**	0
Corn Germ, toasted	**245**	13
Cornmeal: Whole-grain, 2.2 oz	**220**	2
Self-rising, bolted, 2.2 oz	**205**	2
w/Wheat Flour added, 3 oz	**250**	3
Cornstarch, ½ cup, 2¼ oz	**245**	0
Couscous, dry, 3¼ oz	**345**	<1
cooked, 3.2 oz	**100**	0
Farina, dry, 3 oz	**325**	0
cooked, 4.1 oz	**60**	0
Flax Seeds, 2 oz	**280**	20
Garbanzo (Chick Pea), ½ c., 2 oz	**200**	3
Matzo Meal, ½ cup	**260**	1
Millet, raw, ½ cup, 3½ oz	**380**	4
cooked, ½ cup, 4¼ oz	**145**	1
Oats, ½ cup, 2¾ oz	**305**	5
Oat Bran, raw, ½ cup, 1.7 oz	**115**	3
cooked, ½ cup, 4 oz	**115**	1
Oats, rolled/oatmeal, dry	**155**	2
cooked, ½ cup, 4.2 oz	**75**	1
Polenta, ½ cup	**220**	2
Potato Flour, ½ cup, 3.2 oz	**315**	<1
Psyllium Husks, 1 Tbsp	**10**	<1
Quinoa, ½ cup, 3 oz	**320**	5
Rye: Grains, ½ cup, 3 oz	**280**	2
Flakes, ½ cup, 1½ oz	**150**	<1
Flour, dark, 2¼ oz	**210**	2
Medium light, 1.8 oz	**185**	1
Semolina, ½ cup, 3 oz	**305**	1
Sorghum, ½ cup, 3.4 oz	**325**	3
Soybean Flakes, ½ cup, 1½ oz	**190**	8
Soy Flour, ½ cup, 2 oz	**250**	11
Tapioca, pearl, dry, ½ cup, 2.7 oz	**260**	0
3 Tbsp, 1 oz	**100**	0

	CALS	FAT
Teff (Seed) Flour, 2 oz	**200**	<1
Tortilla Flour Mix, ½ cup, 2 oz	**225**	12
Triticale, ½ cup, 3.4 oz	**325**	2
Flour, whole-grain, ½ cup	**220**	1
Wheat: Average, ½ cup, 3½ oz	**320**	2
Wheat Bran, unproc., ½ cup, 1 oz	**65**	1
Wheat Flakes, ½ cup, 1½ oz	**160**	<1
Wheat Germ: Crude, 2 oz	**205**	11
Toasted, ½ cup, 2 oz	**215**	12
Wheat Flour: Whole grain, 2.1 oz	**205**	1
White, all types, ½ c., 2.2 oz	**220**	<1

Also See Arrowhead Mills Cereals — p.63.

RICE

BROWN RICE

	CALS	FAT
Raw: Short grain, 1 cup, 7 oz	**700**	3
Long grain, 1 cup, 6½ oz	**650**	3
Cooked:		
Short grain, hot, ½ c., 3¾ oz	**125**	<1
Cold, ½ cup, 2¾ oz	**95**	<1
Long grain, hot, ½ c., 3½ oz	**120**	<1
cold, ½ cup, 2½ oz	**90**	<1

WHITE RICE (Polished)

	CALS	FAT
Raw: Short/Med. grain, 1 c., 7 oz	**720**	<1
Long grain, 1 cup, 6½ oz	**670**	<1
Cooked (Boiled/Steamed):		
Short/Medium grain,		
Hot, ½ cup, 3¾ oz	**115**	0
1 cup, 7½ oz	**230**	0
Cold, ½ cup, 2¾ oz	**90**	0
Long grain,		
Hot, ½ cup, 3½ oz	**110**	0
Cold, ½ cup, 2½ oz	**80**	0
Parboiled, ckd, hot, ½ cup, 3 oz	**90**	0
Precook./Instant: Dry, ½ c., 3½ oz	**370**	<1
Cooked, hot, ½ cup, 3 oz	**90**	0
Fried, Chinese (egg/veg./pork), 1 cup, 5 oz	**320**	13
Wild Rice: Raw, 1 cup, 5½ oz	**570**	2
Cooked, hot, 1 cup, 5¾ oz	**165**	<1
½ cup, 3 oz	**85**	<1

RICE BRAN/FLOUR

	CALS	FAT
Rice Bran, ⅓ cup, 1 oz	**90**	6
Rice Flour, ½ cup, 2¾ oz	**290**	2
Rice Polish, ½ cup	**220**	7

RICE-A-RONI (Mix), prepared:

	CALS	FAT
Broccoli (Per ¾ cup)	**270**	14
Chicken Florentine; Gdn. Pilaf	**200**	6
Rice Pilaf; Risotto	**290**	9
Stroganoff	**285**	12

PASTA & NOODLES

MACARONI, SPAGHETTI

- Macaroni includes all shapes and sizes; e.g. elbows, shells, tubes, twists, sheets, cannelloni, manicotti, spaghetti, ziti.
- All regular macaroni products have the same calories/fat on a weight basis.
- 1 oz Dry = approx. 2½-3 oz cooked.

	CALS	FAT
Dry Macaroni/Spagh.: 1 oz	105	<1
1 lb box/pkg., 16 oz	1680	7
Elbows, 1 cup, 3¾ oz	395	2
Shells, small, 1 cup, 3¼ oz	340	2
Spirals, 1 cup, 3 oz	315	2
Cooked, Plain (no added fat):		
Firm/Al Dente (8-10 mins.), 1 oz	42	<1
Medium (11-13 mins.), 1 oz	37	<1
Tender (14-20 mins.), 1 oz	32	<1
(Longer cooking increases water absorbed)		
Elbows/Spirals, 1 cup, 5 oz	185	1
Small Shells, 1 cup, 4 oz	150	<1
Spaghetti, ½ cup, 2½ oz	90	<1
Med. serving, 1 cup, 5 oz	185	1
Large (restaurant), 2 c., 10 oz	370	2
Corn: Cooked, 1 cup, 5 oz	175	<1
Protein-fortified: Dry, 1 oz	107	<1
Cooked, 1 cup, 5 oz	230	<1
Spinach/Vegetable: Dry, 1 oz	105	<1
Cooked, 1 cup, 5 oz	180	<1

MACARONI, SPAGH. (CONT.)	CALS	FAT
Whole-wheat: Dry, 1 oz	100	<1
Cooked, 1 cup, 5 oz	175	<1
FRESH PASTA (Refrigerated)		
Plain/Spinach/Tomato, average:		
As purchased, 4 oz	325	2.5
Cooked, 1 cup, 5 oz	190	1
Home-made, without egg:		
Cooked, 1 cup, 5 oz	175	1

Other Spaghetti/Pasta Listings:
Froz. Foods, Pp. 40-47; Canned, Pp. 48-49.
Restaurant Dishes — Italian, Pp. 102.
Spaghetti Sauces — Sauces, Pp. 56-57.

NOODLES

Plain/Egg:		
Dry, 1 oz	108	1
1 cup, 1⅓ oz	145	1.5
Cooked, 1 oz	38	<1
½ cup, 2¾ oz	105	1
1 cup, 5½ oz	210	2
'No Yolks' (Foulds), ckd, 1 cup	210	2
Chinese: Celloph./Rice, dry, 1 oz	100	0
Chow Mein/Hard, dry, 1 oz	150	5
Japanese: Soba, dry, 1 oz	95	<1
cooked, 1 cup, 4 oz	110	<1
Somen, dry, 1 oz	100	<1
cooked, 1 cup, 6 oz	225	<1

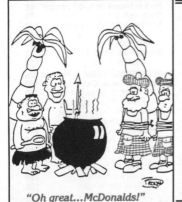

"Oh great...McDonalds!"

BREADS

Note: All breads have similar calories on a weight basis. However, volume may vary. For example, 1 oz of bread may equal 1 slice regular bread or 2 slices of a lighter bread. It is best to weigh bread used and calculate on 1 oz bread = 70 calories.

	CALS	FAT (g)
Average of All Varieties: (White/Brown/Wheat/French/Italian Oat/Buttermilk/Sourdough)		
Thin slice (¼"), 1 oz	**70**	1
Extra thin slice, ¾ oz	**55**	<1
Light thin slice, 0.6 oz	**40**	<1
Toasting slice, 1.2 oz	**85**	1
Thick slice (⅜"), 1½ oz	**105**	1.5
Large thick (½"), 2 oz	**140**	2
1-lb Loaf, 16 oz	**1120**	6
Toast has same calories as bread used.		
1 thin slice + 1 tsp of fat	**105**	5
1 thick slice (⅜") + 2 tsp fat	**175**	10
Bran-style, 1 oz slice	**70**	1
Buttermilk, average, 1 oz slice	**80**	2
Challah, 1 oz slice	**85**	2
Cinnamon, 1 oz slice	**85**	2
Corn Bread, aver., 1 pce., 3 oz	**180**	7
Dark Bread, 1 oz slice	**70**	1
Date & Nut, 1 oz slice	**90**	1
'Enriched' Breads, aver., 1 oz sl.	**75**	1
French Bread, 1 oz slice	**70**	1
French Toast, 1 slice, 2¼ oz	**160**	7
Garlic Bread, 1 pce. w/fat, 1 oz	**125**	6
Italian Bread, 1 oz slice	**75**	1
Light Bread, aver., 0.8 oz slice	**40**	<1
1 oz slice	**70**	1
Nut/Health Nut, 1 oz slice	**85**	2
Oatmeal Bread, 1 oz slice	**70**	1
Party Breads: (Pepperidge Farm):		
Dijon; Pumpernickel, 1 slice	**18**	<1
Rye Slices, 1 slice	**15**	<1
Pita Bread, aver. all types, 2 oz	**150**	2
Mini/Pocket, 1 oz	**75**	1
Poppyseed (Vienna), 0.8 oz sl.	**55**	1
Pumpernickel, 1 oz slice	**75**	1
Cocktail size, 0.4 oz	**30**	<1
Raisin Bread, 1 oz slice	**80**	1
Roman Meal, 1 oz slice	**70**	1
Rye, average, 1 thin slice, 1 oz	**75**	1
1 thick slice, 2 oz	**150**	2
Cocktail size, 0.4 oz	**25**	<1
Sandwich Bread, 1 oz slice	**70**	1
Sourdough, 1 oz slice	**70**	1
Wheat/Cracked Wheat, 1 oz sl.	**75**	1
Weight Watchers, ½ oz slice	**40**	<1

BAGELS

	CALS	FAT (g)
Average all types:		
1 small/bagelette, 1 oz	**80**	<1
1 medium bagel, 2 oz	**160**	1.5
1 large bagel, 3 oz	**240**	2
Burger King: Regular, 3¼ oz	**270**	6
with Cream Cheese, 4¼ oz	**370**	16
Sara Lee, aver. all types, 3 oz	**220**	2
Lender's, average, 2 oz	**160**	1
Bagel Chips (New York Style), 4 slices, ¾ oz	**90**	2
Bagel Crisps (Burns/Ricker), 1 oz	**150**	9

BREAD ROLLS & BUNS

	CALS	FAT (g)
Brown 'n Serve, average, 1 oz	**80**	2
Challah Roll, 2 oz	**150**	2
Dinner Rolls: 1 medium (2½" diam. x 2" high), 1 oz	**85**	2
1 extra med. (3" diam.), 1½ oz	**130**	3
Frankfurter/Hot Dog: 1¼ oz	**100**	2
1½ oz size	**120**	2
French: 1 medium, 1.3 oz	**110**	1
1 large, 3 oz	**240**	2
Hamburger: Regular, 1½ oz	**120**	2
Large, 3 oz	**240**	4
Hoagie/Submarine, average (11½" x 3" x 2½" high), 4¾ oz	**400**	8
Kaiser Roll, 2 oz size	**170**	3
Onion Roll, 2 oz size	**170**	2
Parker House Roll, 0.7 oz size	**65**	1
Party Roll, 0.6 oz	**55**	1
Sandwich Roll, 1.6 oz size	**120**	2
Soft Pretzel Bun, 3 oz	**235**	3
Sweet Rolls, 1 oz	**100**	2
Wheat Roll: Small, 1 oz	**75**	<1
Medium, 1½ oz	**110**	1
PEPPERIDGE FARM — Per Roll/Bun		
Brown 'n Serve: Club	**100**	1
French (3 per pkg), 1 roll	**240**	2
French (2 per pkg), 1 roll	**360**	4
Dinner Rolls: Dinner/Finger	**60**	2
Old Fashioned	**50**	2
Fancy Rolls: Crescent/Twist	**110**	6
Frankfurter Roll	**140**	3
French: 9 per pkg, 1 roll	**110**	1
4 per pkg, 1 roll	**240**	4
Sandwich Rolls: Onion	**150**	3
Buns with Sesame	**160**	3
Sliced Hamburger	**130**	2
Soft Family Rolls	**110**	2
Sourdough (French style)	**100**	1

BREAD PRODUCTS

	CALS	FAT (g)
Bread Crumbs, dry:		
Plain or seasoned, 1 oz	110	1
1 rounded Tbsp, 10g	35	<1
1 cup, 3½ oz	390	5
Corn Flake Crumbs, 1 oz	110	1
Graham Cracker Crumbs, 1oz	115	1
Keebler, 1 cup, 4¼ oz	520	14
Bread Dough: Frozen, 1 slice	75	<1
Refrigerated, French, 1" sl.	60	1
Wheat/white, 1" slice	80	2
Breadsticks:		
Stella D'oro: Sesame, 1 pce.	50	2
Plain/Onion/Wheat, 1 pce.	40	1
Keebler/Lance, 2 sticks	30	<1
Salt Sticks, plain, 1 oz	110	1
Croutons: Aver. all brands, 1 oz	130	6
¼ cup, 11g	50	2
Coating Mixes, seasoned:		
Average, 1 oz	110	3
Featherweight, 1.4 oz pkg	72	<1
English Muffins, aver., 2 oz	140	2
Pretzels: See Snacks (Page 85).		
Stuffing: Average, dry mix, 1 oz	110	1
Made-up, ½ cup, 4 oz	180	9

CROISSANTS

	CALS	FAT (g)
Average All Brands		
Plain/All Butter, petite, 1 oz	120	7
1 Medium, 1½ oz	180	10
1 Large, 2½ oz	300	18
Burger King: 1½ oz croissant	180	10
(Croissan'wiches — See Fast Foods Sect.)		
Dunkin' Donuts: Plain, 2½ oz	310	19
Almond, 3½ oz	420	27
Chocolate, 3¼ oz	440	29
Pepperidge Farm: All Butter	240	14
All Butter Petite	140	9
Sara Lee: All Butter, 1½ oz	180	9
All Butter Petite, 1 oz	120	6

RICE CAKES

	CALS	FAT (g)
Average All Types/Brands,		
Regular size, 1 cake, 9g	35	0
Lundberg, all types, 15g each	60	<1
Hain, Mini, average, 3g each	12	<1

TACO SHELLS

	CALS	FAT (g)
Regular size	50	2
Super size	100	4
Salad shell, flour (Azteca)	200	5

CRACKERS

	CALS	FAT (g)
Average All Brands		
(Brands — See following pages.)		
Cheese Crackers: Per cracker		
Plain, 1" square	5	<1
Small, octagonal	10	<1
Round (2" diam.)	15	<1
Sandwich (peanut butter)	35	1
Graham, 2½" square, 1 cracker	30	0.5
Melba Toast, plain, 1 piece	20	0
Oyster & Soup crackers, ½ oz	60	2
(40 small oysters/20 lge hexagons)		
Rice crackers: 1 small	9	<1
Rice Snax (Amsnack), ½ oz	60	1
Saltines, 2 crackers	25	1
Snack-type, 1 round cracker	15	<1
Soda, 1 cracker, ½ oz	60	2
Uneeda, 1 cracker	30	1
Water (Carr's), regular, 1 cr.	32	<1
Bite-size, 1 cracker	13	<1
Wheat, thin, 1 cracker	9	<1
Zweiback Toast, 1 piece	30	<1

CRISPBREADS

	CALS	FAT (g)
Per Crispbread/Cracker		
Finn Crisp: Original, rye	35	<1
Other types	19	<1
Kavli Norwegian: Thin	17	<1
Thick	20	<1
Malsovit, meal Wafers	75	4
Rykrisp: Natural, 1 crispbread	20	0
Seasoned	23	1
Sesame	25	1
Ryvita: Dark/Light, 1 piece	26	<1
High Fiber	23	<1
Wasa: Breakfast; Sesame	50	<1
Extra Crisp; Rye (Light)	25	<1
Fiber Plus	35	<1
Rye (Hearty)	45	<1

MAZTO (MANISCHEWITZ)

	CALS	FAT (g)
American Matzos, 1 board, 1 oz	115	2
Passover Matzos, 1 board, 1.1 oz	130	<1
Passover Egg Matzos, 1.1 oz	130	2
Egg 'n Onion Matzo, 1 oz	112	1
Thin Salted Tea Matzos, 0.9 oz	100	1
Unsalted; Whole Wheat, 1 oz	110	1
Dietetic Matzo Thins, 0.83 oz	90	<1
Crackers: Miniatures, 1 cr.	9	<1
Passover Egg Matzo, 1 cr.	11	<1
Matzo Meal, 1 cup, 4¾ oz	515	2
Matzo Farfel, 1 cup, 2.7 oz	180	<1

Other Crackers/Tams — Page 71.

CRACKERS & COOKIES

AUSTIN

CRACKERS — Per Package	CALS	FAT
Cheese Peanut Butter: Regular	200	10
50% more Peanut Butter	250	14
Cream Cheese & Chives	200	10
Cheese on Cheese	180	7
Combo Cheese	190	8
Cheedar Ch. Smackers, ¼ pkt	47	2
Rye Cheese; Toast P'nut Butter	200	10
Wheat Crackers/S.Cream/On.	210	12
Wheat 'n Cheddar	200	11
Wheat Smackers Crackers	200	10

BAKERY WAGON

Original Oatmeal (per cookie)	100	5
Peanut Butter Oatmeal	110	7
Oatmeal Walnut; Iced Molasses	100	4
Other Varieties, average	100	3

BARBARA'S

Chocolate Chip: Regular, ½ oz	65	3
Tray, 1 cookie, ¾ oz	87	4.5
Chocolate Crisps, each	23	1
Date Walnut	50	3
Fruit & Nut: Regular, ½ oz	62	1
Tray, 1 cookie, ¾ oz	85	1.5
Oatmeal Raisin: Regular, ½ oz	50	1
Tray, 1 cookie, ¾ oz	70	7.5
Peanut Butter	50	4
Toasted Almond	50	2
Tropical Coconut	32	1
Crisps: Chocolate/Vanilla, each	23	<1
Animal Cookies, each	18	1
Calif. Lem./Orange; Ginger Snap	20	<1
Chocolate/Carob Swirl	25	1
French Vanilla Cookies	20	1
Sandwich Cookies, all types	65	3

BREMNER

Wafers: All varieties, 1 wafer	10	<1
Soup/Chili Crackers, ¼ c. (20), ¼ oz	26	<1

ESTEE

Crackers: All varieties, ½ oz	70	4
Cookies: All flavors	30	1
Choc Chip Mix, 2" cookie	50	3
S/wich Cookies, all flavors	50	2
Wafers: Assorted, Creme filled	30	2
Chocolate; Vanilla	20	1
Snack Wafers: All flavors	80	4
Chocolate coated	130	7
6-Calorie	6	<1

FEATHERWEIGHT

Per Cookie	CALS	FAT
Choc. Chip Cookies	45	2
Other varieties, average	45	2
Creme Wafers, each	20	1

FROOKIE

Cookies: Average all types	45	2
Animal Frackers	10	0
Fruitins: Apple; Fig	60	1
Large Frooks: All types	120	4

GRANDMA'S

Candied Animal	140	6
Glazed Gingerbread	120	3
Big Cookies & S/wiches: Snacks (p.85).		

HEALTH VALLEY

Per Cracker/Cookie		
Crackers: Amaranth Graham	16	<1
Fancy Honey Graham	14	<1
Oat Bran Crackers	17	<1
Rice Bran	19	<1
Stoned Wheat: All types	4	<1
7-Grain Vegetable	4	<1
Cookies: Amaranth	70	3
Fancy Fruit Chunks:		
Apr. Almond; Date Pecan	45	2
Raisin Oat Bran	35	1
Other varieties	45	1
Fat Free Cookies	25	<1
Fat Free Jumbos	70	<1
Fiber Jumbos	100	3
Fruit & Fitness	40	1
Fruit; Honey Jumbos, aver.	70	3
Oat Bran: Fruit Jumbos	70	2
Animal Cookies	16	<1
Fruit & Nut	55	2
The Great Tofu	45	1
The Great Wheat Free	40	1

KEEBLER

Crackers (Retail): Town House, 4	70	4
Alpha Grahams, 6 pieces	70	2
Club, Reg./Low Salt, 4 pces.	60	3
Clubettes, 22 pieces	70	4
Deluxe Grahams, 2 pieces	90	4
Toasteds: Sesame/Wheat, 4	60	3
Sun Wheats, 10 pieces	70	4
Wheatables, Reg./Low Salt, 12	70	3
White Cheddar/Ranch, 11	70	4
Zesta Saltine, 5 pieces	60	2

KEEBLER (CONT)

	CALS	FAT (g)
Crackers (Food Service):		
Club Crackers, (2)	30	2
Graham Crackers:		
Kitchen Rich Grahams, (2)	60	2
Fiber Enriched Honey, (3)	90	2
Multigrain Crackers, (2)	30	1
Oyster Crackers,		
50 small/26 lge, 18g	80	2
Town House Crackers, (2)	35	2
Wholegrain Wheat Cr., (2)	30	1
Waldorf Sodium Free, (2)	30	1
Zesta Saltine: Reg; Unsalt., (2)	25	1
Melba Toasts, aver., 2 pces.	25	<1
Toasted Snack: All types, (2)	30	2
Pretzels: 1 pkg, ½ oz	55	<1
Cookies (Retail):		
Baby Bear Cookies, 3	70	2
Choc. Chip, P'nut Butt./Walnut	80	5
E.L. Fudge, 2	80	4
E.L. Fudge S/wiches, aver., 1	60	3
Fudge Sticks, 2 pces.	100	6
Fudge Stripes, 1 piece	50	3
Magic Middles, all types	80	5
Mim Middles, aver., 4	80	4
Pecan Sandies	80	5
Softbatch: Choc. Chip	80	4
Oatmeal Raisin	70	3

LADY-J

	CALS	FAT (g)
Average all varieties	115	4

LANCE

	CALS	FAT (g)
Soft Chocolate Chip	65	3
Fudge/Chocolate Chip	65	3
Oatmeal	65	3
Apple-Cinnamon	60	2
Blueberry; Strawberry	60	2
Cracker Sandwiches: See Snacks (p. 85).		
Crackers (Food Service):		
Saltines, 2-pak	25	1
Other Crackers, average, 2	30	1
Melba Toast, aver., 2 slices	25	1
Bread Sticks, 2	30	0

> '*You can begin to control what you eat when you write it down everyday*'

LU MARIE LU

	CALS	FAT (g)
Per Cookie		
Butter Twist; Marie LU	50	2
Crokine	18	0
Chocolatiers	42	2
Creme Wafer	37	2
Dipped Chocolatiers	52	3
Little Schoolboy	65	3.5
Marie LU, Wheat & Cinnamon	45	1
Mini Marie LU	10	<1
Petit Beurre	40	1
Pims	48	1
Prince	67	3

MANISCHEWITZ

	CALS	FAT (g)
Matzo Boards — See Page 69.		
Matzo Cracker, Miniatures	9	0
Whole Wheat Crackers	9	0
Tam Tams	15	1
Onion/Garlic/Wheat Tams	15	1

MOTHER'S BRAND

	CALS	FAT (g)
Almond Shortbread	60	4
Butter Flav.; Vanilla Wafers	24	1
Checkerboard Wafers	17	1
Chocolate Chip: Cookies	70	3
Cookies (bag)	30	2
Angel Cookies	60	4
Chocolate Creme Sandwich	55	2
Circus Animal Cookies	28	2
Cocodas Coconut Cookies	30	2
Dinosaur Grrrahams: Average	75	3
Double Fudge; Duplex S/wich	50	2
English Tea Sandwich	100	4
Fig Bars: Regular; Wheat	57	1
Flaky Flix Fudge Wafer	65	5
Flaky Flix Vanilla Wafer	58	2
Fudge 'n Chips Cookies	30	2
Fudge Swirl Cookies	74	6
Gaucho Peanut Butter S/wich	90	5
Iced Raisin; Macaroon	80	4
Mini Dinosaurs: Average, each	10	0
Mint Patties	60	2
Oatmeal Cookies: Regular	60	3
Iced; Chocolate Chip	70	3
Oatmeal Raisin Cookies	30	2
Royal Grahams; Walnut Fudge	70	4
Striped Shortbread Cookies	50	2
Sugar Cookies	65	4
Taffy Sandwich	97	6

(Continued Next Page)

NABISCO

CRACKERS — Per Cracker

	CALS	FAT (g)
American Classic: All types	17	1
Bacon Flavored Thins, each	10	1
Better Cheddars: Reg; Low Salt	7	<1
Toasted Bran Thins, each	9	<1
Cheddar Wedges, ½ oz (31)	70	3
Chicken in a Bisket, ½ oz (7)	80	5
Crown Pilot	70	2
Dandy: Soup & Oyster, ½ oz, (20)	60	2
Escort	23	1
Harvest Crisps: 5-Grain/Oat	10	<1
Meal Mates: Ses. Bread Wafers	23	1
Nips Cheese, ½ oz, (13)	70	3
Oysterettes, ½ oz, (18)	60	1
Premium: Saltines, all types	12	<1
Fat Free Saltine	10	0
Premium Bits, ½ oz, (16)	70	3
Ritz: Regular; Low Salt	17	1
Ritz Bits: All types, ½ oz (22)	70	4
S/wiches: Chse./P'nut But., (1)	13	1
Royal Lunch	60	2
Sociables	12	<1
Swiss Cheese	10	<1
Tid Bits, cheese, ½ oz, (16)	70	4
Triscuit Wafers: All types	20	1
Triscuit Bits Wafers	7	<1
Twigs Snack Sticks	14	1
Uneeda, Unsalted Tops	30	1
Vegetable Thins	10	<1
Waverly: Reg; Low Salt	17	1
Wheat/Oat Thins: All types	9	<1
Wheatsworth; Stone Ground	17	1
Zwieback Toast	30	<1

COOKIES — Per Cookie

	CALS	FAT (g)
Almost Home: Real Choc. Chip	60	3
Other varieties	70	3
Baker's Bonus: Oatmeal	80	3
Barnum's Animal Crackers	12	<1
Biscos: Sugar Wafers	17	1
Waffle Cremes	35	2
Bugs Bunny Graham Cookies	12	<1
Cameo Creme Sandwich	70	3
Chips Ahoy: Chewy	60	3
Choc. Chip; Sprinkled	50	2
Mini	12	<1
Other types, average	95	5
Cookie Break; Van. Crm. S/wich	50	2
Cookies 'n Fudge: Party Grahams	45	2
Striped Shortbread	60	3
Striped Wafers	70	4

COOKIES (CONT.): Per Cookie

	CALS	FAT (g)
Giggles Sandwich Cookies	60	3
Heyday Bars: All types	110	6
Honey Maid: Grahams	30	<1
Graham Bites: All types	5	<1
Ideal Bars: Chocolate & Peanut	90	5
Lorna Doone: Shortbread	23	1
Mallomars: Chocolate Cakes	60	3
Mystic Mint Sandwich	90	5
Nabisco: Per Cookie/Wafer		
Brown Edge Wafers	28	1
Chocolate Chip Snaps	23	1
Chocolate Grahams	60	3
Chocolate Snaps	17	<1
Devil's Food Cakes	70	1
Famous Chocolate Wafers	28	1
Fudge Cakes	90	4
Grahams	30	<1
Marshmallow Puffs	90	4
Marshmallow Twirls	140	6
Old Fash. Ginger Snaps	30	1
Pure Chocolate Middles	80	5
National Arrowroot Biscuit	20	1
Newtons: Fig; Cinn. Raisin	60	1
Apple, Strawb., Raspberry	70	2
Variety Pack, each	120	3
Nilla Wafers: Regular; Cinnamon	17	<1
Nutter Butter: P'nut Butter S/wich	70	3
Peanut Creme Patties, 1	40	2
Oreo: Chocolate Sandwich	50	2
Fudge Chocolate Sandwich	110	6
Big Stuf Choc. Sandwich	250	12
Double Stuf Choc. S/wich	70	4
Pantry: Molasses Cookies	80	3
Pecan Shortbread	80	5
Pinwheels: Choc./Marshmallow	130	5
Social Tea Biscuits	20	1
Suddenlys' Mores	100	4
Teddy Grahams Bearwich's	17	1
Teddy Grahams Snacks: All types	5	<1

72

CRACKERS & COOKIES (CONT)

PEPPERIDGE FARM

	CALS	FAT (g)
CRACKERS — Per Cracker		
English Wafer Biscuit	17	<1
Goldfish Cheese Thins	17	1
Butter Flavored; Sesame	20	1
Cracked Wheat	30	1
Hearty Wheat; 3 Crack. Assort.	25	1
Toasted Wheat with Onion	20	1
Tiny Goldfish: All flavors	3	0
COOKIES — Per Cookie		
Almond Supreme	70	5
Apricot Raspberry	50	2
Assortment: Champagne	32	2
Chocolate Laced Pirouette	35	2
Seville	50	3
Southport	75	3
Beacon Hill Brownie Nut	120	7
Bordeaux	35	2
Brownie Chocdate Nut	55	3
Brussels	55	3
Brussels Mint	65	3
Cappucino	55	3
Capri	80	4
Chesapeake Choc. Chunk Pecan	130	7
Chessman	45	2
Chocolate Chip	50	3
Chocolate, Chocolate Chip	55	3
Chocolate Chunk Pecan	65	4
Date Pecan	55	3
Geneva	65	4
Gingerman	35	1
Hazelnut	55	3
Lemon Nut Crunch	55	3
Lido	95	6
Milano: Regular	60	3
Mint; Orange	75	4
Milk Chocolate Macadamia	70	4
Molasses Crisps; Orig. Pirouettes	35	2
Monte Carlo	45	3
Nantucket Chocolate Chunk	120	7
Nassau; Tahiti	85	5
Oatmeal: Irish	45	2
Raisin	55	3
Orleans: Regular	30	2
Sandwich	60	4
Paris	50	4
Raisin Bran	55	3
Sante Fe Oatmeal Raisin	110	4
Sausalito Milk Choc. Macadamia	110	7
Shortbread	75	4
Strawberry, Sugar	50	2

STELLA D'ORO

	CALS	FAT
Almond Toast (Mandel)	60	1
Angel Bars	80	5
Anisette Sponge/Toast	50	1
Castelets, regular/chocolate	70	3
Coconut Cookies	50	2
Dutch Apple Bars	110	3
Egg Biscuits, sugared	80	1
Golden Bars; Love Cookies	110	4
Hostess/Lady Stella Assorted	40	2
Margherite, chocolate/vanilla	70	3
Peach Apricot/Prune Pastry	90	4
Swiss Fudge	70	3

SALERNO

	CALS	FAT
Crackers: Graham	17	<1
Oyster Crackers, ¼ cup, (20)	30	<1
Royal Graham: Small	47	2
Large	70	4
Saltines: All varieties	12	<1
Cookies: Almond Crescent	20	1
Animal Cookies	8	<1
Bonnie Shortbread	32	1
Butter Cookies: Regular	28	1
Mini, each	6	<1
Dinosaurs: Large	70	2
Mini, each	8	<1
Gingerbread; Gingles	23	1
Iced Oatmeal	65	2
Patties; Peanut; Mint Creams	75	4
Royal Stripes	70	3
Vanilla Wafer	19	<1
WWF Superstars; Super Mario	13	<1

SUNSHINE

	CALS	FAT
Crackers: Krispy Saltine	12	<1
Cheez-It Crackers	6	<1
Wheats Snack Crackers	9	<1
Animal Crackers	10	<1
Oyster & Soup, 16 crackers	60	1
Honey Graham, 1 whole	60	2
Cinnamon Graham	70	3
Cookies: Grahamy Bears	14	<1
Ginger Snaps	20	1
Oatmeal Cookies	55	3

WESTBRAE

	CALS	FAT
Dino Snaps: Aver., 4 snaps	70	2
Snaps: Aver., 3 snaps	130	5
Cocoa Chip; Peanut Butter	140	7
Carob; Ginger	130	5

CAKES, PASTRIES, DONUTS

CAKES & PASTRIES

	CALS	FAT
Angel Food: Plain, 2 oz	160	0
with Cream Icing	230	7
Banana w/Butter Cream, 3 oz	300	13
Black Forest, 3 oz	230	10
Carrot Cake: Plain, 3 oz	230	8
with Cream cheese icing	380	21
Cheesecake: 3 oz serving	260	18
Large serving, 5 oz	430	30
w/lowfat cheese/fruit, 3 oz	150	8
Chocolate Cake: Plain, 2 oz	220	11
with Cheese Icing, 3 oz	320	15
& Cream Filling, 3½ oz	360	21
Coffee Cake, 2½ oz	230	7
Cream Puff (custard fill.), 4½ oz	300	18
Cupcake: Plain, 1½ oz	140	6
with icing	170	7
Danish Pastry: Average		
Small, 2 oz	220	10
Large, 4 oz	440	20
(McDonald's, Arby's, Carl's, Hardie's		
— See Fast Foods Section)		
Date Nut Roll, ½" slice	80	2
Eclair, Choc., Cust. fill., 3½ oz	240	14
Rich's, 2 oz	205	10
Fruit Cake, Dark/Light, 1½ oz	165	7
Gingerbread: From mix, 3" sq.	200	6
Homemade, 2½ oz	270	0
Lemon Cake, 2½ oz	220	9
Meringues: Page 77.		
Plain Cake, 3 oz	310	12
with White Icing, 4¼ oz	450	14
Pineapple Upside Down, 2½ oz	230	9
Peach Melba, 3½ oz	300	8
Pound Cake, 1 oz	130	67
Sponge: Plain, 2½ oz	190	3
with Cream & Strawb.	325	8
with Chocolate Icing	300	12
Raising Bun, 1 bun, 2¼ oz	180	2
Strudel, fruit, average, 3 oz	280	8
Sweet Roll, average, 1½ oz	155	7
Toaster Pastry, 1¾ oz	200	6
Turnovers, fruit, aver., 3 oz	270	12
White Cake, homemade, 2½ oz	260	11
w/Choc. Icing, 2¾ oz	300	12
Yellow Cake, h/made, 2½ oz	270	12
w/Choc. Icing, 2¾ oz	310	13
FROZEN & MIXES — See Pages 76-77.		

DONUTS

	CALS	FAT (g)
DUNKIN' DONUTS (Per Donut)		
Apple w. Cinn. Sugar, 2¾ oz	250	11
Blueberry filled, 2½ oz	210	8
Glazed Yeast Ring, 2 oz	200	9
Glazed Chocolate Ring, 2½ oz	325	21
Glazed Coffee Roll, 2¾ oz	280	12
Jelly Filled, 2½ oz	220	9
Lemon Filled, 2¾ oz	260	12
HOSTESS (Per Donut)		
Family Pack: Cinn./Plain/Powd, 1 oz	110	1
Assorted: Cinn/Plain/Powd, 1⅔ oz	190	10
8's Pack: Plain, 1.1 oz	130	7
Cinn/Powdered, 1.2 oz	140	7
Donettes: Cinn/Plain/Powd, ½ oz	60	3
TASTYKAKE (Per Donut)		
Assorted: Aver. all types, 1⅔ oz	200	9
Choco-Dipped	180	10
Premium: Aver. all types, 2½ oz	350	20
Powdered Sugar (12/pkg), 1 oz	125	6
Mini: Aver. all types, 0.4 oz	60	3
WINCHELL'S DONUTS (Per Donut)		
Apple Fritter	580	37
Cinnamon Roll	360	21
Devil's Food; Cinnam. Crumb	240	12
French Iced (Choc.)	220	13
Glazed Jelly	300	13
Glazed Round/Twist; Plain	210	12
Iced (Choc.) Bar/Raised/Cake	220	11

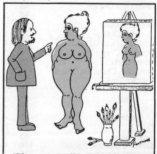

"You went off your diet while I was on vacation, didn't you?"

74

MUFFINS & PIES

MUFFINS

READY-TO-EAT	CALS	FAT (g)
Average All Types:		
Small, 1 oz	80	3
Medium, 2 oz	160	6
Large, 3 oz	240	9
Jumbo/Extra Large, 4 oz	320	12
English: Average, 1 muffin	150	2
Arby's: Blueberry Muffin	200	6
Carl's: Blueberry Muffin	340	9
Bran Muffin	260	6
Dunkin Donuts: Per Muffin		
Apple 'n Spice	300	8
Banana Nut; Bran w/Raisins	310	10
Blueberry; Cranberry Nut	280	8
Oat Bran; Corn	330	11
Health Valley: Per Muffin		
Fat-Free Fruit Muffin, average	135	<1
Oat Bran Fancy Fruit, average	180	4
Rice Bran Fancy	210	7
Hostess:		
Average all types, 1½ oz	155	6
2 oz Muffin	250	14
McDonald's: Apple Bran	190	0
Pepperidge Farm:		
Stone Ground Wheat	130	1
Other types, average	175	6
Sara Lee: Apple Oat Bran	190	6
Golden Corn	240	13
Other types	210	8

MUFFIN MIXES:	CALS	FAT (g)
Prepared — Per Muffin		
Betty Crocker: Bake Shop, av.	200	7
Apple; Banana; Blueberry	120	4
Cinn. Streusel, Oat Bran	200	9
Choc., Carrot, Oatmeal	150	5
Duncan Hines: Blueberry, reg.	120	3
Bakery Style Blueberry	190	6
Oat Bran Blueberry	110	4
Cinn. Topp. O/Bran Honey	140	5
Bakery Style: Cinn. Swirl	200	7
Cranberry Orange Nut	200	8
Pecan Crunch	220	11
O/meal & Apples/Walnuts	210	9
Estee: Oat Bran	100	4
Whole Foods: All types, aver.	110	5

PIES & TARTS

Average All Brands	CALS	FAT (g)
⅛ of 9″ Pie, 4 oz:		
Apple; Blueberry; Cherry	290	13
Boston Cream Pie	330	14
Chocolate Pie	300	18
Custard; Coconut Custard	250	13
Lemon Chiffon Pie	360	14
Lemon Meringue	270	11
Mince Pie	300	13
Pecan Pie	470	24
Pumpkin Pie	240	13
Strawberry Pie	230	9
Sara Lee/Weight Watchers Frozen Pies		
— Next Page		

SNACK PIES	CALS	FAT (g)
Hostess, Fruit, average, 5 oz	400	18
Pudding Pies, average, 5 oz	480	18
TastyKake, Fruit, average	370	14
French Apple	420	12
Coconut Creme	510	32

PASTRY & PIECRUSTS

PIECRUST	CALS	FAT (g)
Baked, 9″ diameter shell		
1 Pie Shell, 6½ oz	900	60
2-Crust Pie, 9″, 11¼ oz	1500	93
Keebler Dessert Shells:		
Ready Crust, 9″, ⅛	100	5
3″ Shell	110	5
Pet-Ritz, Deep Dish, ⅙, 1 oz	130	8
Pillsbury (All Ready):		
⅛ of 2-Crust Pie	240	15
Piecrust Sticks, 8 oz	960	64
Choux Pastry, raw, 1 oz	60	4
Filo Pastry, 4 sheets, 2½ oz	210	?
Flaky Pastry, 1 sheet, 6 oz	780	72
Puff (Pepp. Farm), ½ sheet	520	34
Shell	210	15
Pastry Pockets (Pillsb.), each	230	13
Pizza Crust (Pillsb.), ⅛ whole	90	1

PIE FILLINGS

Canned — Per 3½ oz or ⅙ Pie	CALS	FAT (g)
Fruit: Regular, average	110	0
Reduced Calorie	75	0
Chocolate, Coconut	130	3
Mincemeat, ⅓ cup	150	1

CAKES — FROZEN

SARA LEE

Calories Per Slice	CALS	FAT (g)
All Butter Pound:		
Original, 1/10 whole	130	7
Family Size Original, 1/15	130	7
All Butter Coffee: Per 1/8 Whole		
Butter Streusel, Pecan	160	7
Cheese, 2 oz	210	11
Single Layer Iced: Per 1/8 Whole		
Banana, 1.7 oz	170	6
Carrot, 2.4 oz	250	13
Two Layer: Per 1/8 Whole		
Black Forest; Strawb. Short.	190	8
Three Layer: Per 1/8 Whole		
Double Chocolate	220	11
Lights: Per Whole Cake		
Carrot Cake	170	4
Double Chocolate	150	5
Lemon Cream Cake	180	6
Indiv. Wrapped Coffee: Per Whole		
Apple Cinnamon	290	13
Butter Streusel	230	12
Pecan	280	16
Original Cheesecake: Per 1/6 Whole		
Cherry Cream, 3.2 oz	243	8
Plain Cream, 2.8 oz	230	11
Strawberry Cream, 3.2 oz	220	8
Classics: Per 1/8 Whole		
Choc. Mousse; Fr. Cheesecake	260	17
Strawb. Fr. Ch/Cake, 3.2 oz	240	13
Classic Lights: Per Whole Cake		
Chocolate Mousse	170	8
French Cheesecake	150	4
Strawberry French Ch/Cake	150	2
Snacks: Per Cake		
All Butter Pound; Carrot	200	11
Chocolate Fudge Cake	190	10
Classic Cheesecake	200	14
Country Apple Pie	230	9
Fudge Brownie; Pecan	270	14
Danish Twist: Per 1/8 Whole		
Apple; Raspberry	190	10
Cheese	200	12
Individual Danish: Per 1 Roll		
Apple	120	6
Cheese; Cinnam. Raisin	140	8

SARA LEE (CONT)

Homestyle Pies (9") Per 4 oz Serving (1/10 of Pie)	CALS	FAT (g)
Apple; Cherry; Peach; Raspb.	280	12
Pumpkin	240	10
Blueberry; Dutch Apple; Mince	300	13
Pecan	400	18

HOSTESS LIGHTS

	CALS	FAT
Choc./Choc. Frost, 1½ oz	110	1
Creme filled, 1¾ oz	180	6
Other Flavors, 1½ oz	130	1
Creme filled, 1¾ oz	180	6

PEPPERIDGE FARM

Cakes Supreme: Per 3 oz Slice	CALS	FAT
Boston Cream, Lemon Cocon.	290	14
Chocolate	310	17
Peach Melba	270	7
Raspberry Mocha	310	14
Cream Cakes Supreme:		
Pineap./Strawb. Cr., 2 oz sl.	190	7
Layer Cakes: Per 1½ oz Slice		
Butterscotch Pecan	160	7
Choc. Fudge; German Choc.	180	10
Chocolate Mint	170	9
Devil's Food; Coconut; Golden	180	9
Vanilla	190	8
Old Fashioned Cakes: Per 1 oz Sl.		
Butter Pound	130	7
Carrot w. Cream Cheese Icing	140	8
Cholesterol Free Pound Cake	110	6
Fruit Squares: Single		
Apple; Blueberry; Cherry	220	12

WEIGHT WATCHERS

	CALS	FAT
Apple Pie, 1 serving	200	5
Apple Sweet Roll	190	4
Black Forest Cake	180	5
Boston Cream Pie	190	4
Brownie Cheesecake	200	6
Carrot Cake	170	5
Cheesecake	220	7
Chocolate Brownie, each	100	3
Chocolate Cake	190	5
Chocolate Mocha Pie	160	5
German Chocolate Cake	200	7
Strawberry Cheesecake	180	5

CAKE & COOKIE MIXES

PACKET CAKES & COOKIES

Made as directed	CALS	FAT (g)
AUNT JEMIMA		
Coffee, 1/8 cake	160	5
BETTY CROCKER		
Per 1/12 Package		
Cherry Whip	190	3
Choc. Chip Golden Vanilla	280	14
Sour Cream White	180	3
Butter Chocolate	270	13
Other flavors, average	250	11

If using No Cholesterol Recipe,
deduct 40 calories; and 4 grams fat.

MicroRave: Per 1/6 Package		
Apple Streusel	240	11
Choc Fudge & Frosting	310	16
Cinnamon Pecan Streusel	290	13
Devils Food & Frosting	310	16
German Chocolate & Frosting	320	17
Golden Vanilla & Frosting	320	17
Lemon; Yellow & Frosting	300	16

If using No Cholesterol Recipe,
deduct 40 calories; and 4 grams fat.

Angel Food Cakes:		
All flavors, 1/12 mix	150	0
Brownie Mixes:		
Caram. Swirl; Supreme Fudge	120	4
Choc; Fudge; Walnut	140	6
Frosted, German Chocolate	160	6
MicroRave Brownies:		
Fudge; Walnut	160	7
Frosted	180	7
DUNCAN HINES		
Angel Food, 1/12 whole	140	0
Other Flavors, average, 1/12	265	13
Frostings: Average, 1/12 serv.	160	7
Cookies: All flavors, 1 cookie	55	2
Brownies: 1 Piece		
Fudge	130	5
Plus Double Fudge	150	6
Plus Milk Chocolate	160	8
Plus Peanut Butter	150	8
Plus Walnuts	150	7
Gourmet Turtle	200	9
ESTEE		
Brownie, 1 pce, 2" x 2"	50	2
All cakes, 1/10 cake	100	2

PILLSBURY

	CALS	FAT (g)
Plus: Per 1/12 Cake		
All flavors, average	250	12
Microwave: Per 1/8 Cake		
Lemon; Yellow; Chocolate	220	13
Double Chocolate Supreme	330	19
Double Lemon Supreme	300	15
Streusel Swirl Cinnamon	240	11
Tunnel of Fudge	290	17
Microwave with Frosting: 1/8 Cake		
All flavors	300	17
Streusel Swirl: Per 1/16 Cake		
Cinnamon; Lemon	270	11
Bundt Brand Ring: Per 1/16 Cake		
Tunnel of Fudge	260	12
Tunnel of Lemon	270	9
Boston Cream; Pineapple Cr.	270	10
Choc. Mac.; Black Forest	240	8
Brownies: Per 2" Square		
The Ultimate, all flavors	170	7
Deluxe Fudge, all flavors	150	7
Microwave Fudge	190	9

CAKE FROSTINGS

	CALS	FAT (g)
Average All Flavors, 2 Tbsp	160	8
BETTY CROCKER		
Creamy Deluxe (Ready-to-Spread)		
All flavors, aver., 1/12 tub	160	7
Creamy Frosting Mix:		
Made as directed, 1/12 mix		
Coconut Pecan	150	8
Other flavors, aver.	180	6
Fluffy Frosting Mix:		
White, 1/12 mix	70	0
ESTEE		
Frosting Mix, 1½ Tbsp	50	1
Whipped Topping, 1 Tbsp	4	<1
PILLSBURY — Per 1/12 Tub		
Cream Cheese; Lemon	160	6
Dble. Dutch; Milk Choc.; Fudge	150	6
Coconut Pecan; Almond	160	10
Coconut Almond	150	9
Choc Chip	150	5
Fluffy White; Frost It Hot	60	0
All other flavors	160	8
Decorators, Choc., 1 Tbsp	70	2

PANCAKES & WAFFLES

PANCAKES

	CALS	FAT (g)
Average All Types		
Small (3" diam.), ¾ oz	50	1
Medium (4" diam.), 1¼ oz	80	2
Large (5" diam.), 2½ oz	160	4
(Syrups & Toppings — Extra)		

FAST FOOD OUTLETS

	CALS	FAT
Carls: Hot Cakes (w/marg./syr.)	360	12
Hardees: 3 Pancakes (no fat)	280	2
with Sausage Patty	430	16
with 2 Bacon Strips	350	9
Syrup	120	0
Margarine/Butter Blend	35	4
Jack In The Box:		
Pancake Platter	610	22
Pancake Syrup	120	0

PANCAKE MIXES

Per 3 Pancakes (4" diam.)

	CALS	FAT
Aunt Jemima:		
Pancake & Waffle: Original	200	7
Buttermilk, Buckwheat	220	8
Whole Wheat	270	9
Complete	250	4
Buttermilk Complete	230	3
Microw. Pancake: (3½ oz Serv.)		
Original; Blueberry	210	4
Buttermilk	210	3
Lite	140	3
Betty Crocker:		
Buttermilk (3 x 4" pancakes)	280	10
Complete Buttermilk	210	3
Bisquick (Shake 'N Pour):		
(Pancake & Waffle Mixes)		
Average all types, 3	260	5
Estee: 3 x 4" pancakes	160	<1
Featherweight: 3 x 4" p'cakes	140	2
Hungry Jack:		
Buttermilk (3 x 4" pancakes)	240	11
Complete	180	1
Complete Packets	180	3
Blueberry	320	15
Extra Lights	210	7
Complete	190	2
Panshakes	250	6
Pillsbury:		
Average all types, 3	250	4

WAFFLES

	CALS	FAT
Homemade: 7" waffle, 2½ oz	245	13
From Mix: 7" waffle, 2½ oz	205	8
Aunt Jemima (Per 2½ oz Waffle):		
Blueberry	175	5
Wholegrain Wheat/Oat	155	3
Other flavors	175	6
Eggo: Average all types	120	5

SYRUPS (PANCAKE & WAFFLE)

Per 1 fl.oz (2 Tbsp)

	CALS	FAT
Aunt Jemima: Orig., 2 Tbsp	110	0
Butter Lite/Lite, average	55	0
Estee, 2 Tbsp	16	0
Featherweight, Lite Syrup, 2 T.	32	0
Golden Griddle, 2 Tbsp	110	0
Honey, 2 Tbsp	130	0
Jam/Preserves: See Page 80.		
Karo, 2 Tbsp, 1 fl.oz	115	0
Log Cabin: Reg./Buttered	110	0
Lite	60	0
Maple/Molasses: See Syrups (p.80).		
Vermont Maid, 2 Tbsp	100	0

BISCUITS

	CALS	FAT
Mixes/Refrig. Dough,		
Average all brands, 1 oz	90	4
Homemade, 1 oz	100	5

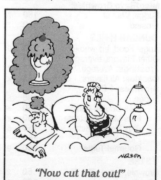

"Now cut that out!"

PUDDINGS, CUSTARDS, GELATIN

PUDDINGS

	CALS	FAT (g)
INSTANT PUDDING & PIE MIXES		
Per ½ Cup		
Regular, average all flavors	170	4
Reduced Calorie: D-Zerta	70	<1
Estee	70	<1
Featherweight	80	0
Jell-O, sugar free	90	2
Royal, sugar free	100	2
Weight Watchers:		
Inst. Puddings	90	1
Mousse, all flavors	60	3
READY-TO-SERVE		
Del Moule Pudding Cup, 5 oz:		
Average all flavors	180	5
Hunt's Snack Pack, 5 oz:		
Average all flavors	210	9
Jell-O Pudd. Snacks, 4 oz cup:		
Regular, aver., all flavors	170	6
Jell-O Light, average	100	2
Swiss Miss, average, 4 oz	150	6
Thank You, average, ½ cup	170	4
PUDDING BARS (FROZEN)		
Bullwinkle Pudd. Stix, 2½ fl.oz:		
All flavors	120	2
Good Humor Pudding Stix	90	2
Jell-O Pudding Pops: Regular	80	2
Chocolate covered	130	8
WEIGHT WATCHERS (FROZEN)		
Chocolate Mousse	170	6
Praline Pecan Mousse	190	7
Raspberry Mousse	150	6
HOMEMADE PUDDINGS		
Apple Tapioca, ½ cup	150	<1
Bread Pudding, ½ cup	250	8
Blancmange, ½ cup	140	5
Chocolate, ½ cup	190	6
Corn Pudding, ½ cup	135	7
Rennin Dessert, ½ cup	115	5
Rice with Raisins, ½ cup	200	4
Tapioca Cream, ½ cup	110	4
Trifle, ½ cup	180	7

MERINGUES

Meringue Swirl, ½ oz	50	0
Meringue Shell, 1 oz shell	100	0
(Add extra for fillings.)		

CUSTARDS

	CALS	FAT (g)
CUSTARD MIX		
Jell-O (Americana) Gldn. Egg:		
Prep. w/whole milk, ½ cup	160	5
Prep. w/skim milk, ½ cup	125	1
Royal, ½ cup	150	5
HOMEMADE CUSTARD		
Baked, plain, ½ cup, 4½ oz	150	7
w/skim milk, artif. sweetened	70	3
Boiled, ½ cup	165	7

GELATIN DESSERTS

Regular, all flavors, ½ cup	80	0
Sugar Free/Low Cal., ½ cup	8	0

DESSERT TOPPINGS

CREAM: See Page 29.

SYRUPS — Per 1 Tbsp		
Kraft: Chocolate; Caramel	60	0
Hot Fudge	70	3
Pineapple; Strawberry	50	0
Estee: All flavors, 1 Tbsp	4	0
Magic Shell: Chocolate Nut	100	8
Chocolate; Choc. Fudge	85	8
Smuckers: Average all flavors	65	1
Light Hot Fudge	35	<1
(Other Syrups — See Page 80.)		
NUTS: Chopped Nuts, 1 Tbsp	40	4

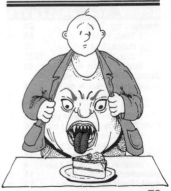

79

SUGAR

	CALS	FAT (g)
White Sugar, granulated:		
1 level teaspoon, 4g	15	0
1 heaping teaspoon, 6g	25	0
1 cube, ½"	24	0
Single portion, 1 packet	25	0
1 tablespoon, 12g	46	0
1 ounce, 1 oz	110	0
1 cup, 7 oz	770	0
1 pound	1760	0
Brown Sugar: 1 Tbsp, 13g	50	0
1 ounce, 1 oz	109	0
1 cup, not packed, 5 oz	540	0
1 cup, packed, 7¾ oz	845	0
Powdered/Confectioners:		
Sifted, 1 cup, 3½ oz	385	0
Unsifted, 1 cup, 4¼ oz	460	0
Other Sugars:		
Cinnamon Sugar, 1 tsp	15	0
Date Sugar, 1 oz	110	0
Dextrose, 1 oz	110	0
Fructose, 3 Tbsp, 1 oz	110	0
Glucose, 1 oz	110	0
Sorbitol, 1 oz	110	0
Turbinado Sugar, 1 oz	110	0
Unrefin. Cane Sugar, 1 oz	110	0
Artificial Sweeteners:		
Tablet/Liquid	Negl.	
Granulated, equiv. to 2 tsp	4	0
Sugar Delight (Light Cane Sugar)		
1 pkt (½ tsp)	8	0

HONEY, JAM, PRESERVES

	CALS	FAT (g)
Honey: 1 tsp, ¼ oz	22	0
1 Tbsp, ¾ oz	65	0
1 ounce, 1 oz	86	0
1 cup, 12 oz	1030	0
Single Portion, ½ oz pkg	45	0
Jams/Jellies/Preserves:		
Regular, 1 tsp, ¼ oz	18	0
1 Tbsp, ¾ oz	55	0
1 ounce	75	0
Single Portion, ½ oz pkg	38	0
Fruit Spreads: Regular, 1 tsp	16	0
Low Sugar, 1 tsp	8	0
Low Cal. (Featherwt.), 1 tsp	4	0
Jelly: Regular, average, 1 tsp	18	0
Imitation, Low Calorie, 1 tsp	4	0
Marmalade, citrus, 1 tsp	18	0
Apple/Fruit Butters, 1 tsp	12	0

BAKING & COOKING INGREDIENTS

	CALS	FAT (g)
Almond Paste (Marzipan), 1 oz	125	7
Baking Powder: Regular, 1 tsp	3	0
Cream of Tartar, 1 tsp	2	0
Butter/Margarine: ½ cup, 4 oz	820	91
Carob Flour, ½ cup	90	<1
Chocolate, cooking/baking:		
Sweetened, 1 oz	140	10
Unsweetened, 1 oz	140	15
(Bakers Brand — See next page.)		
Cocoa Powder, 1 Tbsp	14	1
Coconut, desiccated:		
Shredded/grated, ⅓ c., 1 oz	140	9
(Coconut Products — See Page 86.)		
Cornstarch, 1 Tbsp	30	0
Flour: All Purpose, 1 cup, 5 oz	500	<2
Flavor Extracts, average all brands:		
Imitation, 1 tsp	15	0
Pure Extract, 1 tsp	20	0
Almond, Vanilla, 1 tsp	10	0
Fruit Pectin: Swtnd, 1 Tbsp, ½ oz	35	0
Unsweetened, 1 Tbsp	2	0
Gelatin, dry, ¼ oz packet	30	0
Lemon/Orange Peel, ¼ cup	30	0
Nuts & Seeds: See Pages 86-87.		
Rennin, 1 packet (11 g)	12	0
Vinegar, aver. all types, 1 oz	4	0
Whey, sweet, dry, 1 oz	90	<1
Yeast: Active, dry, ¼ oz pkg	20	0
Fresh/household, Fleischmann's, 0.6 oz pkg	15	0
Bakers, compressed, 1 oz	25	0
Brewers; Torula, 1 oz	80	<1

SYRUPS

Per Tablespoon (approx. ¾ oz)

	CALS	FAT (g)
Blueberry (Featherweight), 1 Tbsp	16	0
Cane; Fruit; Strawberry, aver.	50	0
Chocolate Syrup, 1 Tbsp	40	<1
Corn, light/dark (Karo)	60	0
Maple: Regular, 1 Tbsp	50	0
Imitation (Karo)	60	0
Low Calorie (S&W)	12	0
Molasses, light/med/dark, aver.	45	0
Pancake Syrup: Regular	55	0
Lite, 1 Tbsp	30	0
(Brands: See Page 78.)		
Single Portion, 1 oz package	116	0
1½ oz package	175	0

CANDY, CHOCOLATES

CHOCOLATE READY RECKONER

	CALS	FAT
Average All Brands		
Milk Chocolate, regular:		(g)
Plain/Nuts/Fruit, aver., 1 oz	150	10
1½ oz Bar	225	15
2 oz Bar	300	20
4 oz Block	600	40
8 oz Block	1200	80
1 Pound, 16 oz	2400	160
Dark/White Chocolate, 1 oz	150	10
Chocolate-coated:		
Almonds, 5-6, 1 oz	160	11
Macadamias, 2-3 pces., 1 oz	180	13
Peanuts, 12 medium, 1 oz	160	11
Clusters, nut, 2, 1 oz	160	11
Raisins, 30 medium, 1 oz	120	4
Mints, 1 medium, 11g	45	1
Fudge, 1 oz	125	5
Nougat & Caramel, 1 oz	120	4
Creme/Cordial Centers, 1 oz	120	4
Cooking Chocolate, Baker's Brand:		
Sweet/Semi-sweet, 1 oz	140	10
Chips, ½ cup, 2.8 oz	400	20
Unsweetened, 1 oz	140	15
Big Chip, milk, ½ cup	480	26
CAROB CANDY — See Page 83.		
Carob, plain, 1 oz	160	11

"O.K.! Just for that,
from now on everything
that you like to eat is
going to be fattening!"

BRANDS & GENERIC

	CALS	FAT
After Dinner Mints, 1 small	45	1
Almond Joy, 1.76 oz	250	14
Snack Bar, 1 bar	100	5
Almonds, sugar-coated (7), 1 oz	130	5
Baby Ruth, 2.2 oz bar	300	13
Snack size, 1 bar	110	5
Bar None, 1½ oz bar	240	14
Barley Sugar, 1 piece, 0.2 oz	23	0
Bit-O-Honey, 1¾ oz bar	200	4
Black Cow Sucker	130	3
Blow Pop, all flavors, 1 pop	50	0
Bonkers!, all flavors, 1 piece	20	0
Bounty Bars, 1 pkg (2 bars)	300	16
Breath Savers, all flavors, 1 pce.	8	0
Butterfinger, 2 oz bar	260	12
Snack size, 1 oz bar	130	6
Butternut, 2 oz bar	270	13
Butterscotch, 6 pieces	115	5
Chips, 1 oz	150	7
Cadbury's: Per 2 oz bar		
Almond; Brazil Nut; Hazelnut	310	18
Fruit & Nut; Milk Chocolate	300	16
Caffioca Mocha Parfait, 4 pieces	120	3
Candy Corn (Brach's), 1 piece	7	0
Caramels, Plain/Choc, 3 pces, 1 oz	115	3
Caramello, 1.6 oz bar	220	11
Certs: Regular, 12 pieces	60	0
Sugar-free, 12 pieces	70	1
Charleston Chew!, 2 oz piece	240	6
Chips Away, 1 pkt	200	9
Choc Fudgie, 3 pieces	110	3
Choc Stars, 7 pieces	145	7
Chocolate Parfait, 1 piece	30	1
Chuckles, all varieties, aver., 1 oz	95	0
Chunky Fruit & Nut, 1 oz	150	8
Clark Bar, 1½ oz bar	200	8
Coffee/Caramel Nip, 4 pieces	120	3
Cough Drops/Lozenges — Page 87.		
Creme de Menthe (Andes), 1 pce.	25	2
Creme Eggs, 1 oz	136	6
Crunch, 1.4 oz bar	210	10
Dum Dum Drops, 1 drop	20	0
European Chocolates: Per Piece		
Baci (Perugina)	80	5
Ferrero Rocher	70	4
Lindor (Lindt)	70	4
Marcipan Brod (Anthon Berg)	120	7
Neuhaus, average all types	80	5
Seashells (Guylian)	65	4

Continued Next Page

81

CANDY, CHOCOLATES (CONT)

BRANDS & GENERIC (CONT.)	CALS	FAT
5th Avenue, 2.1 oz bar	290	13
Fudge: Chocolate/Vanilla, 1 oz	115	3
with Nuts, 1 oz	120	4
Fruit Leathers, average, ½ oz	40	0
Fruit Rolls (Sunkist), 1 roll	80	0
Fruit Roll-Ups/Ripples, ½ oz	50	<1
Fruit Wrinkles, 1 pouch	100	1
Fudge (Nabisco) Bar	85	3
Golden Alm. Choc., ½ bar, 1.6 oz	260	17
Golden III Choc., ½ bar, 1.6 oz	250	15
Gum (Per Pce.): Beechies	6	0
Bazooka Bubble	18	0
Beech-Nut	10	0
Bubble Gum, sugarless	10	0
Bubble Yum: Regular	25	0
Sugarless	20	0
Care Free (sugarless)	10	0
Dentyne	6	0
Estee, bubble/regular	5	0
Extra (sugarfree), average	8	0
Featherweight	4	0
Freedent, all flavors	10	0
Fruit Stripe	10	0
Hubba Bubba, regular	23	0
Sugarfree, average	14	0
Orbit	8	0
Trident (sugarless)	5	0
Wrigley's, all types	10	0
Gum Drops, 28 pieces, 1 oz	100	0
Gummi Bears (Brachs), each	8	0
Halvah: Plain or with nuts, 1 oz	160	7
Chocolate-coated, 1 oz	160	8
Hard Candy, all flavours, 1 oz	110	0
1 regular piece	18	0
Hershey's: Milk Choc., 1.55 oz	240	14
w/Almonds, 1.45 oz bar	230	14
Special Dark, 1.45 oz bar	220	12
Holidays, 1 oz package	140	6
Honeycomb: Plain, 1 oz	113	<1
Choc-coated, 1 oz	125	5
Hot Tamales, Mike & Ike, 1 pce.	9	0
Jellies, 3 medium, 1 oz	120	3
Jelly Beans, 10 small, 1 oz	100	0
Jelly Rings (Chuckles), each	37	0
Jujubes (Chuckles), each	55	0
Junior Mints, 12 pieces, 1 oz	120	3
Ju Jus: Assorted, 1 piece	7	0
Coins or raspberries, 1 pce.	15	0
Kisses (Hershey's): Plain, 1 kiss	24	2
with Almonds, 1 kiss	25	2
Kit Kat, 1.63 oz bar	250	13
Snack size, 3 oz bar	85	5

	CALS	FAT
Kraft: Caramels	35	1
Chocolate Fudgees	35	1
Toffees	30	1
Krackel, 1.55 oz bar	230	13
Snack size, 0.35 oz bar	55	3
Licorice: Aver. all types, 1 oz	100	0
Twists, black, 1 piece	27	0
red (Amer. Lic. Co.), 1 pce.	33	0
Life Savers, all flavors, 1 piece	8	0
Lollipops: Life Savers	45	0
Blow Pops, 1 oz size	110	0
Flat Pops, 1 oz size	120	0
Junior size	60	0
Icecream Pops, 1 oz	120	0
Tootsie Roll Pops	55	0
M & M's: Peanut, 1.74 oz pkg	250	13
Fun size, 0.8 oz	120	6
1 M & M	10	0
Plain, 1.69 oz pkg.	240	10
Fun size, 0.6 oz	110	5
1 M & M	4	<1
Malted Milk Balls (Brach's), 1 ball	10	<1
Mars Bar, reg./almond, 1.7 oz	240	11
Marshmallows: Firm/Soft, 1 oz	90	0
Regular size, 1 piece	25	0
Miniature, 1 piece	2	0
Marshmallow Eggs, 1 egg	110	0
Milky Way: Regular, 2.1 oz	280	11
Fun size, 0.8 oz	110	4
Dark bar, 1.7 oz	220	8
Mints, uncoated, 1 oz	100	<1
1 small mint (¾" diam.)	7	0
1 large mint (1½" diam.)	30	0
Peppermint Pattie (Nabisco)	55	0
Butter/Party (Kraft), each	8	0
Mounds, 1.9 oz	260	14
Snack size, 1 bar	100	6
Mr Goodbar, 1.75 oz bar	290	19
Munch Bar, 1.42 oz bar	220	14
Necco Sky Bar, 1.38 oz bar	175	8
Nestle Milk Chocolate, 1.45 oz	220	13
Snack size, 0.35 oz bar	55	3
Nonpareils (Nestle Sno-Caps), 1 oz	140	0
Nougat, 2 pieces, 1 oz	115	1
Chocolate covered, 1 oz	120	4
Oh Henry!, 2 oz	280	14
PB Max, 1½ oz bar	240	16
Park Avenue (Tom's), 1.8 oz bar	230	9
Payday (Hollyw. Brands), 1.9 oz	250	12
Peanut Bar (Planters), 1.6 oz bar	240	11
Chocolate-coated, 2 oz bar	320	18
Peanut Brittle, 1 oz	130	5

CANDY, CHOCOLATES (CONT)

BRANDS & GENERIC (CONT.)	CALS	FAT
Peanut Butter: Cups, 2 cups	280	17
Flav. Chips, ¼ cup, 1½ oz	230	13
Peanut Butter Sesame, 1 oz	150	9
Peanut Crunch Bar (S'hadi), ¾ oz	110	6
Peanut Parfait (Andes), 1 piece	28	2
Peanut Roll (Tom's), 1.75 oz pce.	230	11
Peppermints, 7 small, ½ oz	50	<1
Pepp. Pattie (Nabisco)	55	<1
Pollen Drops (Queen Bee), 1 pce.	20	<1
Popcorn — See Snacks (next page).		
Powerhouse (Peter Paul), 2 oz	260	11
Pralines, average, 1 piece	35	2
Raisinets, 1 oz	120	4
Reese's P/nut But. Cups, 1.8 oz	280	17
Reese's Pieces, 1.85 oz pkg.	260	11
Rolo (Hershey's), 1 piece	35	2
Rum Wafers, 1 wafer	150	7
Skittles, 2.3 oz package	265	3
Skor Toffee Bar, 1.4 oz	220	14
Smarties Candy Rolls, 1 roll	30	0
Snickers, 2.07 oz bar	280	14
Fun size, 0.8 oz bar	110	5
Solitaires, ½ bag, 1.6 oz	260	17
Spearmint Leaves, 1 oz	110	0
Starburst Fruit Chews, 2 oz	240	5
Sugar Babies, 1.6 oz package	180	2
Sugar Daddy (Juniors), 1 pop	50	4
Symphony (Hershey's), 1.4 oz	220	14
3 Musketeers, 2.1 oz bar	260	8
Snack size, 0.8 oz bar	100	3
Taffy, average, 1 piece, ¼ oz	30	<1
Ting-A-Ling (Andes), 1 piece	25	1
Toblerone, dark/white, 1 piece	40	2
Toffees: Regular, 1 oz	150	9
Kraft, ¼ oz	30	2
Tootsie Rolls: 1 midgee	25	<1
Chocolate, 1 oz bar	115	3
Snack Bars (½ oz)	60	2
Pops, 1 pop	55	0
Truffles, average: 1 small, ½ oz	75	5
1 medium, ¾ oz	100	7
1 large, 1 oz	155	10
Turtles (Queen Bee), 1 pce., 1 oz	240	17
Twix, Caramel, 2 oz pkg (2 bars)	280	14
Twizzlers (Y & S), 1 oz	100	1
Snack size, ½ oz	50	<1
Whatchamacallit, 1.8 oz bar	260	13
Willy Wonka's, fun-size, average	100	4
Y & S Bites/Nibs, 1 oz	100	1
Yogurt Candy: Plain, 1 oz	120	6
Coated Raisins, 1 oz	120	4
York Peppermint Pattie, 1½ oz	180	4

(Snack & Granola Bars — Page 85)

DIETETIC CANDY

	CALS	FAT
		(g)
Estee (Per Piece):		
Caramels, all flavors	30	1
Chocolate Bars, 1 square	30	2
Chocolate-coated Raisins	3	<1
Estee-ets	7	<1
Fruit & Nut Mix, 4 pieces	35	2
Gummy Bears; Gum Drops, 1 pce.	7	0
Lollipops	25	0
Peanut Butter Cups	40	3
Peanut Brittle, ¼ oz	35	1
Featherweight (Per Piece):		
Candy (Fruit Blends)	12	0
Chocolate Bars: Almonds, 1 sect.	90	6
Milk/Crunch, 1 section	80	7
Peppermint Swirls	20	5
Cool Blue Mints; Butterscotch	25	6
Caramels	30	5
Fruit Drops, all flavors	30	8

Note: Sorbitol and fructose sweetened candy have similar calories to regular candy.

CAROB CANDY

	CALS	FAT
Carob: Plain/Natural, 1 oz	160	11
Carob-coated: Raisins, 1 oz	130	8
Almonds/Peanuts, 1 oz	150	10
Malt Balls, 1 oz	135	8
Caramels, 1 oz	110	4
Dates, 1 oz	125	5
Soybeans	145	9
Trail/Party Mix, 1 oz	140	9
Carob Chips, unsweetened, 1 oz	140	7
Carob Bars, average all brands:		
Plain/Nut, 1 oz	160	11
Fruit & Nut, 1 oz	155	10
Mint/Orange, 1 oz	160	11
Caroby Natural Touch, 3 oz	450	27
Joan's Natural Bars (3 oz):		
Coconut; Peanut, average	520	35
Fruit & Nut	560	38
Honey Bran	490	33
Nature Snacks (Sun Maid):		
Carob Crunch, 1 oz	145	8
Carob Peanuts, 1¼ oz	190	12
Carob/Yogurt Raisins, 1¼ oz	160	12
Tahitian Treat; Yogurt Cr., 1 oz	125	7
Queen Bee: Carob Turtles, 1 pce.	230	15
Fantasy Truffles, 1 piece	225	12
Tiger's Milk, carob-coated bar	160	6
with Peanut Butter	160	7

SNACKS, CHIPS, PRETZELS

Per 1 oz (unless indicated)	CALS	FAT (g)
Bacon Cheese Crackers	140	6
Beef Jerky: Average, 1 oz	120	5
6" Stick, 0.2 oz	25	1
8½" Stick, 0.3 oz	35	2
Beef Sticks (Frito-Lay's), ½ oz	80	7
Bugles, 1 oz	150	8
Carrot Chips (Hain)	150	9
Cheddar Sticks/Lites	160	4
Cheese Balls, 1⅛ oz package	190	13
Cheese Crackers, 1 oz	130	6
Cheese Filled (Frito-Lay's)	210	10
Cheese Curls, 1 oz	150	8
Cheese Straws, 4 pieces	110	1
Cheese Twists, 1½ oz pkg.	260	13
Cheetos: Regular, all flavors	160	10
Light, cheese flavored	140	6
Cheez Balls (Planters)	160	10
Cheez Curls (Planters)	160	10
Cheez Doodles	160	10
Cheez Waffies	140	8
Churros, 10" stick, 1.2 oz	140	6
Corn Chips: Average all varieties,		
½ oz bag	80	5
1 oz bag	160	10
2 oz bag	320	20
8 oz bag	1280	80
Corn Crunchies/Spirals, 1 oz	160	10
Corn Crisps (Pringle), 1 oz	140	7
Corn Nuggets (Fr. Lay's), 1.38 oz	170	5
Corn Snackers (Wt. Watchers),		
1 bag, ½ oz	60	2
Funyun's Onion flav'd., 1 oz	140	6
Gold-N-Chee (Lance), 1⅜ oz pkg	180	9
Hot Sausage (Frito-Lay's)	80	7
Nuts & Seeds — Pages 86-87.		
Munchies (Skinny Haven):		
Chocolate Fudge, ½ oz	66	2
Other flavors, aver., ½ oz	59	2
PB&C Crackers (Eagle), 1 pce.	280	16
Popcorn, popped:		
Air-popped (no oil), plain, 1 oz	90	<1
1 cup (6g)	23	0
Oil-popped, plain, 1 oz	220	13
1 cup (11g)	55	3
Microwave, aver. all brands:		
Regular, 1 cup	50	4
Light, 1 cup	27	<1

Popcorn (Cont.):	CALS	FAT (g)
Packaged: Reg./flav'd., ½ oz	80	5
1 oz pkg.	160	10
Light, ½ pkg.	60	3
Caramel-coated, 1 oz	130	3
Popcorn Oil, 1 Tbsp	120	14
Pork Skins, fried: Baken-ets, 1 oz	160	10
½ oz package (Lance)	80	5
Potato Chips, aver. all brands:		
Reg. or flavored, 1 oz bag	150	10
4 oz bag	600	60
Pringle, all flavors, 1 oz	170	12
CrunchTators, 1 oz	140	7
Kettle Fry (Eagle), 1 oz	150	8
Light: Ruffles, 1 oz	130	6
Pringle, 1 oz	150	8
Pretzels: Aver. all types, 1 oz	110	2
Sticks, thin, 2¼" (90/oz), 1	1	0
Twisted, thin, ¼" (5/oz), 1	25	0
Dutch, 2¾"x2⅝" (2/oz), 1	55	1
Soft Pretzels (J & J Snack):		
Bites, ½ oz bite	40	<1
Mini Twist, 1 oz	75	1
Regular Twist, 2½ oz	190	3
King Size Twist, 5½ oz	420	7
Soft Pretzel Bun, 3 oz	285	3
Rice Chips (Amsnack):		
Bar-B-Q/Onion, ½ oz	70	3
Sesame Sticks, 1 oz	155	8
Toast/Cheese Crackers		
(Planters), 1 package	140	7
Tortilla Chips: Average, 1 oz	150	8
(3 oz = approx. 11 chips or 12 strips)		
Doritos: 18 chips, 1 oz	140	6
Light, 1 oz	120	4
Keebler Suncheros Light	150	8
Weight Watchers Snacks:		
Apple Chips, ¾ oz pkg.	70	0
Apple Snacks, ½ oz pkg.	50	<1
Corn Snackers, ½ oz pkg.	60	3
Fruit Snacks, ½ oz pkg.	50	<1
Great Snackers, ½ oz pkg.	60	2

QUIZ QUESTION

How many cups of air-popped popcorn have the same calories as 1 cup of roasted peanuts?
(Answer — Page 86.)

SNACKS & GRANOLA BARS

	CALS	FAT (g)
(Carob Candy & Bars: Page 83)		
Carnation Breakfast Bars	200	11
Diet Workshop Energizer	150	2
Fi·Bar: Strawberry/Raspberry	100	3
Cranberry & Wild Berries	100	3
Almond/Peanut, average	130	5
Figurines (Pillsbury), 1 bar	100	5
Frito Lay's:		
Cheese filled crackers, 1½ oz	210	10
P'nut But. filled crackers, 1½ oz	210	10
Fudge Nut Brownie, 2 oz	240	9
Peanut Butter Bar, 1¾ oz	270	16
Fruit & Nuts/Trail Mixes:		
Average all brands, 1 oz	130	6
3 oz pkg.	390	18
Grandma's Cookies:		
Big Cookies (2), 2.75 oz:		
Choc. Chip, 2 cookies	370	17
Fudge Chocolate	350	13
Oatmeal Apple Spice	330	12
Molasses; Raisin	320	9
Peanut Butter	410	30
Sandwich Cremes: Per Serv.(1.8 oz)		
Chocolate; Vanilla	260	12
Peanut Butter	260	13
Health Valley: Per Bar		
Bakes: All flavors	100	3
100% Org. Fat Free Fruit	140	<1
Fruit & Fitness, 1 pkg/2 bars	200	5
Oat Bran: Apricot Bake	100	3
Fig & Nut Bake	110	3
Oat Bran Jumbo Fruit Bars:		
Alm. & Date; Fruit & Nut	170	5
Raisin & Cinnamon	160	2
Rice Bran Jumbo Fruit	160	5
Kellogg's Smart Start:		
Oat Bran with Raspberry	170	6
Corn Flakes w/Mixed Berry	170	7
Nutri Grain Blueb./Strawb.	180	8
Raisin Bran	160	5
Rice Krispies w/Almonds	130	6
Kudos Snack Bars: Raisin	170	9
Other varieties, average	190	11
Lance Sandwiches: Per Pkg. (1¼-1½ oz)		
Fig Bar	150	2
Captain's Wafers w/Crm. Chse.	170	9
Other varieties, average	190	10

	CALS	FAT
Meal On The Go: Apple, 1½ oz	150	6
Original; Banana w/Pecans	145	5
Nature Valley Granola Bars:		
Cinnamon, Oats 'n Honey	120	5
Oat Bran — Honey Graham	110	4
Peanut Butter	120	6
Rice Bran	90	4
Pathway Granola Bars (Matol)		
Crunchy Oat & Peanut	190	6
Matola: Wild Berry	285	3
Honey Oats & Raisin	285	3
Planters: Peanut Bar, 1.6 oz	230	11
Honey Roasted Bar	230	13
Sweet 'n Crunchy Bar	250	15
Old Fashioned Bar, 1 oz	140	9
Crackers (4 s/wiches), 1 oz	140	7
Power Bars, all types, 2¼ oz	225	2
Quaker Granola Bars:		
Chewy: Apple; Strawberry	120	3
Other varieties, average	130	5
Dipps: Caramel Nut	150	6
Chocolate Chip	140	6
Chocolate Fudge	160	8
P'nut Butter/Choc. Chip	170	9
Spicers Wheat Snacks: 1½ oz	150	7.5
Ultra Slim-Fast: Average	110	3
Yogurt Raisins, 1 oz	120	4

"My new diet allows me a small saucer of anything I want for lunch."

85

Shelled, Per 1 oz (unless shown):

	CALS	FAT
Acorns, raw, 1 oz	105	7
Almonds, Dried/Dry roasted:		
Whole, 24-28 med., 1 oz	170	15
½ cup, 2½ oz	420	37
Chopped, ½ cup, 2¼ oz	380	34
Sliced, ½ cup, 1²/₃ oz	280	25
Choc.-coated (5-6), 1 oz	160	11
Oil rstd. (Blue Diamond), 1 oz	175	16.5
Almond Meal (partially defatted)		
1 cup (not packed), 2¼ oz	260	10.5
Honey roasted, 1 oz	170	13
Brazil Nuts, 8 medium, 1 oz	185	19
Cashews, Dry or Oil roasted:		
14 large/18 med./26 small, 1 oz	165	14
½ cup, 2.4 oz	400	33
Honey roasted, 1 oz	170	12
Chestnuts, average all types:		
Raw/Fresh, 5-6 nuts, 1 oz	60	<1
Dried, 1 oz	105	1
Canned, water chestnuts,		
sliced/whole, drained, 1 oz	23	<1
Coconut: Flesh (no shell), 1 oz	100	9.5
Raw: 1 pce. (2"x2"x½"), 1.6 oz	160	15
½ medium (4½" diam.)	650	62
Dried (Desiccated):		
Unsweetened, 1 oz	187	18
Sweetened, shredd., 1 oz	140	9
Grated, ½ cup, 1.3 oz	185	12
Cream (can.), ½ c., 5.2 oz	285	26
Milk (canned), ½ c., 4 oz	225	24
Water (center liq.), ½ c., 4¼ oz	23	<1
Filberts or Hazelnuts:		
Shelled, 18-20 nuts	180	18
Chopped, ¼ cup	180	18
Ground, ¼ cup	120	12
Ginko Nuts, can., 14 med., 1 oz	32	<1
Hickory, 30 small nuts	190	18
Macadamia Nuts, shelled:		
Raw, 7 med./14 small, 1 oz	200	21
½ cup, 2.3 oz	460	48
Oil roasted, 1 oz	205	22
½ cup, 2.4 oz	490	52
Choc.-coated, 2-3 pces., 1 oz	180	13
Mixed Nuts: 18-22 nuts, 1 oz	175	13
Planters: Dry roasted	160	14
Dry roasted, unsalted	170	15
Honey roasted (dry rst'd)	170	13
Oil roasted, all types	180	16

	CALS	FAT
Nut Toppings, chop., 1 T., ¼ oz	40	4
Peanuts:		
Raw/Dried, in shell, 1 oz	117	10
Shelled, 1 oz	160	14
Boiled, ½ cup, 1.1 oz	102	7
Roasted, 30 lge./60 sml., 1 oz	165	14
1 cup, 5.1 oz	840	71
Chopped, 3 Tbsp, 1 oz	165	14
Planters: Oil roasted, 1 oz	170	15
Dry roasted, 1 oz	160	14
Honey roasted, 1 oz	170	13
Honey/Dry rst'd., 1 oz	160	13
Cocktail, oil rst'd., 1 oz	170	14
Sweet 'N Crunchy, 1 oz	140	8
Pecans, kernel halves, 1 oz	190	19
(20 Jumbo or 31 large halves)		
1 cup halves, 3.8 oz	720	73
Chopped, ½ cup, 2 oz	380	30
Oil roasted, 1 oz	195	20
Honey roasted, 1 oz	200	18
Pilinuts, dried, ¼ cup, 1 oz	205	23
Pinenuts, dried, 1 Tbsp, 10g	50	5
Pistachios:		
Unshelled, ½ cup, 2 oz	165	14
Shelled, ¼ c., 45 nuts, 1 oz	165	14
Lance, 1⅛ oz package	180	14
Planters: Dry roasted, 1 oz	170	15
Fruit 'n Nut Mix, 1 oz	150	9
Nut Topping, 1 oz	180	16
Tavern Nuts, 1 oz	170	15
Sesame Nut Mix (Planters), 1 oz	160	12
Soybean Nuts:		
Dry roasted, 1 oz	130	6
½ cup, 3 oz	390	18
Oil roasted, 1 oz	140	7
Walnuts:		
Black, 15-20 halves, 1 oz	175	16
Chopped, ¼ cup	190	18
Ground, ¼ cup	120	12
English/Persian:		
14 halves, 1 oz	185	18
Chopped, ¼ cup	195	19

> *Answer To Quiz (Page 84)*
>
> *36½ cups of air-popped popcorn have the same calories as 1 cup of roasted peanuts (840 cals.).*

SEEDS

	CALS	FAT
Caraway; Fennell, 1 tsp	10	<1
Cottonseed Kernels, rst., 1 Tbsp	50	4
Lotus Seeds, dried, ½ c., ½ oz	50	<1
Pumpkin & Squash Seeds, whole:		
Roasted, 1 oz	125	5.5
½ cup (32g)	140	6
Dried, 1 oz	155	13
Safflower Kernels, dried, 1 oz	150	11
Sesame Seeds: Dried, 1 Tbsp, 9g	50	4.5
Roasted/Toasted, 1 oz	160	14
Sunflower Kernels/Seeds:		
Dry roasted, 1 Tbsp, 8g	45	4
¼ cup, 1 oz	160	14
Oil roasted, ¼ cup, 1 oz	180	17
Watermelon, dried, ¼ cup, 1 oz	160	13.5

NUT & SEED BUTTERS

Per 1 Tbsp (Approx. ½ oz)

Almond Butter	105	9
Honey & Cinnamon	95	8
Cashew Butter	92	7
Hazelnut Butter	100	10
Peanut Butter: Average, 1 oz	170	14
Chunky/Creamy, 1 Tbsp, 16g	95	8
Smucker's: Honey Swtnd., 1 T	100	8
Goober Grape/Strbry, 1 Tbsp	90	5
Skippy, honeynut, 1 Tbsp, 16g	95	8
Sesame Butter/Tahini, 1 tsp	30	3
1 Tbsp	90	8
Sunflower Butter, 1 Tbsp	97	7

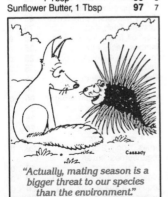

"Actually, mating season is a bigger threat to our species than the environment."

Cassady

VITAMINS, SUPPLEMENTS

Vitamins/Minerals:	CALS	FAT
Tablets/Capsules, aver. each	<3	0
Vitamin E Capsules, each	5	<1
Fiber Supplements:		
Tablets, average, each	1	0
Metamucil, 1 packet	5	0
Regular, 1 rounded Tbsp	34	0
1 heaping tsp	14	0
Sugar-Free, 1 med. Tbsp	6	0
Aloe Vera Juice, undil., 2 fl.oz	4	0
Cod Liver Oil, 1 Tbsp	120	13
Fish Oil Capsules, aver., each	10	1
Garlic Tablets/Capsules, each	3	0
Km (Matol), 1 Tbsp	<2	0
Lecithin Granules, 1 Tbsp	40	5
Capsules, each	11	<1
Oyster Tablets/Pearls, each	3	0
Pollen Granules/Meal, 1 Tbsp	35	<1
Protein: Powders, aver., 1 oz	100	<1
Tablets, 20 tabs., ½ oz	70	0
Seaweed: Dried, 1 oz	85	<1
Soaked, drained, 1 oz	15	<1
Spirulina, 1 tablet	2	0
Yeast: Tablets, 2 tabs.	4	0
Flakes, 1 heaping Tbsp, ⅓ oz	30	<1
Powder, 1 heaping Tbsp, ½ oz	50	<1

COUGH & PHARMACEUTICAL

Cough/Cold Syrups: 1 tsp	36	0
Regular, average, 1 Tbsp	120	0
Sugar-free, 1 Tbsp	<1	0
Cough Drops/Lozenges:		
Beech Nut, 1 tablet	10	0
Hall's, 1 tablet	15	0
Hall's Plus, 1	78	0
Helps Cough, all flavors, 1	14	0
Listerine Loz. (Amer. Chicle)	9	0
Luden Throat, all flavors, 1	8	0
Pine Bros, 1 cough drop	8	0
Squibb Cough/Throat Loz.'s, 1	16	0
Sucrets (Beecham) Lozenges:		
Cough/Cold/Throat, 1	10	0
Antacids: Average, 1 tablet	4	0
Liquid, 1 Tbsp	6	0
Sudafed Syrup, 1 tsp	14	0
Tylenol Liquid: Child, 1 tsp	17	0
Extra Strength, 1 tsp	11	0
Pharmaceutical Drugs:		
Average, 1 tablet/capsule	<1	0

FRESH FRUIT

WEIGHTS AS PURCHASED	CALS	FAT
Acerola, 1 cup, 20 pcs, 3½ oz	**30**	0
Atemoya, ⅓ cup	**95**	<1
Apples, whole, average all varieties:		
1 small (4 per lb), 4 oz	**70**	0
1 medium (3 per lb), 5½ oz	**90**	0
1 large (2 per lb), 8 oz	**135**	<1
1 extra large, 11 oz	**170**	1
without skin, ½ medium	**35**	0
Apricots: 1 small (12 per lb)	**17**	0
1 medium (8 per lb), 2 oz	**25**	0
1 large (5-6 per lb), 3 oz	**35**	0
Avocado (wt. w/out seed):		
Average, ½ medium	**160**	15
California, ½ medium, 3 oz	**150**	15
Mashed/Puree, ½ c., 4 oz	**200**	20
Florida, ½ medium, 5½ oz	**170**	13
Mashed/Puree, ½ c., 4 oz	**125**	10
½ cup cubed, 3 oz	**95**	8

Note: Avocados are nutritious with no cholesterol. Fat is mainly monounsaturated and benefits blood cholesterol.

	CALS	FAT
Banana: 1 small (4/lb), 4 oz	**55**	0
1 medium (3 per lb), 5 oz	**80**	<1
1 large (2½ per lb), 7 oz	**105**	<1
W/out skin, 1 med., 3¼ oz	**80**	<1
½ cup, mashed, 4 oz	**105**	<1
Berries, average all types: (Black/Boysen/Blueberries)		
½ cup, 2½ oz	**40**	0
1 pint, 14 oz	**220**	1
Breadfruit, ½ cup, 4 oz	**115**	<1
Cantaloupe, ½ med. (5″ diam.)	**100**	<1
1 slice, 2½ oz (w/out skin)	**20**	0
1 cup pieces/balls, 5½ oz	**55**	<1
Carambola (Star Fruit), 1 med.	**50**	<1
Cassava, ⅓ cup	**120**	0
Cherimoya (Custard Apple), ¼ only, 5 oz	**130**	<1
Cherries: Sweet, 8 fruit, 2 oz	**40**	1
½ lb (30 cherries)	**145**	2
Sour, 8 fruit, 2 oz	**25**	0
½ lb (30 cherries)	**100**	<1
Coconut: Fresh, 1 piece, 1 oz	**100**	10
Shredded, fresh, ½ cup	**140**	14
Sweetened, dried, ½ cup	**235**	16
Cream, can, ½ cup	**285**	26
Milk, can, ½ cup	**225**	24
Water, ½ cup	**20**	<1

	CALS	FAT
Crab Apples, ½ cup slices, 2 oz	**40**	0
Cranberries, ½ cup, 2 oz	**20**	0
Currants (per ½ cup):		
European Black, raw, 2 oz	**35**	0
Red & White, raw, 2 oz	**30**	0
Dates — See Dried Fruits.		
Durian, flesh, 4 oz	**140**	2
Elderberries, ½ cup, 2½ oz	**55**	0
Feijoas, 1 medium, 2½ oz	**35**	0
Figs, green/black: 1 med., 2 oz	**40**	0
1 large, 3 oz	**60**	0
Fruit Salad, fresh, average,		
½ cup, 3½ oz	**60**	0
1 cup, 7 oz	**120**	0
Gooseberries, raw, ½ c., 2½ oz	**30**	0
Grapefruit, average all types,		
½ fruit, 8½ oz (4½ oz flesh)	**40**	0
1 cup sections w/juice, 8 oz	**75**	0
Grapes: Aver., 1 cup, 5½ oz	**100**	<1
1 small bunch, 4 oz	**70**	0
1 medium bunch, 7 oz	**125**	<1
1 large bunch, 1 lb	**285**	1
Granadilla, flesh, 3½ oz	**95**	2
Groundcherries, ½ cup, 2½ oz	**35**	0
Guava: 1 fruit, 4 oz	**80**	<1
½ cup, 3 oz	**40**	<1
Honeydew, 1 wedge (7″x2″ wide), 8 oz (with skin)	**45**	0
1 cup cubes/balls, 6 oz	**60**	0
Honey Murcots, 1 only, 5 oz	**45**	0
Jabotica, flesh, 4 oz	**75**	2
Jackfruit, flesh, ⅛ aver., 4 oz	**105**	0
Jambos, flesh, 4 oz	**35**	0
Java-Plum, 4 plums, ½ oz	**25**	0
Jujube, 3 oz	**65**	0
Kiwifruit, 1 medium, 3 oz	**45**	0
1 large, 4 oz	**60**	0
Kumquats, 5 medium, 3½ oz	**60**	0
Kiwano, ½ medium, 5 oz	**35**	0
Langsat, Duku, 1 medium, 2 oz	**25**	0
Lemon, 1 medium, 4 oz	**20**	0
1 wedge, 1 oz	**5**	0
Limes, 1 only, 2 oz	**20**	0
Loganberries, frozen,		
½ cup, 2½ oz	**40**	0
Logans, 5 fruit, ½ oz	**10**	0
Loquats, 4 fruit, 2¼ oz	**20**	0
Lychees, 4 fruit, 2¼ oz	**25**	0

WEIGHTS AS PURCHASED	CALS	FAT (g)
Mamey Apple, 1 whole, 3 lb	430	4
¼ fruit (1 cup flesh), 7 oz	100	1
Mandarin: 1 small, 3 oz	25	0
1 medium, 4 oz	35	0
1 large, 6 oz	55	0
Mango, flesh, ½ cup sl., 3 oz	55	0
1 whole, medium, 11 oz	140	<1
Melons: Average all types:		
1 cup, cubes/balls, 6 oz	60	0
Monstera Deliciosa (Taxonia),		
Edible part, 4 oz	50	0
Mulberries, 20 fruit, 1 oz	15	0
Nashi Fruit (Asian Pear),		
1 medium, 4½ oz	50	0
Nectarines, 1 medium, 4 oz	50	0
1 large, 5½ oz	70	0
Oheloberries, ½ cup, 2½ oz	20	0
Olives, Pickled:		
Green, 10 large, 1½ oz	45	5
Ripe, Grk. Style, 10 med., 1 oz	70	7
Ripe (Black), Californian:		
1 Small/Medium	4	<1
1 Large/Extra Large	6	<1
1 Jumbo	7	<1
1 Colossal	9	1
1 Super Colossal	13	1
Oranges, average all varieties:		
1 Small, 5 oz	50	0
1 Medium, 8 oz	80	0
1 Large, 10 oz	95	0
Californian: Valencias, 8 oz	85	0
Navels (thick skin), 8 oz	70	0
Flesh only, 1 cup, 6 oz	80	0
Florida, 1 medium, 7 oz	70	0
Papaya, ½ cup, cubed, 2½ oz	30	0
1 medium, 16 oz	120	<1
Passionfruit, 1 medium, 1¼ oz	20	0
Peaches: 1 med. (4 per lb), 4 oz	35	0
1 large, 6 oz	55	0
Pears: Bartlett, 1 small, 4 oz	60	0
1 medium, 6 oz	90	<1
1 large, 8 oz	120	<1
Bosc, 6 oz	90	<1
D'Anjou, 1 medium, 8 oz	120	<1
Red Pear, 5 oz	80	<1
Seckel (Wash'ton), 2¼ oz	35	0
Asian (Nashi), 1 large, 7 oz	80	0
Pepino, ½ medium, 4 oz	20	0

	CALS	FAT
Persimmons: Native, 1 oz	30	0
Japan. (2½″ d. x 3½″ h.), 7 oz	120	0
Seedless (Maui), 1 md., 5 oz	100	0
Pineapple (flesh only): 1 slice,		
(¾″ thick, 3½″ diam.), 3 oz	40	0
1 cup, diced, 5½ oz	80	1
1 medium, 4½ lb	525	5
Pitanga, 3 fruit, 1 oz	6	0
Plaintains, ½ cup slices, 2½ oz	90	0
Plums, average all types:		
Mini/Damson, (1″ dm.), ½ oz	8	0
Small, (1¾″ diam.), 2 oz	30	0
Medium, (2¼″ diam.), 3 oz	45	0
Large, (2½″ diam.), 4 oz	65	0
Pomegranates, ½ fruit, 5 oz	55	0
Pummelo, flesh, ½ cup, 4 oz	35	0
Prickly Pears, 1 fruit, 5 oz	40	<1
Quinces, 1 fruit, 5 oz	50	0
Rambutan (Rambotang),		
Red/Yellow, 1 med., 2 oz	15	0
Raspberries, ½ cup, 2 oz	30	0
Rhubarb, raw, ½ cup, 2 oz	15	0
Sapodilla (Chico), 1 md., 7½ oz	140	2
Sapotes, 1 medium, 11 oz	300	1
Soursop, 1 cup pulp, 8 oz	150	<1
Strawberries: 1 cup, 5½ oz	45	<1
6 medium/3 large, 2 oz	15	0
1 pint, 12 oz	95	1
Sugar Apples, ½ cup pulp, 4 oz	120	0
Tamarind: 1 fruit, ¼ oz	5	0
Tangelo: 1 Small, 4 oz	30	0
1 Medium, 5 oz	40	0
1 Large, 7 oz	55	0
Tangerine, 1 fruit, 4 oz	35	0
Tangor, 1 medium, 4 oz	35	0
Tomato: Cherry, 1 med., ¾ oz	5	0
1 Small, 3 oz	25	0
1 Medium, 5 oz	35	0
1 Large, 7 oz	45	0
1 medium slice	5	0
Canned Tomatoes/Products — Page 95.		
Tree Tomato (Tamarillo), 1 md., 3 oz	20	0
Ugli Fruit, Tangelo type, 5 oz	40	0
Watermelon (flesh only):		
1 slice, 8 oz	70	0
1 cup cubed, 5½ oz	50	0
Wax Jambu (Rose Apple),		
1 medium, 2 oz	10	0

FRUIT — DRIED, SNACKS, CANNED

DRIED FRUIT

	CALS	FAT
Apples, 5 rings, 1 oz	75	0
Apricots, 8 halves, 1 oz	65	0
Banana Chips, ½ cup, 1½ oz	160	5
Banana Flakes, 4 Tbsp, 1 oz	80	0
Currants, ¼ cup, 1¼ oz	100	0
Dates, 5 medium dates, 1½ oz	120	0
Large Calif., 3 dates, 2 oz	160	0
½ cup, chopped, 3 oz	240	<1
Figs, 3 medium figs, 2 oz	145	0
Longans; Lychees, 1 oz	80	0
Mango Slices, 4 strips, 1 oz	70	0
Mixed Fruit, 1 oz	70	0
Papaya Spears, 1 oz	75	0
Peaches, 2 halves, 1 oz	60	0
Pears, 3 halves, 2 oz	75	0
Pineapple, 1 oz	80	0
Prunes, dried: With pits, 1 oz	60	0
1 Medium (60/lb)	16	0
1 Large (50/lb)	22	0
1 Extra Large (40/lb)	27	0
Without pits, 4 med., 1 oz	70	0
Cooked: w/sugar, ½ c., 5 oz	200	0
w/out sugar, ½ c., 4½ oz	125	0
Raisins, 2 Tbsp, 1 oz package	85	0
½ cup, 2½ oz	215	0

CANDIED GLACE FRUIT

Apricot, 1 medium, 1 oz	100	0
Cherry, 3 large, ½ oz	50	0
Citron/Fruit Peel, 1 oz	90	0
Fig, 1 piece, 1 oz	90	0
Ginger, 1 oz	95	0
Pineapple, 1 slice, 1¼ oz	120	0

FRUIT ROLLS & CANDY

Berry Bears, 1 pouch	100	1
Fruit Leathers, aver., 1 pce., ½ oz	40	<1
Fruit Rolls: Betty Crocker, 1 pce.	50	<1
Flavor Tree, ¾ oz roll	80	<1
Fruit Roll-ups, ½ oz	50	<1
Fruit Wrinkles (Betty Cr.), 1 pch.	100	1
Garfield Frt. Snacks: 1 roll, ½ oz	50	<1
1 pouch	90	1
Shark Bites Frt. Corners, 1 pch.	100	1
Weight Watchers Fruit Snacks	50	<1
Other Snack Bars w/Fruit — See Pp. 83-85		

FRUIT SNACKS

	CALS	FAT
Fruit In Juice:		
Apple Sauce: Mott's, 4 oz	100	0
Hunt's Snack Pack, 4¼ oz	80	0
Fruit Cup (Del Monte):		
Mixed Fruits, 5 oz pkg	110	0
Peaches, 5 oz pkg	115	0
Fruit Paks (Mott's), 4 oz pak	100	0

CANNED FRUITS

SOLIDS & LIQUIDS
½ Cup (Approx. 4 oz)

Apples, sweetened	70	<1
Apricots: In water	35	0
In juice	60	0
In syrup	105	0
Blackberries; Blueberries; Boysen,		
In heavy syrup, 4½ oz	115	0
Cherries, pitted, sweet: In water	55	0
In light syrup	85	0
In heavy syrup	110	0
In extra heavy syrup	130	0
Fruit Cocktail: Water pack, 4½ oz	40	0
In juice, 4½ oz	55	0
In light syrup, 4½ oz	80	0
In hvy. syrup, ½ c, 4½ oz	95	0
Fruit Salad: In water, 4½ oz	35	0
In juice, 4½ oz	60	0
In heavy syrup, 4½ oz	95	0
Gooseberries: Light syrup	90	0
Grapefruit: Juice pack	45	0
In light syrup	75	0
Oranges (Mandarin): In water	40	0
In light syrup	75	0
Peaches: In water	30	0
In juice	50	0
In light syrup	70	0
drained, ½ peach	40	0
In heavy syrup	100	0
Pears: In water, ½ cup, 4 oz	35	0
In juice	60	0
In heavy syrup	90	0
Pineapple: In juice, ½ cup	70	0
In heavy syrup	95	0
1 slice (½" th.) + 1 Tbsp liq.	35	0
Plums: Unsw., in juice, 4½ oz	75	0
In heavy syrup, 4½ oz	115	0
Prunes, in heavy syrup	125	0
Raspberries, in heavy syrup	120	0
Strawberries: Unsw., in water	25	0
In heavy syrup, 4½ oz	115	<1
Mixed Fruit, hvy. syrup, 4½ oz	90	0

FRUIT & VEGETABLE JUICES

FRUIT & VEGE. JUICES

AVERAGE OF BRANDS

Per 6 fl.oz (unless indicated)	CALS	FAT
Aloe Vera Juice	12	0
Apple, fresh/can/bottle, 6 fl.oz	90	0
8½ fl.oz box	130	0
10 fl.oz bottle	150	0
11½ fl.oz can	170	0
Blackberry, fresh	70	0
Blueberry; Blackcurrant	100	0
Carrot Juice: Fresh, 6 fl.oz	60	0
Sweetened	70	0
Cranberry	85	0
Green Mix (Ferraro's), 6 oz	12	0
Grape, white/red/purple	110	0
10 fl.oz bottle	180	0
Grapefruit: Unsweetened, fresh	70	0
Sweetened	80	0
Lemon Juice: Fresh, 6 fl.oz	35	0
Lime Juice, fresh	50	0
Loganberry, fresh	80	0
Orange: Fresh/canned/frozen:	90	0
8½ fl.oz box	130	0
10 fl.oz bottle	150	0
11½ fl.oz can	170	0
Pineapple; Passionfruit	100	0
Prune, 6 fl.oz	130	0
Strawberry/Raspberry	75	0
Tangerine	90	0
Tomato Juice, 6 oz	35	0
V8 Vegetable (Campbells), 6 oz	35	0
Fruit Nectars: Average	110	0
Fruit Blends: Average	95	0

FRUIT DRINKS, BLENDS ADES & PUNCHES

Average All Varieties		
1 small glass, 6 fl.oz	110	0
8½ fl.oz box	155	0
10 fl.oz bottle	180	0
11½ fl.oz bottle/can	210	0
BRANDS — 6 oz (unless indicated)		
Bama Punch, all flavors	90	0
Boku Fruit Juice Coolers	90	0
Capri Sun: Maui Punch, 6¾ fl.oz	110	0
Fruit Drinks, aver., 6¾ fl.oz	110	0
Crystal Geyser: Juice Squeeze	70	0
Light Seltzer w/Juice, aver.	60	0
10 fl.oz bottle	100	0
Five Alive, average all flavors	90	0
Hawaiian Punch, average	100	0
Low Sugar	30	0

FRUIT DRINKS (CONT)

Per 6 fl.oz (unless indicated)	CALS	FAT
Hi-C: Average all flavors, 6 fl.oz	95	0
8½ fl.oz box	135	0
Kerns Nectars: Strawb./Banana	100	0
Apricot; Guava; Pear	110	0
Banana/Coconut; Pineapple	120	0
Kool Aid Koolers, 8.45 oz box, aver.	130	0
Knudsen (8 fl.oz box): Lemonade	100	0
Apple Cranb.; Peach Nect.	70	0
Apple; Cherry; Tropical	110	0
Raspb. Nect; Grape, aver.	125	0
Spritzers: 12 fl.oz can		
Blk. Cherry, Cranb; Grape	120	0
Lem./Mand. Lime; Strawb.	120	0
Cola; Or. Passfrt.; Raspb.	140	0
Oran.; Boysenb.; Trop. Lime	160	0
Libby's Juicy Juice Tropical	100	0
Mauna Lai: Guava; Passionfruit	100	0
Mott's: Apple blends, 8½ fl.oz box	130	0
9½ fl.oz cans: Grapefruit	120	0
Apple Cranb./P'app., aver.	170	0
Other flavors, average	150	0
Minute Maid Juices, average:		
10 fl.oz bottle	155	0
10 fl.oz can	175	0
Ades/Punches: Lemonade	80	0
Fruit Punch, 6 fl.oz	90	0
Citrus Punch; Grpade	95	0
Ocean Spray: Grapefruit	70	0
Cranapple; Cran. Grape	130	0
Cranicot, Cran. Raspb./Tastic	110	0
Low Cal. Cran Apple/Berry	40	0
Orange Julius: Orange, 16 fl.oz	265	1
Strawberry, 16 fl.oz	340	1
Recharge, aver., 8 fl.oz	60	0
Squeezit, aver. 6¾ fl.oz	110	0
Sundance Jce Sparklers, 10 oz	125	0
Tang Fruit Box, 8½ fl.oz	130	0
Tropicana Twister: P/app Grpfrt.	95	0
Orange Apric./Cranb.; Grpfrt.	85	0
Or. Passfrt; Strawb. Banana	70	0
Welch's: Sparkling Apple, 6 fl.oz	100	0
Grape Jce. Varieties, 6 fl.oz	120	0
Juice Cocktail, 10 fl.oz bottle:		
Apple	190	0
Orange	160	0
Grape; Other blends	120	0
Cocktails-In-A-Box (8½ fl.oz)		
Average all varieties	150	0
Fruit Drinks, 11½ fl.oz, aver.	210	0

Orange flavor Bkfst Drinks — Page 97

VEGETABLES — FRESH OR FROZEN

	CALS	FAT
Alfalfa Sprouts, ½ cup, ½ oz	5	0
Artichokes, Globe/French:		
1 medium, 4½ oz	65	0
Artichoke Heart, ½ cup, 3 oz	40	0
Asparagus, raw/frozen:		
4 medium spears, 2 oz	15	0
Cuts & Tips, ½ cup, 3 oz	25	<1
Bamboo Shoots, ckd, ½ c., 4 oz	15	0
Beans: Green/Snap, ½ c., 2 oz	20	0
Broadbeans, ckd, ½ cup, 3 oz	90	0
Butterbeans, ½ cup, 3 oz	90	0
Lima, baby, ½ cup, 3 oz	90	0
Dry Beans, average all types:		
(Kidney, Brown, Haricot, Lima, Mung, Navy, Pinto, Red, White)		
Raw, 2 Tbsp, 1 oz	95	<1
1 cup, 7 oz	665	3
Cooked, 1 oz	35	0
½ cup, 3 oz	105	<1
Soybeans: Mature, dry, 1 oz	110	5
Dry, ½ cup, 3½ oz	385	18
Cooked, ½ cup, 3 oz	105	5
Bean Sprouts, aver., ½ c., 3 oz	25	0
Beets, cooked: ½ c., slices, 3 oz	25	0
1 beet, 2″ diam., 2 oz	17	0
Beet Greens, ckd, ½ c., 2½ oz	20	0
Black Eyed Peas, ckd, ½ c., 2 oz	160	<1
Bok Choy (Chinese Chard), 3 oz	12	0
Broccoli: Raw, ½ cup, 1½ oz	12	0
1 spear (5 oz edible)	40	<1
Cooked, ½ cup, 3 oz	25	0
Brussels Sprouts, ckd, ½ c, 3 oz	35	0
Cabbage, average all varieties:		
Raw, shred., ½ cup, 1¼ oz	8	0
Cooked, ½ cup, 2½ oz	15	0
Carrots: Ckd, ½ c. slices, 2¼oz	35	0
Raw, 1 medium, (7½″), 3 oz	33	0
Raw, 1 lb, (5-6 med)	175	<1
4 sticks (4″), 1½ oz	15	0
Shredded, ½ cup, 2 oz	25	0
Cauliflower, cooked:		
3 flowerettes/½ c. 1″ pces, 3 oz	15	0
½ medium (15 oz raw)	100	0
Celeriac, ½ cup, raw, 2¾ oz	30	0
Celery, 1 stalk, 7½″, 1½ oz	5	0
Diced, ½ cup, 2¼ oz	10	0
Chard (Swiss), ½ cup, ckd, 3 oz	20	0
Chick Peas (Garbanzo Beans):		
Dry, 1 cup, 6 oz	550	10
Cooked, 1 cup, 6 oz	270	4

	CALS	FAT
Chicory/Witloof — See Endive.		
Chicory, Greens, ½ cup, 3 oz	20	0
Chives, chopped, 1 Tbsp	1	0
Collards, ½ cup, 3 oz	15	0
Corn, yellow/white:		
Raw, kernels, ½ c., 2¾ oz	65	1
Ear (5″x1¾″), 5½ oz	80	1
Trimmed to 3½″ long	60	1
Cooked, kernels, ¼ c., 1½ oz	35	<1
(Also see Frozen & Canned Corn Pp. 94-95)		
Cress, Garden, ½ cup, 1 oz	10	0
Cucumber: 1 whole, 11 oz	40	0
½ cup slices, 2 oz	5	0
Dandelion Greens, ½ cup, 1 oz	15	0
Eggplant: 1 whole, 4½ oz	30	0
½ cup, 1″ pieces, 1½ oz	10	0
1 slice, fried, 1 oz	40	4
Endive, Belgian/French:		
1 med. head (6″), 2½ oz	12	0
Fennel, 2 oz	10	0
Garlic, 1 clove	4	0
Ginger: ¼ cup slices, 1 oz	20	0
Crystallized (sugared), 1 oz	95	0
Horseradish, 1 pod, ¾ oz	4	0
Jerusalem Artichoke, ½ cup	60	0
Jicama, raw, ½ cup	25	0
Kale, ½ cup, 2 oz	20	0
Kohlrabi, ½ cup, cooked, 3 oz	25	0
Leeks, cooked, 1 whole, 4 oz	40	0
Lentils, green/brown: Dry, 1 oz	95	0
Dry, 1 cup, 6½ oz	620	0
Cooked, ½ cup, 3½ oz	115	0
Lettuce: 1 c., chop./shred., 2½ oz	10	0
Butterhead, 2 leaves, ½ oz	2	0
Cos/Romaine, ½ c, shred., 1 oz	4	0
Iceberg: 1 leaf, ¾ oz	3	0
1 medium head, 15-16 oz	60	0
Lotus Root, 10 slices, ckd, 3 oz	60	0
Mung Bean Sprouts, ½ cup	15	0
Mushrooms: Raw, ½ cup, 1 oz	10	0
Cooked, ½ cup, 2½ oz	20	0
Mustard Greens, ½ cup, 1 oz	7	0
Okra, ckd., ½ cup, slices, 2¾ oz	25	0
Onions: Raw, 1 medium, 4 oz	45	0
½ cup, chopped, 3 oz	30	0
Dehydrated flakes, ¼ c, ½ oz	45	0
Rings, breaded/fried, 2 rings	80	5
Scallions, ½ cup, 2 oz	15	0
Spring, ¼ cup, chopped, 1 oz	6	0

VEGETABLES — FRESH OR FROZEN

	CALS	FAT
Parsley, chopped, ½ cup, 1 oz	10	0
Parsnips, 1 medium, 4 oz	80	0
Cooked, ½ cup slices, 2¾ oz	65	0
Peas: Green, ¼ cup, 1½ oz	35	0
raw, with pods, ½ lb	70	0
Snow Peas (8-9 pods), 1 oz	10	0
Split, dry, hulled, 1 oz	50	0
cooked, 1 cup, 7 oz	230	1
Peppers: Bell, 1 med., 5 oz	25	0
½ cup, chopped, raw, 1¾ oz	12	0
1 ring (3″ diam. x ¼″ thick)	2	0
Sweet, 1 medium, 5 oz	35	0
Chili: Green/Red, 1½ oz	18	0
Habanero, 1 only, 8g	11	0
Pigeon Peas, cooked, ½ cup	85	1
Pimientos, 3 medium, 3½ oz	25	0
Potatoes: Raw (with skin)		
1 Baby, Gourmet, 2 oz	45	0
1 Small, 3 oz	65	0
1 Medium, 5 oz	110	0
Peeled, 4 oz	90	0
1 Large, 8 oz	180	0
1 Extra Lge.(Russet), 12 oz	270	0
Mashed with milk & fat,		
½ cup, 3½ oz	110	4
Baked (no fat); Large, 10 oz raw:		
Plain, with skin, 7 oz	220	0
without skin, 5½ oz	145	0
With Toppings:		
+ 2 tsp fat	290	8
+ Sour Cr./Chives, 2 T.	270	6
+ Plain Yogurt, 2 Tbsp	240	1
+ Grated Cheese, 1 oz	330	9
+ Cottage Cheese, 2 oz	280	2
Roasted with fat, 3 oz	155	8
French Fries:		
Small serving, 2½ oz	220	12
Medium serving, 4 oz	350	20
Frozen, uncooked:		
18 fries, 4 oz	185	7
Oven-heated, 18 fries, 4 oz	185	7
Fried, 18 fries, 3 oz	275	15
Hash Browns:		
Homemade, ½ cup, 2½ oz	165	10
with Butter Sauce, 2½ oz	125	6
Au Gratin, ½ cup, 4.3 oz	160	9
Pancakes, 1 only, 2½ oz	495	13
Puffs, fried, 4 puffs, 1 oz	65	3
Scalloped, ½ cup, ¼ oz	105	4
Potato Salad, ½ c., 4½ oz	180	10
Poi, ½ cup, 4¼ oz	135	0

	CALS	FAT
Pumpkin, mashed, ½ c., 4 oz	25	0
Purslane, cooked, ½ cup, 2 oz	10	0
Radish: aver., 10 only, 1½ oz	10	0
Oriental, ½ c. slices, 1½ oz	10	0
Rutabagas, ckd., ½ c. cubes, 3 oz	30	0
Salsify, ckd, ½ cup slices, 2½ oz	45	0
Sauerkraut, ½ cup, 4 oz	25	0
Seaweed, average all types:		
Dried, 1 oz	50	<1
Soaked, drained, 1 oz	15	<1
Nori/Laver, dried, 6 sheets, ½ oz	35	<1
Shallots, chopped, 1 Tbsp	7	0
Soybeans — See Beans.		
(Soy Products/Tofu/Tempeh: Pages 50-51)		
Sorrel, raw, ½ cup, 4 oz	20	0
Spinach, cooked, ½ cup, 3 oz	20	0
Squash: Summer, average		
raw, ½ cup slices, 2¼ oz	13	0
cooked, ½ cup slices, 3 oz	18	0
Winter, cooked, 3½ oz		
Acorn, ½ cup cubes	55	0
½ medium (10 oz raw wt.)	85	0
Butternut, ½ cup cubes	40	0
¼ medium (9 oz raw wt.)	95	0
Hubbard, ½ cup cubes	50	0
Spaghetti, ½ cup, 2¾ oz	23	0
Succotash, ckd., ½ cup, 3⅓ oz	110	1
Sweetcorn — See Corn.		
Sweet Potatoes: Cooked with Skin		
No fat, 1 only, 4 oz	120	0
No skin, mash., ½ c, 5½ oz	170	0
Swedes, ½ cup, 3 oz	45	0
Taro, cooked, ½ cup, 2 oz	95	0
Tomatoes: See Fruit, p.89		
1 Medium, 5 oz	35	0
1 Large, 7 oz	45	0
Cooked, ½ cup, 4¼ oz	30	0
Fried, 1 small, 3 oz	60	4
Tomatillo, 1 oz	7	0
Turnips: White, ckd, ½ cup, 3 oz	15	0
Greens, ckd, ½ cup, 2½ oz	15	0
Water Chestnuts, 4 nuts	40	0
½ cup slices, 2¼ oz	65	0
Watercress, 10 sprigs, 1 oz	4	0
Yam, cooked, ½ cup, 2½ oz	80	0
Mountain (Hawaii), ckd, ½ cup	60	0
Yardlong Bean, 1 pod, ½ oz	7	0
Zucchini, 1 medium, 10 oz	45	0
½ cup slices, cooked, 3 oz	13	0

FROZEN VEGETABLES

BIRDS EYE

	CALS	FAT
Combination Vegetables: Per Serve		
French Beans w/Almonds, 3 oz	50	2
Peas with Pearl Onions, 3½ oz	70	0
Peas & Potatoes w/Cr. Sce, 5 oz	190	12
Cheese Sauce Combination Veges:		
Average all types, 5 oz	130	6
International with Sauces: Per 3½ oz		
Bavarian; Italian; San Francisco	100	5
Japanese Style	90	5
New England; Pasta Primavera	125	6
Oriental Style	70	4
Stir Fry: Average 3.3 oz	35	0
International Rice: Country	90	0
French; Spanish, 3.3 oz	110	0
Farm Fresh Mixtures: Per 4 oz		
Broccoli/Carrots/W. Chestnuts	45	0
Broccoli/Corn/Red Peppers	60	1
Broccoli, Other mixes, average	35	0
Brussels Sprouts/Cauli./Carrots	40	0
Cauliflower/Carrots/Snow Peas	40	0
Sugar Snap Peas/Carr./Chestn.	50	0
Zucchini/Carrots/Onions/Mushr.	30	0
Farm Fresh Whole Vegetables:		
Broccoli Spears, Beans, 4 oz	30	0
Custom Cuisine: Per 4½ oz Serving		
Chow Mein Vegetables	80	2
Pasta & Veges/Stroganoff Sauce	120	4
Pasta & Veges/Wh. Cheese Sce	150	6
Veges with Mushroom Sauce	60	2
with Herb or Oriental Sauce	90	4
w/Savory Tomato Basil Sce	110	3
w/Wild Rice in Wine Sauce	100	0
Birds Eye For One:		
Broccoli/Cauli./Carr. in Chs. Sce	110	5
Cheese Tortellini in Tomato Sce	210	5
Potatoes Au Gratin	240	13
Rice and Broccoli Au Gratin	180	6
Butter Sauce Combination: Per 3½ oz		
Sweet Corn	90	2
Broccoli Varieties	45	2
Portion Pack: Per 3 oz		
Broccoli; Spinach; Beans	20	0
Mixed Vegetables	50	0
Green Peas; Corn	70	0
Birds Eye Deluxe: Per Serving		
Baby Carrots, whole, 3¼ oz	40	0
Baby Cob Corn, 2½ oz svg.	25	0
Snow Pea Pods, 3 oz	35	0
'Sugar Snap' Peas, 2½ oz	45	0

MRS PAUL'S

	CALS	FAT
Corn Fritters, 2 fritters	250	12
Eggplant Parmigiana, 5 oz	260	17
Fried Eggplant Sticks, 3½ oz	240	12
Crispy Onion Rings, 2½ oz	180	10
Light Batter Zucchini Sticks, 3 oz	200	12

GREEN GIANT

	CALS	FAT
In Butter Sauce: ½ Cup		
Brocc./Bruss. Spr./Spinach	40	2
Corn, Lima Beans	100	2
Green Beans	30	1
Mixed Vegetables	60	2
Le Sueur Peas, Sweet Peas	80	2
In Cheese Sauce: ½ Cup		
All variet. (Brocc./Cauli./Carr.)	60	2
In Cream Sauce: ½ Cup		
Cream Style Corn	110	1
Creamed Spinach	70	3
ONE SERVE — Per Whole Package		
Broccoli/Cauliflower/Carrots	25	0
in Cheese Sauce	70	3
Broccoli in Butter Sauce	45	2
in Cheese Sauce	70	3
Beans in Butter Sauce	60	2
Corn: All varieties	120	2
Peas in Butter Sauce	90	2
Cheese Sauce: Cauliflower	80	2
Rice 'n Broccoli	180	6
Potatoes & Broccoli	130	5
Broccoli/Carrots/Rotini	120	3
Potatoes Au Gratin	200	10

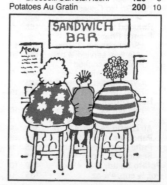

CANNED & BOTTLED VEGETABLES

CANNED/BOTTLED Drained Weight	CALS	FAT (g)
Asparagus, ½ cup, 4 oz	25	0
Bamboo Shoots, 1 cup, 4½ oz	25	0
Bean Salad, ½ cup, 3 oz	90	0
Bean Sprouts, ²/₃ cup	10	0
Beans:		
Baked Beans, ½ cup, 4½ oz	120	<1
Kidney Beans, ½ cup, 4½ oz	105	<1
Lima Beans, ½ cup, 3 oz	90	0
Pinto Beans, ½ cup, 3 oz	100	1
Snap/French Style, ½ c., 4½ oz	15	0
(Also see Canned Products — Pp. 48-49)		
Beets, ½ cup, 3 oz	30	0
Butter Beans, ½ cup, 3 oz	90	0
Carrots, ½ cup, 2½ oz	17	0
Corn, per ½ cup:		
Solids & Liquid, 4½ oz	80	<1
Drained Solids, 3 oz	65	<1
Cream Style, 4½ oz	95	<1
Dill Cucumber/Pickles - See Page 57.		
Garbanzo/Chick Peas, 3 oz	100	2
Mushrooms: ½ cup, 2½ oz	20	0
in Butter Sauce, 2 oz	30	10
Onions: Pickled, 1 med., ¾ oz	10	0
Cocktail, 1 onion	2	0
Peas, ½ cup, 3 oz	60	0
Peppers: Hot Chili, 1 only, 1 oz	8	0
Sweet, undrained, 2½ oz	15	0
Jalapeno, w/liq., ½ cup chopped	17	0
Potatoes, ½ cup, 3 oz	55	0
Salsa: Average all types, 2 Tbsp	15	0
Sauerkraut, undrained, ½ c. 4 oz	25	0
Spinach, ½ cup, 3½ oz	25	<1
Succotash: W/Cream Style Corn,		
½ cup, 4½ oz	100	<1
With whole kernels,		
undrained, ½ cup, 4½ oz	80	<1
Sweetcorn: Kernels, ½ cup, 3 oz	70	<1
Creamed Style, ½ cup, 4½ oz	95	<1
Sweet Potato, ½ cup, 3½ oz	105	0
Tomatoes: Whole/chopped,		
1 cup, 8½ oz	50	1
w/Green Chili, 1 c., 8½ oz	45	<1
Tomato Puree: 1 cup, 8¾ oz	105	<1
Tomato Paste, 1 cup, 9¼ oz	220	2
Tomato Sauce, 1 cup, 8¾ oz	75	<1
Vegetables, mixed, ½ cup, 4 oz	45	0
Yams in Light Syrup, ½ cup, 4 oz	105	0
Zucchini in Tom. Sce., ½ c., 4 oz	30	0

DELI-STYLE SALADS

Per 4 oz (Approx. ½ Cup)	CALS	FAT (g)
Ambrosia Salad	230	15
Bean Salad	110	5
Bulgar Salad	70	2
Carrot & Raisin	60	5
Caesar Salad	40	2
Coleslaw, traditional	150	8
w/reduced calorie dressing	60	1
Corn, Mexican	240	12
Cucumber, non-oil dressing	60	<1
with oil dressing	140	12
Eggplant Salad	75	5
Fresh Fruit Salad	90	0
Fettucini with Vegetables	110	5
Greek Vegetables	125	12
Macaroni Salad	140	8
Pasta, average all types	160	8
Potato Salad: With mayonnaise	170	10
With yogurt dressing	140	3
Rice Salad	150	9
Saffron Rice	130	3
Tomato & Mozzarella	180	14
Tabouli	150	6
Waldorf with mayonnaise	150	12

ORVAL KENT

(Supplier to Deli's & Institutions)

SIGNATURE SALADS — 6 oz Serving		
Antipasto Salad	510	50
Artichoke Salad, marinated	400	41
California Medley	120	7
Cheese Agnolotti	250	8
Cheese Tortellini, Marinara	210	10
Vinaigrette	300	17
Chicken Salad	420	33
Chicken 'n Pasta Mafalda	230	11
Crabmeat flavored	450	38
Egg Salad	300	23
Fresh Button Mushroom	190	16
Garden Olive	630	67
Ham Salad	400	32
Our Prima Pasta Salad	360	29
Potato & Herb Salad	200	41
Seafood Pasta Del Mar	170	10
Seafood with Crab & Shrimp	420	34
Shrimp Salad	360	32
Tuna Salad	450	36

FAST-FOOD SALADS

See Fast-Foods Section
Hardees, Jack In The Box, McDonald's, Subway, Wendy's (Salad Bar).

BEVERAGES — COFFEE, TEA, COCOA

COFFEE

	CALS	FAT (g)
Coffee, instant powder, Regular or Decaffeinated:		
1 level tsp	2	0
1 rounded tsp	4	0
w/Chicory, 1 rounded tsp	6	0
Coffee, instant/brewed, 6 fl.oz:		
Black, no sugar	4	0
+ 1 tsp sugar (rounded)	25	0
+ 2 tsp sugar	50	0
White, whole milk, 2 Tbsp	25	1
+ 1 tsp sugar	50	1
+ 2 tsp sugar	75	1
2% milk, 2 Tbsp	20	<1
skim milk, 2 Tbsp	15	0
Half & Half, 1 Tbsp	25	2
2 Tbsp	50	4
Coffee Shop: Cappucino	80	4
Coffee Mocha, 1 cup	90	5
Coffee Latte (no cream top)	60	3
Hot Chocolate	180	7
International Coffees (Gen. Foods) (Includes Cafe Amaretto/Francais/Vienna; Double/Dutch Choc; Suisse Mocha; Orange Cappucino) — Average:		
Regular, 1 cup	60	3
Sugar-free, 1 cup	30	2
Coffee Whiteners — See Page 29.		
Powder: Reg., 1 med. tsp	16	<1

COFFEE SUBSTITUTES

Roasted Cereal Grains:
(Includes Cafix, Kafree, Pioneer, Postum)

	CALS	FAT
Average all types, 1 tsp	10	0
Carob-flavored mix, 1 tsp	15	0

COCOA & CHOC. DRINKS

Cocoa Mixes, dry:	CALS	FAT
Alba, all flavors, 1 envelope	60	<1
Carnation, all flav., 1 env. (1 oz)	110	1
'70 Calorie', 1 envelope	70	<1
'Sugar Free', 1 envelope	50	<1
Hershey's, 1 oz	120	1
Malted Milk, choc., ¾ oz	80	1
Quik (Nestle): Reg., heap. tsp	36	<1
Sugar-Free, 1 heaping tsp	18	<1
Swiss Miss Creme Cocoa, 1¼ oz	140	4
Ovaltine, choc./malt, 1 T., ¾ oz	80	<1

96

TEA

	CALS	FAT (g)
Regular: Loose or bags,		
Average all types, 1 cup	2	0
Herbal: Average, 1 cup	3	0
Instant, powder, 1 tsp	2	0
Iced Tea: Per Cup (8 fl.oz)		
Plain, unsweetened	2	0
Sweetened, Shasta, 12 fl.oz	125	0
Sipps, 8½ fl.oz	100	0
Lipton, Fruit Tea Frt. Cooler, as prepared, 8 fl.oz	85	0
Nestea Iced Tea Mix, w/Sugar 1 Tbsp (20g), 8 fl.oz	70	0
Sugar-Free, decaf., 2 tsp	6	0
Iced Teasers, all flav., 8 fl.oz	6	0
Nestea, Ready-To-Drink, Lemon w/Sugar, 8 fl.oz	70	0
Sugar-Free, 8 fl.oz	2	0
Snapple, Diet Iced Tea, 8 fl.oz	4	0
St. Thomas: Sweetened	43	0

SHAKE MIXES

	CALS	FAT
Joe Weider's: Sup. Prot., 1 oz	100	0
90-Plus, 1 oz	100	1
Pathway (Matol), 1 scoop	105	1.5
Slim-Fast, all flavors, 1 oz	90	<1

'SPORTS' DRINKS

Made as directed: Per 8 fl.oz	CALS	FAT
Body Fuel (with Nutrasweet)	4	0
Breakthrough (Weider)	40	0
Exceed: Powder, 2 Tbsp	70	0
12 fl.oz box	105	0
16 fl.oz bottle	140	0
Gatorade: Regular, 8 fl.oz	50	0
GatorLode	140	0
GatorPro	360	7
Max, made-up, 8 fl.oz	96	0
Recharge (Knudsen): Orange	50	0
Lemon	70	0
The Juice, 11½ fl.oz	260	0
Water, plain/mineral	0	0

Dehydration limits sporting performance. **Drink adequate water** before, during and after strenuous exercise. **Plain water is best.** (Lightly sweetened drinks may benefit endurance athletes.)

SOFT DRINKS & SODA

(Nil Fat Content)	CALS 8 fl.oz	CALS 12 fl.oz	(Nil Fat Content)	CALS 8 fl.oz	CALS 12 fl.oz
Birch Beer (Canada Dry)	110	165	Mountain Dew	120	180
Bitter Lemon: Canada Dry	100	150	Mr Pibb	95	145
Schweppes	110	165	Orange: Crush	120	180
Bubble Up	97	145	Fanta	116	170
Cactus Cooler (Can. Dry)	120	180	Hi-C	100	150
Cherry: Crush; Fanta	120	180	Shasta	125	185
Black (Shasta)	105	160	Sunkist	130	195
Wild (Canada Dry)	130	195	Sunrise (Canada Dry)	130	195
Citrus Mist (Shasta)	130	195	Peach (Nehi)	135	200
Club Soda	0	0	Pineapple (Canada Dry)	110	165
Colas: Coca Cola (new)	102	153	Crush	120	180
Coca Cola (classic)	95	145	Root Beer: Regular, aver.	110	165
Caffeine-free	100	150	Diet/Sugar-free, aver.	4	6
Diet Coke	<1	1	Sassparilla (White Rock)	120	180
Cherry Cola	100	150	7-Up; Cherry 7-Up	95	145
Diet Rite	0	0	Slice: Regular	105	160
Jamaica (Can. Dry)	105	160	Low Calorie	17	25
Pepsi Cola	105	160	Sprite: Regular	95	145
Diet Pepsi	<1	1	Diet Sprite	3	5
Royal Crown	110	165	Squirt	105	160
Shasta	105	160	Strawberry: Crush	120	180
Collins Mix (Canada Dry)	80	120	Shasta	100	150
Cream: Can. Dry (Vanilla)	130	195	Schweppes	90	135
Crush (Brown/Red)	110	165	Tab	<1	1
Schweppes	115	170	Tahitian Treat (Canada Dry)	130	195
Shasta (creme)	110	165	Tonic Water: Canada Dry	95	145
Dr Diablo (Shasta)	105	160	Schweppes	90	135
Dr Nehi (Royal Crown)	110	165	Shasta	85	130
Dr Pepper	95	145	Upper Ten (Royal Crown)	110	165
Fresca	2	3	Welch's Sparkling Sodas	120	180
Fruit Punch: Nehi	130	195			
Shasta Plus	110	165	**Club Soda,** plain	0	0
Ginger Ale: Canada Dry	95	145			
Schweppes	90	135	**Diet Soft Drinks:** Average	<2	<4
Shasta	90	135			
Sugar-free (Can. Dry)	3	4	**Seltzers:** Plain/Diet	0	0
Ginger Beer (Schweppes)	95	145	Sweetened, average	100	150
Grape: Crush	120	180	w/Fruit Juice	80	120
Fanta	115	170			
Hi-C	105	160	**Mineral Water:** Plain	0	0
Nehi, Schweppes	130	195	Sweetened/flavored	100	150
Grapefruit: Schweppes	105	160	w/Fruit Juice	80	120
Shasta	117	175			

SOFT DRINK MIXES & BREAKFAST DRINKS

(Nil Fat Content)	CALS 8 fl.oz	CALS 12 fl.oz		CALS	FAT
Half & Half (Canada Dry)	110	165			
Hi-Spot (Canada Dry)	100	150	**Bright & Early,** 6 fl.oz	90	0
Lemonade (Shasta Plus)	115	170	**Kool-Aid,** per 8 fl.oz:		
Lemon Lime (Shasta)	100	150	All flavors, unsweetened	2	0
Lime (Canada Dry)	130	195	Sugar sweetened	80	0
Mello Yello	115	170	Sugar free (NutraSweet)	4	0
Minute Maid Orange	116	170	**Tang:** All flavors, 6 fl.oz	90	0
Diet Minute Maid	4	6	Sugar-free, 6 fl.oz	6	0

BEERS

Beer contains negligible fat.

	CALS 1 Glass 8 fl.oz	CALS Can/Bot. 12 fl.oz
REGULAR		
Average all brands	100	150
Specific Brands:		
Anchor Steam	103	155
Anheuser; Augsberger	115	170
Beck's	97	145
Blatz (Heileman)	90	135
Brauhaus	100	150
Budweiser	95	140
Bud Dry	85	130
Busch	97	145
Carlsberg	100	150
Carling Black Label	110	165
Country Club	105	160
Coors	95	140
Corona; Dos Equis Dark	100	150
Falstaff	100	150
Hamm's	90	135
Heidelberg	100	150
Heileman: National Prem.	105	155
Black Label	87	130
Special Export	97	145
Old Style	100	150
Heinekin; Henry Weinhard	100	150
Grand Union; Kirin	100	150
Knickerbocker	95	140
Kronenbourg	113	170
Labatt's Blue	97	145
Lowenbrau	105	160
Malt Duck Apple	165	250
Malt Duck Grape	140	210
Michelob	100	150
Michelob Dry	87	130
Mickeys	105	160
Miller	100	150
Molson	103	155
Old Dutch	100	150
Old Milwaukee	97	145
Old Ranger	100	150
Olympia	103	155
Pabst Blue Ribbon	97	145
Pilsner's Original	100	150
Rainier; Rolling Rock	97	145
Ruper Knickerbock; Schaefer	105	160
Schlitz; Schmidt	100	150
Stag; Sterling; Stroh's	100	150
Tuborg; Tudor	100	150
Weidemann	100	150

BEERS (CONT)

	CALS 1 Glass 8 fl.oz	CALS Can/Bot. 12 fl.oz
LIGHT & LOW ALCOHOL BEERS		
Amstel Light	63	95
Blatz Light; Black Label Light	65	100
Blatz L.A.	50	75
Bud Light; Busch Light	73	110
Carlsberg Light	73	110
Coors Light; Corona Light	70	105
Gablinger's	65	100
Heidelberg	87	130
Heileman Light	63	95
Henry's Private Res. Light	80	120
Herman Joseph's Light	87	130
Labatt's Blue Light	77	115
Lowenbrau Light	65	100
Michelob Light	90	135
Miller Lite	63	95
Molson Light; Natural Light	73	110
Nordik Wolf Light	73	110
National Prem. Light (Hlmn.)	65	100
Old Milwaukee Light	80	120
Old Style L.A. (Heileman)	50	75
Old Style Light (Heileman)	73	110
Olympia Gold Light	50	75
Pearl Light	60	90
Rainier Light; Schlitz Light	65	100
Special Export Light (Hlmn.)	77	115
Stroh's Light	75	115
NON-ALCOHOLIC/NEAR BEERS		
Birell Non-alcoholic Brew	50	75
Cheers (Pabst)	36	55
Odoul's	50	75
Texas Select	43	65
Near Beers:		
Average all brands	43	65
ALES & MALT LIQUORS		
Blatz Cream Ale	103	155
Champale: Regular	105	160
Extra Dry	113	170
Colt 45 Malt Liquor	103	155
Elephant Malt Liquor	140	210
King Cobra	120	180
Tiger Head Ale	110	165
Non-Alcoholic Malt Beverages:		
Carling; Kingsbury; Schmidt	40	60
Firestone; Sharp's Prem.	50	75
Kaliber Non-alcohol. Brew	33	50
Schmidt Select	40	60

CIDER

	CALS	FAT (g)
Alcoholic Cider, aver. all brands 1 glass, 6 fl.oz	70	0
Sparkling Apple Cider (Welch) Non-Alcoholic, 6 fl.oz	90	<1

TABLE WINES

Average of Brands — Per 4 fl.oz

	CALS	FAT
Bordeaux: Red	95	0
White	95	0
Burgundy: Red	95	0
Sparkling	110	0
White	100	0
Chablis: Regular	95	0
Light	60	0
Champagne: Bollinger, 3 fl.oz	72	0
Great Western, Regular	70	0
Brut, 3 fl.oz	75	0
Pink, 3 fl.oz	80	0
Taylor, Dry, 3 fl.oz	80	0
Chardonnay	80	0
Chianti	90	0
Claret	95	0
Kosher (Manischewitz):		
Dry, all varieties	90	0
Medium, all varieties	110	0
Sweet, all varieties	170	0
Leibfraumilch	90	0
Moselle	95	0
Rhine	95	0
Rose	90	0
Sauterne	110	0
Non-Alcoholic Wine:		
Ariel Dealcoholized Wines:		
Cabernet Sauvignon	25	0
Chardonnay	27	0
Brut; Blanc de Noirs	32	0

Mulled Wine: Calories same as wine used. (Insufficient heat to evaporate alcohol.)

WINE COOLERS

	CALS	FAT
Wine Coolers: Average all brands 12 fl.oz Bottle or Can	200	0

COOKING WITH WINE

Regular Wines (Unsweetened): Negligible calories if sufficient heat and cooking time for alcohol to evaporate.

Sweetened Wines (e.g. Sherry): Residual calories after cooking — 10 calories per fl.oz.

APERITIF & DESSERT WINES

Average of All Brands **Per Wine Glass, 3½ fl.oz**	CALS	FAT (g)
Asti Spumante; Madeira	145	0
Muscatel; Port	160	0
Sherry: Sweet, 2 fl.oz	85	0
Dry, 2 fl.oz	75	0
Vermouth: Dry	125	0
Sweet	160	0
White Tokay	170	0

SPIRITS

All spirits with the same proof (alcoholic content) have similar calories and no fat. Includes Bourbon, Brandy, Gin, Rum, Scotch, Whiskey, Tequila, Vodka.

Spirits:	CALS 1 fl.oz	CALS 1½ fl.oz	CALS 750ml Bottle
80 proof	65	100	1650
86 proof	70	105	1780
90 proof	74	110	1880
100 proof	83	125	2110
Southern Comfort (80 pr.)	80	120	2000

COCKTAILS

Per Cocktail	CALS	FAT
Bloody Mary; Daiquiri	120	0
Bourbon & Soda	105	0
Gin & Tonic; Gin Rickey	160	0
Golden Cadillac	250	11
Mai Tai	200	0
Manhattan; Planter's Punch	170	0
Martini	150	0
Pina Colada	300	10
Screwdriver	175	0
Tequila Sunrise	190	0
Tom Collins	120	0
Whiskey Sour	140	0
White Russian	200	6
Bacardi Frozen Conc. Fruit Mixers:		
Per 8 fl.oz (Made with 1 fl.oz Rum/Tequila)		
Margarita	165	0
Peach/Raspb./Strawb. Daiquiri	200	0
Pina Colada	220	2

BITTERS & CAMPARI

	CALS	FAT
Angostura Bitters, ¼ tsp	3	0
Lemon, Lime & Bitters, 6 fl.oz	90	0
Campari (45 proof), 1 fl.oz	65	0

LIQUEURS

	CALS	FAT
Average all types, 1 fl.oz	90	0

HEALTH HAZARDS

● **Excess alcohol** contributes to obesity, high blood pressure, stroke, heart and liver disease and some types of cancer.

● **Excess alcohol** also reduces mental abilities and sporting performance, increases the risk of accidents, worsens insomnia, and is commonly linked to domestic violence and family breakups. Sexual performance is lessened, and impotency is more common.

● **Extra health hazard for dieters.** Alcohol is potentially more harmful while on a low calorie diet. Blood sugar levels may drop to very low levels with resultant tiredness, weakness, headaches and nausea. Mental abilities, reflexes and driving skills are further impaired.

SAFE ALCOHOL LIMITS
(Dietary Guidelines for Americans, 1990)

Women: No more than **1 drink** per day.
Men: No more than **2 drinks** per day.

1 Drink = 12 fl.oz regular beer, **or** 5 fl.oz wine, **or** 1½ fl.oz spirits (80 proof). Each drink contains approx. **14g alcohol.**

Do not drink alcohol at all, if you are:
● pregnant or trying to conceive
● taking medication
● planning to drive or do anything that requires full attention or skill
● a child or adolescent.

Note: Even 2-3 drinks daily has been linked to **brain shrinkage** and damage in some social drinkers.

ALCOHOL COUNTER

BEER, ALE & MALT LIQUOR	Alcohol (grams)
Beer: Regular (Average, 4.5% alc.)	
5 fl.oz glass	5.5
8 fl.oz glass	8.5
12 fl.oz glass/can	13
25 fl.oz bottle	27
Light Beer (Average, 4% alc.):	
8 fl.oz glass	7
12 fl.oz glass/can	11.5
Low Alcohol Beer (<2.5% alcohol):	
8 fl.oz glass	4
12 fl.oz glass/can	6.5
No Alcohol/Near Beers (<0.5% alcohol)	
12 fl.oz glass/can	<1
Malt Liquor: Average, 12 fl.oz	15
Non-Alcoholic, 12 fl.oz	<1
Cider, 1 glass, 8 fl.oz	8

WINES	
Table Wines (11.5% alcohol):	
Red/Rose/White, 3½ fl.oz glass	10
Champagne, 1 glass	10
Dessert Wines (19% alcohol):	
Dry/Sweet, 2 fl.oz	9
Wine Coolers, average, 6 fl.oz	6

DISTILLED SPIRITS	
(Includes Gin, Rum, Vodka, Whiskey)	
Per 1½ fl.oz Jigger	
80 Proof (40% alcohol)	14
86 Proof (43% alcohol)	15
90 Proof (45% alcohol)	16
94 Proof (47% alcohol)	17
100 Proof (50% alcohol)	18
Cocktails, average all types	18
Liqueurs: Aver. all types, 1 fl.oz	9

"Alcohol provides calories, stimulates the appetite, and weakens the dieter's resolve ...and so should play no part in weight reduction."

CALCULATING ALCOHOL CONTENT

Percent alcohol refers to volume.
To convert to grams (wt.) of alcohol, multiply volume by 0.8
(since 1ml alcohol weighs 0.8 gram)
Example: 12 fl.oz Beer (4% alcohol)
4% vol. = 4% of 360ml (1 fl.oz = 30ml)
= 14.4ml alcohol
(x 0.8) = 11.5g alcohol

Note: Calories of these dishes are only a guide. Large variations occur with serving size, recipe ingredients and cooking methods.

CHINESE & ASIAN DISHES

APPETIZERS

	CALS	FAT
Curried Meat Triangles, 1 pce	150	5
Dim Sum (Dumplings), 1 ball	65	2
Egg Rolls, mini, 3 rolls	100	3
Spring Roll, fried, each:		
Small, 1½ oz	100	7
Medium, 3 oz	200	12
Large, 5 oz	350	15
Soup: Clear, 1 bowl	30	1
with Noodles	100	3
Chicken & Corn	150	8
Wonton, 1 only	55	3

ENTREES & MAIN DISHES
Per Whole Dish (2-3 Serves)

Beef with Broccoli, 16 oz	650	30
Beef in Black Bean Sce, 17 oz	530	33
Chicken & Almonds, 18 oz	685	49
Chop Suey: Chicken, 20 oz	560	37
Pork, 20 oz	680	49
Chow Mein: Beef/Chick., 24 oz	940	59
Crispy Fried Chicken, 8 oz	485	33
Lemon Chicken, 10 oz	580	32
Omelet: Chick./Shrimp, 16 oz	990	82
Sweet & Sour: Fish, 20 oz	1160	58
Pork, 18 oz	950	49
Duck, 18 oz	1120	71
Vegetable Combination	250	17

Extra Listings: See Frozen Entrees/Meals.

RICE: Plain: 1 cup, 5 oz	170	0
Fried: 1 cup, 5 oz	320	13
Large dish, 16 oz	1010	40
Noodles: Chinese Egg,		
boiled, 1 cup	200	3

CAJUN — CREOLE

Per Serving

Baked Herb Chicken	850	53
Bouillabaisse	350	11
Cajun Fried Turkey	630	25
Crawfish Bisque	500	10
Creole Jambalaya	550	29
Jambalaya, Shrimp & Crabmeat	520	14
Roasted Quail, w/Bacon on toast	550	25
Stuffed Smothered Steak	630	46
with 1 cup Rice	890	49

FRENCH

	CALS	FAT
Blanquette d'Agneau	800	30
(Lamb Stew w/Veg.)		
Brioche, 1 cake	280	14
Bouillabaise (Fish Stew)	400	15
Coq au Vin (Chicken in Wine)	800	30
Coquilles St. Jacques, fried, 6 lge	300	14
Creme Caramel (Caram. Custard)	260	10
Crepe Suzette, 1x6" crepe/sauce	220	10
Duck a l'Orange	780	35
Escargots (Snails), in garlic but., 6	200	18
Frogs Legs, fried, 4 med. pairs	400	20
Lamb Noisettes, fried, 2 chops	500	40
Mousse au Chocolat	380	15
Potage Creme Crecy (Carrot Soup)	360	18
Salade Nicoise (Tuna/Oliv./Veg.)	450	13
Veal Cordon Bleu (Veal/Ham/Ch)	650	25
Vichyssoise (Pot./Leek Soup), 1 c	200	9

GERMAN

Bavarian Brd. Dumpling, 3 sm.	330	9
Beef: Goulash with Veges	520	20
Black Forest Cake, 1 slice	380	16
Chicken: Fried, Viennese-style	520	20
Livers w/Apple/On., 6 oz	460	28
Herring, Pckld: Rollmops, 4 oz	260	16
with Sour Cream, 4 oz	310	7
Hot Sausage Curry	300	7
Kugelhupf (Yeast Cake), 1 lge sl.	400	12
Pastry-wrap. Bratwurst, 1 med.	250	10
Sauerbraten Pork (Pot Roast)	650	35
Sauerkraut (Cabbage), no fat, ½ c	25	<1
Torte: Linzer (Alm./Raspb. Jam)	430	18
Sacher (Choc./Apricot Jam)	260	12
Wiener Schnitzel, 1 medium	750	35

GREEK FOODS

Baklava Pastry, 1 only, 3¾ oz	400	21
Calamari, deep fried, 1 cup	300	13
Galactobureko, 1 only	360	15
(Filo, Custard, Pastry in Syrup)		
Kataifi, (Filo, Nut, Pastry in Syrup)	350	11
Moussaka, 1 serve, 8 oz	350	22
Souvlakia (Lamb), each, 2 oz	120	6
Stuffed Tomatoes, 2 only	250	12
Taramosalata, 1 Tbsp, ½ oz	40	3
Tyropita (Filo/Egg/Cheese Pastry)	350	26
Tzatziki (Cucumb/Yog Dip), 1 Tbsp	20	1
Vine Leaves, stuffd., 3 rolls, 6 oz	200	5

INDIAN (ASIAN)

Per Serving	CALS	FAT
(Meat dishes allow 4 oz meat/serving		(g)
Aloo Samosa, each		
(Savory Pastries w/Potato filling)	150	12
Alu Gosht Kari (Meat/Pot. Curry)	600	40
Bhona Gosht (Mint Brld. Lamb)	560	28
Chicken Pilaf (Murgh Biriyani)	700	53
Chapati/Roti, 7" diam. piece		
(Baked Whole Wheat Bread)	60	<1
Dal (Lentil Puree), 1 cup, no oil	230	1
1 Tbsp Tadka (oil topping)	120	13
Gosht Kari (Meat Curry/Tom./Pot.)	460	25
Lamb Pilaf	520	35
Masala Gosht (Beef/Tom. Gravy)	400	25
Mulligatawney Soup, average	300	15
Pappadom, 1 large/2 small	50	3
Pork Vendaloo Curry	620	47
Rogan Josh (Lamb/Yogurt Sce)	500	30
Saag Gosht (Beef/Spinach Sce)	430	26
Shahi Korma (Braised Lamb)	430	28
Tandoori Chicken: Breast	260	13
Leg/Thigh portion	300	17

ITALIAN DISHES

	CALS	FAT
Cannelloni, 1 tube, 6 oz	280	15
Chicken Cacciatore	370	22
Gnocchi, Spinach	300	18
Lasagne with meat, 10 oz	400	17
Manicotti, cheese/tomato	230	14
Minestrone Soup, 1 cup	260	6
Osso Buco (Veal/Tom./Mushr.)	550	28
Ravioli, 8 oz	300	12
Risotto (Chicken)	420	14
Spaghetti: Plain, 1 cup, 5 oz	185	1
Restaurant: 2 cups	370	2
w/Bolognese (Meat Sce)	650	16
w/Marinara (Seafoods)	700	20
w/Napoletana (Tom. Sce)	540	13
Saltimbocca (Veal/Ham/Cheese)	430	28
Tortellini, 20 pieces	530	20
Veal Marsala	400	20
Veal Parmigiana	350	20
Pizza: Per ½ Pizza (12")		
Vegetarian/Cheese: Thin Crust	650	26
Thick Crust	850	24
Sausage/Pepperoni: Thin Crust	700	42
Thick Crust	900	40
(Also see Pizza Hut, Domino's, Shakey's,		
Godfather's Pizza — Fast Foods Section.)		

JAPANESE

SUSHI	CALS	FAT
Lunch Menu (Assorted Sushi)		(g)
Regular, 1 serving	330	3
Deluxe, 1 serving	430	4
Sushi Rice, ckd, 1 Tbsp	25	<1
1 cup, 5¼ oz	380	3
Nigiri-Zushi: (Fish-wrapped Sushi)		
Per 1 oz Piece		
Ebi-zushi (Jumbo Shrimp)	20	<1
Kani-zushi (Surimi Crab)	30	<1
Maguro-zushi (Tuna)	25	<1
Sake-zushi (Salmon)	35	1
Suzume-zushi (Baby Snapper)	30	<1
Tai-zushi (Red Snapper)	30	<1
Nori-Maki-Zushi: Per Piece		
(Seaweed-wrapped Sushi Rolls)		
Anago-maki (Conger Eel)	20	1
California-maki (Crab/Caviar/Avocado)		
½ roll	70	1
Futo-maki (Egg Omelet, Shellfish, Veg.)		
1 piece	70	1
Kobana-maki		
(Egg Omelet/Cucumber)	35	<1
Kappa-maki (Cucumber)	15	<1
Tekka-maki (Tuna)	20	<1
Uni-maki (Sea Urchin)	20	<1
Inari-Zushi (Bean Curd Pouches w/Sushi)		
1 pouch, 3 oz	130	2
Tamago-Yaki (Omelet-wrapped Sushi)		
1 piece	45	1
Sashimi (Sliced Raw Seafood/Beef)		
Ika (Squid), 4 oz	105	2
Hamachi (Yellowtail), 4 oz	165	6
Naguro (Yellowfin Tuna), 4 oz	120	1
Niku (Beef), 5 oz	200	10
Saba (Mackerel), 4 oz	160	7
Suzuki (Sea Bass), 4 oz	110	<1
Tako (Octopus), 4 oz	95	1
Dipping Sauces: Aver., 2 Tbsp	30	0
Ginger Vinegar Dress., 2 Tbsp	20	0
Miso Soup w/tofu pces, 1 cup	85	3
Sukiyaki (Beef/Tofu/Veg.), 8 oz	400	24
Tempura (Batter-fried Shrimp & Veges.)		
3 large shrimp & veges.	320	18
1 shrimp only	60	4
Teppan Yaki (Steak, Seafood & Veges.)		
10 oz serving	470	30
Teriyaki Beef, 4 oz serving	350	25
Sake Wine (16% alc.), 3 fl.oz	115	0

JEWISH FOODS

	CALS	FAT (g)
Bagel/Bialy, ½ small, 1 oz	80	1
Beiglach (Cheese Knish)	350	17
Blintzes, average, 1 only	120	4
w/Sour Crm. & Preserves	370	10
Borscht, (no cream), 1 cup	85	6
Diet/Reduced Cal., 1 cup	30	1
Cabbage Roll (meat/rice), 5 oz	170	6
Chicken Broth, 1 cup	80	8
with vegetables	100	8
with noodles	150	9
Lowfat, plain, 1 cup	25	1
Cholent, 1 med. serve, 1 cup	350	26
Chopped Liver: 1 serve, 3 oz	110	6
with Egg Salad, ¼ cup	100	7
Farfel, dry, ½ cup	90	<1
Hallah (Yeast Bread), 1 sl., 1 oz	85	2
Gefilte Fish Balls:		
Regular, medium, 2 oz	55	2
with jelled broth	80	2
Cocktail size, 1 oz	30	1
Sweet, medium, 2 oz	65	2
with jelled broth	95	2
Herring: Smoked, 2 oz	120	8
in Sour Cream, 2 oz	150	10
Kasha, cooked, ½ cup	100	<1
Kipfel (Vanilla/Almd. Cookie), 1 pce	60	4
Knaidlach, 1 ball	40	2
Knish: Kasha/Potato, 1 only	130	8
Cheese, 1 only	350	17
Kreplach, beef, 1 piece	40	1
Kugel, potato/noodle, 1 serve	150	7
Latkes (Potato Pancake), 2 oz	200	11
3 Latkes w/Sour Cr./Apple Sce	750	20
Lochshen: Plain, 1 cup	130	5
Pudding, 1 cup	380	13
Lox (Smoked Salmon), 1 oz	33	1
Mandelbrot (Almond Bread),		
1 slice, ¼" thick	45	2
Matzo: 1 board, 1 oz	110	<1
(Also see Matzoh — Page 69)		
Matzo Balls, 2 small/1 large	90	3
Soup, with 1 large ball	180	7
New York Cheesecake, 4 oz	350	24
Pierogi, potato/cheese, 1 pce	90	4
Reuben Sandwich	560	37
Schmaltz (Rend'd chick. fat), 1 Tbsp	90	10

LEBANESE — MIDDLE EAST

	CALS	FAT (g)
Baba Ghannouj, 2 Tbsp, 1 oz (Eggplant/Sesame Dip)	70	6
Baklava, 1 pastry, 1¾ oz (Pastry, Nuts, Syrup)	245	18
Cabbage Rolls, 1 roll, 3 oz (Cabbage Leaves, Meat, Rice)	100	3
Cous Cous, 1 serve (Semolina, Milk, Fruit, Nuts)	400	21
Felafel (Chick Pea Fritter):		
Fried, 1 medium, 1 oz	60	4
Hummus, ¼ Cup, 2.2 oz	105	3
Fried Kibbi, 1 piece, 3 oz (Wheat, Meat, Pinenuts)	180	8
Kafta, 1 skewer, 1½ oz (Ground Lamb Saus. on Skewer)	85	5
Kibbeh Naye, 1 cup, 9 oz (Raw Lamb, Bulgur & Spices)	450	18
Lebanese Omelet, 1 serving, 4 oz (Egg, Spinach, Pine Nuts, Onion)	200	12
Pilaf, 1 cup (Rice, Onion, Raisins, Apr., Spices)	680	11
Shawourma, 1 serve, 4 oz (Spit Roast Beef)	280	15
Shish Kabob, 1 stick, 2½ oz	130	7
Spinach Pie, 1 piece	290	21
Sweet Almond Sanbusak, 1 pce (Pastry, Almonds, Spices)	200	15
Tabouli, 1 serve, 4 oz	170	14
Tahini Sauce, aver., 1 Tbsp	90	8

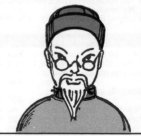

CONFUCIUS SAY:
'*Man who eat with one chopstick never have problem with obesity.*'

MEXICAN FOODS

	CALS	FAT
Black Bean Soup, 1 bowl	200	7
Burritos (Taco Bell): Bean	350	10
Beef	400	17
Chili, plain, ¼ cup	90	6
Chili con Carne, w/Beans, 1 c	310	17
w/out beans, 1 cup	370	28
Corn Chips, ½ cup, 1 oz	160	10
Empanadas, average, 1 small	230	10
Enchilada, average	330	10
Enchirito (Taco Bell)	380	20
Fajitas: Chicken/Steak	200	7
Guacamole, 2 Tbsp, 1 oz	110	12
Margarita (w/1½ oz Tequila)	160	0
Nachos: Taco Bell, regular	350	18
Bellgrande (Taco Bell)	650	35
Cheese (Del Taco)	450	29
Beef & Bean (Del Taco)	585	96
Refried Beans, ¾ cup, 6 oz	210	5
Sopaipillas (flky. pstry. puffs), 1 pc	100	7
w/honey & cream	200	14
Taco (Taco Bell): Regular	185	10
Chicken/Steak, average	220	11
Taco Bellgrande	355	23
Super Combo Taco	285	16
Taco Salad with Shell	940	61
Taco Sauce, average, ¼ cup	15	0
Taco Shell, regular	50	2
Tamales, Van Camp's (can), ½ c	150	8
Tostada (Taco Bell)	240	11
Tortilla, corn, 6″ diam.	70	1
Tortilla Chips, 1 oz	150	8

Extra Listings of Mexican Dishes:
- Frozen Entrees/Meals (Banquet/Patio etc.)
- Fast Foods Section (Taco Bell, Del Taco, Macheesmo Mouse)
- Canned Bean/Chili Products — Pp.48-49

POLISH

	CALS	FAT
Cabbage Rolls w/Sour Cr., 2 sm.	220	10
Chicken Casserole w/Mushr., 1c.	520	17
Kielbasa (Sausages, Onions), fried, 2 large	350	28
Meatballs in Sour Cream, 3 x 1½″ balls	300	16
Pierogi, Fruit/Veg, 3″ ball	80	2
Pork Goulash (Pork, Veg. Stew)	550	21
Pot Roast with Vegetables	630	21

SPANISH

Per Serving	CALS	FAT
Arroz Abanda (Fish with Rice)	340	8
Arroz Con Pollo (Rice/Chick. Sal.)	500	23
Clams Marinera, 8 clams	330	16
Cochifrito (Lamb w. Lemon/Garlic)	650	25
Cochinillo Asado, 2 slices (Roast Suckling Pig)	300	15
Cocido Madrileno (Madrid-Style Boiled Dinner)	450	27
Flan de Leche (Caramel Custard)	325	9
Fritadera de Ternera (Sauteed Veal Strips)	450	27
Gazpacho, 1 bowl	60	3
Paella a la Valenciana (Chicken & Shellfish Rice)	900	42
Pollo a la Espanola (Chicken)	475	30
Ternera al Jerez (Veal w/Sherry)	660	29
Zarzuela (Fish & Shellfish Medley)	530	27

VIETNAMESE

	CALS	FAT
Bo Xao Dau Phong (Per Whole Dish) (Ginger Beef w/Onion + Fish Sce.)	750	30
Bo Nuong (Beef Satay), 2	265	9
Ca Chien Gung (Whole Schnapper w. Ginger)	600	16
Canh Chay (Veg./Tofu Soup)	80	3
Cuu Xao Lan (Curried Lamb, Veges in Coconut)	900	35
Ga Chien (Crsp. Chick.+Plum Sce)	900	40
Ga Nuong (Chicken Satay + Sce.)	240	11
Ga Xao Rau (Marinated Chick. braised w/Veg.)	800	26
Rau Cai Xao Chay (Stir fried Vegetables in Soy Sce.)	400	25
Thit Heo Goi Baup Cai, each (Spicy Cabbg. Rolls stuffed w/Pork)	200	7

GOURMET & MISCELLANEOUS

	CALS	FAT
Ants Eggs/Larvae, 1 Tbsp	20	<1
Ants, Choc. coated, 3 Tbsp	140	7
Bee Maggots, canned, 3 Tbsp	65	2
Caviar, black/red, 1 Tbsp	40	3
Caterpillars, canned, 60g	60	2
Frogs Legs, fried, 1 pair (large)	125	7
Haggis, boiled, 4 oz	350	24
Locusts, raw, 1 oz	35	1
Silkworms, raw, 1 oz	60	2
Snails (Escargots) — See French.		
Snake, roasted, 4 oz	160	6
Turtle, green, canned, 3 oz	90	1

FAST-FOODS SECTION

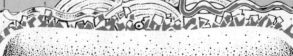

ARBY'S	CALORIES	FAT grams	CHOLEST. mg	CARBOHYD. grams	SODIUM mg	PROTEIN grams
Breakfast Items:						
Toastix	420	25	20	43	440	8
Maple Syrup	120	0	0	29	50	0
Cinnamon Nut Danish	340	9	0	59	230	7
Biscuits: Plain	280	15	0	34	730	6
Bacon	320	18	10	35	900	7
Sausage	460	32	60	35	1000	12
Ham	325	17	20	34	1170	13
Croissants: Plain	260	16	50	28	300	6
Bacon & Egg	390	26	220	30	580	12
Ham & Cheese	345	21	90	30	940	16
Mushroom & Cheese	495	38	115	34	935	13
Platters: Ham	520	26	375	45	1180	24
Sausage	640	41	405	46	860	21
Egg	460	24	345	45	590	15
Blueberry Muffin	200	6	20	34	270	3
Roast Beef Sandwiches:						
Regular Roast Beef	355	15	40	32	590	22
Beef 'n Cheddar	450	20	50	43	955	25
Junior Roast Beef	220	11	25	21	345	13
Giant Roast Beef	530	27	80	41	910	36
Super Roast Beef	530	28	45	46	800	33
Philly Beef 'n Swiss	500	26	90	37	1190	26
Bac n' Cheddar Deluxe	530	33	85	35	1670	29
French Dip	345	12	5	34	680	24
French Dip 'n Swiss	425	18	85	36	1080	30
Chicken Sandwiches:						
Chicken Breast	490	26	45	48	1020	23
Roast Chicken Club	515	29	75	40	1425	31
Roast Chicken Deluxe	375	19	2	37	915	1.7
Chicken Cordon Bleu	660	37	65	50	1825	31
Grilled Chicken Deluxe	425	21	45	39	880	21
Grilled Chicken Barbeque	380	14	45	44	1060	21
Other Sandwiches:						
Sub Deluxe	480	26	45	38	1530	24
Fish Fillet	535	29	80	47	995	21
Turkey Deluxe	400	20	40	36	1045	27
Ham 'n Cheese	330	15	45	33	1350	23
Salads & Salad Dressings:						
Cashew Chicken Salad	590	37	65	23	1140	34
Chef Salad	210	11	115	3	720	21
Garden Salad	150	9	75	2	100	11

	CALORIES	FAT grams	CHOLEST. mg	CARBOHYD. grams	SODIUM mg	PROTEIN grams
Salads & Dressings (cont.):						
Side Salad	25	0	0	4	30	2
Honey French Dressing, 2 oz	320	27	0	22	485	0
Light Italian Dressing, 2 oz	25	1	0	3	1110	0
Thousand Island, 2 oz	300	29	25	10	495	0
Blue Cheese Dressing, 2 oz	295	31	50	2	490	2
Buttermilk Ranch, 2 oz	350	38	5	2	470	0
Croutons, ½ oz	60	2	0	9	155	2
Soups:						
Boston Clam Chowder	205	11	30	18	155	10
Cream of Broccoli	180	8	5	19	1115	8
Pilgrim's Corn Chowder	195	11	30	18	1160	10
Wisconsin Cheese	285	19	30	19	1130	9
French Onion	65	3	0	7	1250	2
Lumberjack Mixed Vegetable	90	4	5	13	1075	2
Chicken Noodle	100	2	25	15	930	6
Split Pea with Ham	200	10	30	21	1030	8
Beef w. Vegetables & Barley	95	3	10	14	995	5
Tomato Florentine	85	1	0	15	910	3
Potatoes & Fries:						
French Fries	245	13	0	30	115	2
Potato Cakes	205	12	0	20	395	2
Curly Fries	335	18	0	43	165	4
Cheddar Fries	400	22	10	46	445	6
Baked Potato: Plain	240	2	0	50	60	6
w. Butter & Sour Cream	465	25	40	53	205	8
Broccoli 'n Cheddar	415	18	20	55	360	10
Deluxe	620	36	60	59	605	17
Mushroom 'n Cheese	515	27	45	57	925	15
Desserts & Shakes:						
Apple Turnover	305	18	0	27	180	4
Cherry Turnover	280	18	0	25	200	5
Blueberry Turnover	320	19	0	32	240	3
Cheese Cake	305	23	95	21	220	5
Chocolate Chip Cookie	130	4	0	17	95	2
Chocolate Shake	450	12	35	76	340	10
Vanilla Shake	330	11	30	46	280	10
Jamocha Shake	370	10	35	59	260	9
P'nut Butter Cup Polar Swirl	515	24	35	61	385	14
Oreo Polar Swirl	480	20	35	66	520	10
Snickers Polar Swirl	510	19	35	73	350	12
Butterfinger Polar Swirl	455	18	30	62	320	12

BURGER KING

	CALORIES	FAT grams	CHOLEST. mg	CARBOHYD. grams	SODIUM mg	PROTEIN grams
Breakfast Items:						
Croissan'wiches:						
with Egg & Cheese	315	20	220	19	605	13
w. Bacon, Egg & Cheese	360	24	230	19	720	15
w. Sausage, Egg & Cheese	535	40	270	22	985	21
with Ham, Egg & Cheese	345	21	240	19	960	19
Croissant	180	10	5	18	285	4
Bagel Sandwiches:						
with Egg & Cheese	405	16	250	46	760	19
with Bacon, Egg & Cheese	455	20	250	46	870	21
w. Sausage, Egg & Cheese	625	36	295	49	1135	27
with Ham, Egg and Cheese	440	17	265	46	1115	25
Bagels: Regular	270	6	30	44	440	10
with Cream Cheese	370	16	60	45	525	12
Biscuits: Regular	330	17	2	42	755	5
with Bacon	380	20	10	42	870	8
with Sausage	480	29	35	44	1005	11
with Bacon and Egg	470	27	215	43	1035	14
with Sausage and Egg	570	36	240	45	1170	17
Scrambled Egg Platter:						
Regular	550	34	365	44	895	17
with Bacon	610	39	375	44	1045	21
with Sausage	770	53	410	47	1270	26
French Toast Sticks	540	32	80	53	535	10
Hash Browns	210	12	5	25	320	2
Danish (Typical)	500	36	5	40	290	5
Burgers: Whopper	615	36	90	45	865	27
Whopper with Cheese	705	44	115	47	1175	32
Double Whopper	845	53	170	45	935	46
Dble. Whopper w. Cheese	935	61	195	47	1245	51
Cheeseburgers: Regular	320	15	50	28	660	17
Deluxe	390	23	55	29	650	18
Double	485	27	100	29	850	30
Bacon Double	515	31	105	26	750	32
Bacon Double Deluxe	590	39	110	28	805	33
Barbecue Bacon Double	535	31	105	31	795	32
Mushroom Swiss Double	475	27	95	27	745	31
Hamburger	272	11	40	28	505	15
Hamburger Deluxe	345	19	45	28	495	15
Sandwiches & Side Orders:						
BK Broiler Chicken S'wich	380	18	55	31	765	24
Chicken Sandwich	685	40	80	56	1415	26
Ocean Catch Fish Filet	495	25	60	49	880	20

	CALORIES	FAT grams	CHOLEST. mg	CARBOHYD. grams	SODIUM mg	PROTEIN grams
Sandwiches & Sides (cont.):						
Chicken Tenders	235	13	45	14	540	16
Fish Tenders	265	16	30	18	870	12
Salads (without dressing):						
Chef Salad	180	9	105	7	590	17
Chunky Chicken Salad	140	4	50	8	440	20
Garden Salad	95	5	15	8	125	6
Side Salad	25	0	0	5	25	1
French Fries (medium, salted)	340	20	20	36	240	4
Onion Rings	300	17	3	34	560	4
Apple Pie	310	14	4	44	410	3
Condiments & Toppings:						
Proc. American Cheese	90	7	25	1	310	5
Processed Swiss Cheese	80	6	20	1	350	6
Cream Cheese	100	10	30	1	85	2
Mayonnaise	195	21	15	2	140	0
Tartar Sauce	135	14	20	2	200	0
BK Broiler Sauce	90	10	5	0	95	0
Bull's Eye Barbecue Sauce	20	0	0	5	45	0
Salad Dressings:						
Thousand Island Dressing	290	26	35	15	400	1
French Dressing	290	22	0	23	400	0
Ranch Dressing	350	37	20	4	315	1
Bleu Cheese Dressing	300	32	60	2	510	3
Olive Oil & Vinegar Dress'g	310	33	0	2	215	0
Red. Cal. Light Italian	170	18	0	3	760	0
Dipping Sauces:						
A.M. Express Dip; Honey	85	0	0	21	20	0
Ranch; Tartar	170	18	0	2	210	0
Barbecue Dipping Sauce	35	0	0	9	400	0
Sweet & Sour Dipp'g Sauce	45	0	0	11	50	0
Beverages:						
Shakes: Vanilla	335	10	35	51	215	9
Chocolate	325	10	30	49	200	9
Chocolate (syrup added)	410	11	35	68	250	10
Strawberry (syrup added)	395	10	35	66	230	9
Pepsi Cola (medium)	195	0	0	47	n.a.	0
Diet Pepsi (medium)	1	0	0	0	n.a.	0
7 Up (medium)	175	0	0	46	n.a.	0
Orange Juice	80	0	0	20	2	1
Milk, 2% low fat	120	5	20	12	120	8
Milk, whole	155	9	35	11	120	8

CARL'S JR.	CALORIES	FAT grams	CHOLEST. mg	CARBOHYD. grams	SODIUM mg	PROTEIN grams
Breakfast Items:						
Sunrise S'wich w. Bacon	370	19	120	32	750	17
w. Sausage	500	32	165	31	990	22
French Toast Dips	480	25	55	54	575	8
Scrambled Eggs	120	9	245	2	105	9
Hot Cakes with Margarine	360	12	15	59	1190	7
English Muffin w. Margarine	180	6	0	28	275	4
Sausage, 1 patty	190	17	25	1	275	7
Bacon, 2 strips	50	4	10	0	200	3
Hash Brown Nuggets	170	9	0	20	350	2
Sandwiches:						
Charbroiler BBQ Chicken	320	5	50	40	955	28
Charbroiler Chicken Club	510	22	85	53	1165	26
California Roast Beef 'n Swiss	360	8	130	43	1070	31
Filet of Fish	550	26	90	58	945	22
Country Fried Steak	610	33	45	54	1290	25
American Cheese	65	5	15	1	290	4
Swiss Cheese	55	4	15	1	220	4
Hamburgers:						
Famous Star	590	36	45	42	890	24
Super Star	770	50	125	44	990	37
Old Time Star	400	17	80	38	760	24
Happy Star	220	8	45	26	445	12
Cheeseburgers: Bacon	630	33	105	49	1415	33
Double Western Bacon	890	53	145	61	1620	42
Potatoes:						
Fiesta	550	23	40	60	1230	25
Broccoli & Cheese	470	17	10	61	690	15
Bacon & Cheese	650	34	45	63	1820	23
Sour Cream & Chive	350	13	10	49	140	8
Cheese	550	22	40	72	785	18
Lite	250	3	0	54	35	8
Soups:						
Cream of Broccoli	140	6	20	14	845	7
Boston Clam Chowder	140	8	20	12	860	6
Old Fash. Chicken Noodle	80	1	14	11	605	4
Lumber Jack Mix Vegetable	70	3	5	10	805	2
Bakery Products:						
Blueberry Muffin	340	9	35	61	300	5
Bran Muffin	260	6	50	44	310	5
Danish (varieties)	300	9	0	49	550	8
Choc. Chip Cookie, 2.5 oz	355	16	15	45	200	3
Chocolate Cake	380	20	70	43	335	7

CARL'S JR. (CONT.)

	CALORIES	FAT grams	CHOLEST. mg	CARBOHYD. grams	SODIUM mg	PROTEIN grams
Side Orders:						
French Fries, regular	420	20	0	54	195	4
Zucchini	380	19	0	44	1120	8
Onion Rings	520	26	0	63	960	9
Salads & Dressings:						
Garden Salad	45	2	5	4	55	2
Chicken Salad	205	8	85	12	455	23
Chef Salad	180	7	65	11	580	19
Taco Salad	355	19	100	18	690	29
Dressings: Italian, 1 oz	120	13	0	1	210	0
House, 1 oz	110	11	10	2	170	1
Blue Cheese, 1 oz	150	15	20	0	255	1
1000 Island, 1 oz	110	11	5	4	200	0
Red. Cal. French, 1 oz	40	2	0	5	290	0
Beverages:						
Carbonated, regular	245	0	0	62	35	0
Orange Juice, small	95	1	0	21	2	2
Shakes, regular	355	7	15	61	255	11

BASKIN-ROBBINS

	CALORIES	FAT grams	CHOLEST. mg	CARBOHYD. grams	SODIUM mg	PROTEIN grams
Deluxe Ice Cream: 1 Scoop						
Chocolate, 1 scoop	270	14	37	32	160	5
Chocolate Chip	260	15	40	27	110	4
Daiquiri Ice	140	0	0	35	15	0
French Vanilla	280	18	90	25	90	4
Jamoca Almond Fudge	270	14	32	30	115	5
Pralines 'n Cream	280	14	36	35	180	4
Rainbow Sherbet	160	2	6	34	85	1
Red Raspberry Sorbet	140	0	0	34	25	0
Rocky Road	300	14	32	39	135	5
Vanilla	240	14	52	24	115	4
Very Berry Strawberry	220	10	30	30	95	3
World Class Chocolate	280	14	36	35	145	5
International Creams:						
Chocolate Raspberry Truffle	310	17	45	35	115	5
Low, Lite 'n Luscious:						
Chunky Banana, ½ cup	100	1	3	20	50	3
Cones: Sugar Cone	60	1	0	11	45	1
Waffle Cone	140	2	0	28	5	3

CHICK-FIL-A

	CALORIES	FAT grams	CHOLEST. mg	CARBOHYD. grams	SODIUM mg	PROTEIN grams
Sandwiches & Nuggets:						
Chicken Sandwiches:						
Chick-fil-A	350	8	65	28	1175	40
Chick-fil-A Deluxe	360	9	65	30	1180	41
Chargrilled	260	5	40	24	1120	30
Chargrilled Deluxe	265	5	40	25	1125	30
Chick-n-Q	205	7	25	22	660	14
Salad (wheat bread)	450	26	50	35	890	10
Chick-fil-A Nuggets, 8 pack	300	15	60	13	1325	28
Chick-fil-A Nuggets, 12 pack	445	23	90	19	1990	42
Salads & Side Orders:						
Carrot & Raisin, cup	120	5	5	18	10	1
Chargrilled Chicken Garden	130	2	30	8	565	20
Chicken Salad, cup	310	28	20	4	545	12
Chicken Salad, plate	580	45	385	17	980	25
Cole Slaw, cup	175	14	10	11	160	1
Potato Salad, cup	200	15	5	14	335	2
Tossed Salad	20	0	0	4	20	1
with Dressing: Ranch	175	16	15	6	205	2
Honey French	245	24	0	7	520	1
1000 Island	230	22	25	9	390	2
Lite Italian	45	2	5	6	355	1
Chicken Soup, small	150	3	45	11	530	16
Waffle Potato Fries, regular	270	14	5	33	45	3
Desserts: Icedream	135	5	25	19	50	4
Fudge Brownie (with nuts)	370	19	n.a.	45	215	5
Lemon Pie, slice	330	5	5	64	300	7
Lemonade, regular	125	0	0	32	0	0

CHURCH'S FRIED CHICKEN

	CALORIES	FAT grams	CHOLEST. mg	CARBOHYD. grams	SODIUM mg	PROTEIN grams
Fried Chicken: Breast	280	17	90	9	560	21
Wing & Side-Breast	305	20	90	9	580	22
Thigh	310	22	120	9	450	19
Drumstick	150	9	65	5	290	13
Chicken Nuggets: 6-Pack	330	18	80	22	750	20
Cole Slaw	90	7	5	6	170	1
Corn w. Butter Oil, 1 cob	240	9	10	33	20	4
Dinner Roll	85	2	0	16	120	1
French Fries, regular	255	13	<10	31	140	3
Hushpuppy, 2	160	6	n.a.	23	110	3

D'LITES	CALORIES	FAT grams	CHOLEST. mg	CARBOHYD. grams	SODIUM mg	PROTEIN grams
Sandwiches:						
(with Multi-Grain Bun)						
¼ lb Fish Filet Sandwich	390	21	95	29	240	22
Chicken Filet Sandwich	280	11	45	24	760	23
Hot Ham 'n Cheese S'wich	280	8	50	26	1160	27
Vegetarian D'Lite	270	14	0	20	610	16
Burgers:						
(with Multi-Grain Bun)						
¼ lb D'Lite Burger	280	12	95	19	240	25
Bacon Cheeseburger	370	18	110	20	730	32
Double D'Lite Burger	450	22	190	19	290	44
Jr. D'Lite	200	7	55	19	210	15
Soups:						
Cream of Broccoli Soup	180	7	10	21	1080	8
Soup D'Lite	130	4	70	10	530	14
Potatoes & Fries:						
Baked, plain, 10 oz	230	1	0	50	1	6
with Bacon & Cheddar	490	20	45	52	1260	25
with Broccoli & Cheddar	410	16	15	51	820	15
French Fries, large	320	15	1	42	120	4
French Fries, regular	260	12	1	34	100	3
Mexican Potato	510	18	60	61	1000	27
Mexiskins, per skin	100	7	15	6	225	4
Potato Skins, per skin	90	6	15	6	225	3
Miscellaneous:						
Litely Breaded Chicken Filet	170	7	35	6	430	20
Litely Breaded Fish Filet	190	10	50	10	95	16
Extra Lean Trimmed Ham	100	3	40	1	800	18
Ground Beef (80% lean)						
2 oz patty	90	5	55	0	30	10
¼ lb patty	170	10	95	0	55	20
Lite Multi-Grain Bun	110	2	0	19	190	5
Lite White Sesame Seed Bun	110	2	0	18	190	5
Bacon, 2 strips	40	4	10	1	200	2
Lite Cheese, 1 slice, ¾ oz	55	3	10	2	310	5
Salad Bar Platter (no dressing)	130	6	0	9	230	10
Lite Mayonnaise, 1 Tbsp	40	4	5	1	85	0
Lite Tartar Sauce, 1 Tbsp	60	6	5	2	150	0
Chocolate D'Lite	200	4	15	36	70	6

DAIRY QUEEN BRAZIER	CALORIES	FAT grams	CHOLEST. mg	CARBOHYD. grams	SODIUM mg	PROTEIN grams
Dairy Queen Products:						
Sandwiches: Chicken	670	41	75	46	870	29
Fish: Plain	400	17	50	41	875	20
with Cheese	440	21	60	39	1035	24
Hamburgers:						
Single Hamburger	360	16	45	33	630	21
with Cheese	410	20	50	33	790	24
Double Hamburger	530	28	85	33	660	36
with Cheese	650	37	95	34	980	43
Triple Hamburger	710	45	135	33	690	51
with Cheese	820	50	145	34	1010	58
Hot Dogs: Regular	280	16	45	21	830	11
with Cheese	330	21	55	21	990	15
with Chili	320	20	55	23	985	13
Super Hot Dog, regular	520	27	80	44	1365	17
with Cheese	580	34	100	45	1605	22
with Chili	570	32	100	47	1595	21
French Fries: Regular	200	10	10	25	115	2
Large	320	16	15	40	185	3
Onion Rings, 3 oz	280	16	15	31	140	4
Brazier Products:						
Fish Fillet	430	18	40	45	675	20
with Cheese	485	22	50	46	870	23
Chicken Breast Fillet	610	34	80	46	725	27
with Cheese	660	38	85	47	920	30
All White Chicken Nuggets	275	18	40	13	505	16
BBQ Nugget Sauces	40	0	0	9	130	0
"DQ" Hounder	480	36	80	21	1800	16
with Chili	575	41	90	25	1900	22
with Cheese	535	40	90	22	1995	19
Desserts:						
Banana Split	540	11	30	103	150	9
Buster Bar	460	29	10	41	175	10
Chipper Sandwich	320	7	15	56	170	5
Dairy Queen Sandwich	140	4	5	24	40	3
Dilly Ba	210	13	10	21	50	3
Health Blizzard	800	24	65	125	325	15
Hot Fudge Brownie Delight	600	25	20	85	225	8
Float	400	7	20	80	90	5
Mr Misty Float	380	7	20	74	95	5
Freeze	500	12	30	89	180	9
Mr Misty Freeze	510	12	30	91	140	9

	CALORIES	FAT grams	CHOLEST. mg	CARBOHYD. grams	SODIUM mg	PROTEIN grams
Desserts (cont.):						
Mr Misty Plain: Large	340	0	0	84	1	0
Regular	250	0	0	63	1	0
Small	190	0	0	47	1	0
Frozen Dessert	180	6	15	27	65	4
Fudge Nut Bar	400	25	10	40	165	8
Kiss	70	0	0	17	1	0
Parfait	430	8	30	76	140	8
Parfait, Peanut Buster	740	34	30	94	250	16
Soft Icecream without Cone	180	6	15	27	65	4
Strawberry Shortcake	540	11	25	100	215	10
Sundae, Chocolate: Large	440	10	30	78	165	8
Regular	310	8	20	56	120	5
Small	190	4	10	33	75	3
Cones:						
Dipped Chocolate: Large	510	24	30	64	145	9
Regular	340	16	20	42	100	6
Small	190	9	10	25	55	3
Double Delight	490	20	25	69	150	9
Queen's Choice; Vanilla	320	16	50	40	75	4
Chocolate Cone	325	16	50	40	85	5
Soft Ice Cream: Large	340	10	25	57	115	9
Regular	240	7	15	38	80	6
Small	140	4	10	22	45	3
Beverages:						
Chocolate Malt: Large	1060	25	70	187	360	20
Regular	760	18	50	134	260	14
Small	520	13	35	91	180	10
Chocolate Shake: Large	990	26	70	168	360	19
Regular	710	19	50	120	260	14
Small	490	13	35	82	180	10
Queen Malt	890	21	60	155	325	16
Queen Shake	830	22	60	140	305	16

~ FEEDBACK WELCOME ~

Please write to the author with your comments on the usefulness or otherwise of this section. Which extra fast-food outlets should be included in future editions? Did this section assist you in making wiser choices?

Author's Address — See last page.

DEL TACO

	CALORIES	FAT grams	CHOLEST. mg	CARBOHYD. grams	SODIUM mg	PROTEIN grams
Burritos:						
Chicken Fajita Burrito	255	11	45	16	845	23
Bean Burrito	310	6	10	51	760	13
Steak & Cheese	340	20	35	19	840	20
Combo Burrito	385	13	35	48	910	18
Del Meat Burrito	430	18	50	42	970	24
Tacos:						
Del Taco	170	11	25	12	220	6
SofTaco	215	10	25	14	625	17
Quarterpound Del Taco	270	17	30	19	355	10
Chicken SofTaco	190	7	35	12	735	19
Nachos:						
Cheese Nachos*	450	29	15	43	1500	4
Beef & Bean Nachos	585	36	35	57	2000	8
Del Nachos*	705	46	50	60	2130	13
(*)Revised figures						
Fajitas:						
Chicken	195	7	35	13	785	21
Steak	200	7	35	13	785	21
Platters:						
Enchilada Platter #1	585	23	40	72	1785	22
Combo Burrito	830	33	55	112	2465	21
Beef Burrito	875	38	70	106	2525	27
Side Dishes:						
Rice	85	2	0	17	425	1
Chips	230	13	5	26	5	2
Beans	210	3	10	19	440	27
French Fries	355	19	5	42	755	4

DOMINO'S PIZZA

Per 2 Slices (16" Pizza):	CALORIES	FAT grams	CHOLEST. mg	CARBOHYD. grams	SODIUM mg	PROTEIN grams
Cheese	375	10	20	56	480	21
Pepperoni	460	17	30	55	825	24
Sausage & Mushroom	430	16	30	55	550	24
Vegi	500	18	35	60	1030	31
Deluxe	500	20	40	59	950	27
Double Cheese & Pepperoni	545	25	50	55	1040	32
Ham	415	11	25	58	800	23

DUNKIN' DONUTS	CALORIES	FAT grams	CHOLEST. mg	CARBOHYD. grams	SODIUM mg	PROTEIN grams
Donuts:						
Apple Filled w. Cinn. Sugar	250	11	0	33	280	5
Bavarian Filled with						
Chocolate Frosting	240	11	0	32	260	5
Blueberry Filled	210	8	0	29	240	4
Choc. Frosted Yeast Ring	200	10	0	25	190	4
Glazed Buttermilk Ring	290	14	10	37	370	4
Glazed Chocolate Ring	325	21	2	34	385	4
Glazed Coffee Roll	280	12	0	37	310	5
Glazed French Cruller	140	8	30	16	130	2
Glazed Whole Wheat Ring	330	18	5	39	380	4
Glazed Yeast Ring	200	9	0	26	230	4
Jelly Filled	220	9	0	31	230	4
Lemon Filled	260	12	0	33	280	4
Plain Cake Ring	270	17	10	25	330	4
Muffins: Apple 'n Spice	300	8	25	52	360	6
Banana Nut	310	10	30	49	410	7
Blueberry	280	8	30	46	340	6
Bran with Raisins	310	9	15	51	560	6
Corn	340	12	40	51	560	7
Cranberry Nut	290	9	25	44	360	6
Oat Bran	330	11	0	50	450	7
Cookies: Chocolate Chunk	200	10	30	25	110	3
Chocolate Chunk with Nuts	210	11	30	23	100	3
Oatmeal Pecan Raisin	200	9	25	28	100	3
Croissants: Almond	420	27	0	38	280	8
Chocolate	440	29	0	38	220	7
Plain	310	19	0	27	240	7

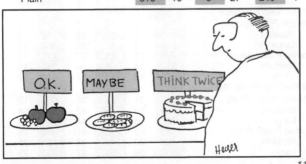

EL POLLO LOCO	CALORIES	FAT grams	CHOLEST. mg	CARBOHYD. grams	SODIUM mg	PROTEIN grams
Combo Meal	720	28	90	70	890	49
Chicken Breast Sandwich	290	7	65	32	370	25
Charbroiled Chicken Salad	200	3	65	11	370	25
Chicken, 2 pieces, 5 oz	310	18	80	2	460	37
Corn Tortillas	210	2	0	42	70	6
Flour Tortillas	280	7	0	45	450	9
Corn	110	2	0	20	110	4
Coleslaw	80	6	10	5	160	2
Potato Salad	140	8	5	15	500	3
Rice	100	1	0	22	250	3
Beans	110	1	1	17	450	8
Dole Whip	90	0	0	19	20	0
Salsa	10	0	0	1	90	0

GODFATHER'S PIZZA

	CALORIES	FAT grams	CHOLEST. mg	CARBOHYD. grams	SODIUM mg	PROTEIN grams
Original Pizza: Per Slice						
Cheese Pizza: Mini	190	4	10	31	260	8
Small	240	7	15	32	400	12
Medium	270	8	15	36	430	13
Large	300	9	20	39	500	15
Large Hot Slice	370	11	25	48	620	18
Combo Pizza: Mini	240	7	10	32	450	10
Small	360	15	30	35	830	18
Medium	400	17	35	39	930	20
Large	440	19	35	42	1020	22
Large Hot Slice	550	24	45	52	1270	27
Thin Crust: Per Slice						
Cheese Pizza: Small	180	6	10	21	370	9
Medium	210	7	15	26	410	10
Large	230	7	15	28	460	11
Combo Pizza: Small	270	13	25	23	710	13
Medium	310	14	25	29	790	15
Large	340	16	30	31	870	17
Stuffed Pie Pizza: Per Slice						
Cheese Pizza: Small	310	11	25	38	560	13
Medium	350	13	25	42	610	14
Large	380	16	30	44	680	16
Combo Pizza: Small	430	20	40	41	1000	19
Medium	480	23	45	45	1100	21
Large	520	26	50	47	1200	23

HARDEE'S

	CALORIES	FAT grams	CHOLEST. mg	CARBOHYD. grams	SODIUM mg	PROTEIN grams
Hamburgers & Sandwiches:						
Hamburger	270	10	20	33	490	13
Cheeseburger: Regular	320	14	30	33	710	16
Quarter-Pound	500	29	70	34	1060	29
The Lean 1	420	18	85	37	760	27
Big Deluxe Burger	500	30	70	32	760	27
Bacon Cheeseburger	610	39	80	31	1030	34
Mushroom 'n Swiss Burger	490	27	70	33	940	309
Big Twin	450	25	55	34	580	23
Regular Roast Beef	260	9	35	31	730	15
Big Roast Beef	300	11	45	32	880	18
Hot Ham 'n Cheese	330	12	65	32	1420	23
Turkey Club	390	16	70	32	1280	29
Fisherman's Fillet	500	24	70	49	1030	23
Chicken Fillet	370	13	55	44	1060	19
Grilled Chicken Sandwich	310	9	60	34	890	24
All Beef Hot Dog	300	17	25	25	710	11
Fries & Special Items:						
French Fries: Regular, 2½ oz	230	11	0	30	85	3
Large, 4 oz	360	17	0	48	135	4
Chicken Stix: 6 pieces	210	9	35	13	680	19
9 pieces	310	14	55	20	1020	28
Big Fry, 5½ oz	500	23	0	66	180	6
Crispy Curls	300	16	0	36	840	4
Salads:						
Side Salad	20	0	0	1	15	2
Garden Salad	210	14	105	3	270	14
Chef Salad	240	15	115	5	930	22
Chicken 'n Pasta Salad	230	3	55	23	380	27
Shakes & Desserts						
Shake: Vanilla	400	9	50	66	320	13
Chocolate	460	8	45	85	340	11
Strawberry	440	8	40	82	300	11
Cool Twist:						
Cone, Vanilla	190	6	15	28	100	5
Cone, Chocolate	200	6	20	31	65	4
Cone, Vanilla & Choc.	190	6	20	29	80	4
Sundae, Hot Fudge	320	12	25	45	270	7
Sundae, Caramel	330	10	20	54	290	6
Sundae, Strawberry	260	8	15	43	115	5
Apple Turnover	270	12	0	38	250	3
Big Cookie	250	13	5	31	240	3

Breakfast Items — Next Page.

HARDEE'S (CONT.)	CALORIES	FAT grams	CHOLEST. mg	CARBOHYD. grams	SODIUM mg	PROTEIN grams
Breakfast Items:						
Rise 'n Shine	320	18	0	34	740	5
Cinnamon 'n Raisin	320	17	0	37	510	4
Sausage Biscuit	440	28	25	34	1100	13
Sausage & Egg	490	31	170	35	1150	18
Bacon Biscuit	360	21	10	34	950	10
Bacon & Egg	410	24	155	35	990	15
Bacon, Egg & Cheese	460	28	165	35	1220	17
Ham Biscuit	320	16	15	34	1000	10
Ham & Egg	370	19	160	35	1050	15
Ham, Egg & Cheese	420	23	170	35	1270	18
Country Ham	350	18	25	35	1550	11
Country Ham & Egg	400	22	175	35	1600	16
Canadian Rise 'n Shine	470	27	180	35	1550	22
Steak Biscuit	500	29	30	46	1320	15
Steak & Egg	550	32	175	47	1370	20
Chicken Biscuit	430	22	45	42	1330	17
Big Country Breakfast:						
Sausage	850	57	340	51	1980	33
Bacon	660	40	305	51	1540	24
Ham	620	33	325	51	1780	28
Country Ham	670	38	345	52	2870	29
Hash Rounds	230	14	0	24	560	3
Biscuit 'n Gravy	440	24	15	45	1250	9
Three Pancakes: Regular	280	2	15	56	890	8
with 1 Sausage Pattie	430	16	40	56	1290	16
with 2 Bacon Strips	350	9	25	56	1110	13
Syrup	120	0	0	31	25	0
Margarine/Butter Blend	35	4	5	0	40	0

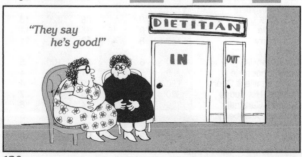

"They say he's good!"

DIETITIAN
IN
OUT

JACK IN THE BOX

	CALORIES	FAT grams	CHOLEST. mg	CARBOHYD. grams	SODIUM mg	PROTEIN grams
Breakfast Items:						
Scrambled Egg Pocket	430	21	350	31	1060	29
Supreme Crescent	550	40	180	27	1050	20
Sausage Crescent	585	43	190	28	1010	22
Breakfast Jack	310	13	200	30	870	18
Scrambled Egg Platter	660	40	350	52	1190	24
Hash Browns	115	7	5	11	210	2
Pancake Platter	610	22	100	87	890	15
Pancake Syrup	120	0	0	30	5	0
Grape Jelly	40	0	0	9	5	0
Hamburgers:						
Hamburger, regular	70	11	25	28	550	13
Grilled Sourdough Burger	710	50	110	34	1140	32
Swiss and Bacon Burger	680	47	90	34	1460	31
Jumbo Jack	580	34	70	42	730	26
Jumbo Jack with Cheese	680	40	100	46	1090	32
Cheeseburger: Regular	315	14	40	33	750	15
Bacon	705	39	85	48	1130	35
Double	470	27	70	33	840	21
Ultimate	940	69	130	33	1180	47
Sandwiches:						
Ham and Turkey Melt	590	36	80	40	1120	27
Chicken Fajita Pita	290	8	35	29	700	24
Grilled Chicken Fillet	410	17	65	33	1130	31
Chicken Supreme	575	36	60	34	1520	27
Fish Supreme	555	32	65	47	1050	20
Sirloin Cheesesteak	620	30	80	51	1450	36
Salads & Dressings:						
Chef Salad	325	18	140	10	900	30
Taco Salad	500	31	90	28	1600	34
Side Salad	50	3	<1	<1	85	7
Dressings: Buttermilk House	360	36	20	8	700	<1
Bleu Cheese	260	22	20	14	920	<1
1000 Island	310	30	25	12	700	<1
Reduced Calorie French	175	8	0	26	600	<1
Fingerfoods:						
Egg Rolls: 3 piece	405	19	30	42	900	15
5 piece	675	32	50	70	1500	26
Chicken Strips: 4 piece	350	14	70	28	750	29
6 piece	525	20	100	42	1120	43
Shrimp: 10 piece	270	16	85	22	670	10
15 piece	400	24	125	34	1000	15

Continued Next Page

JACK IN THE BOX (CONT.)

	CALORIES	FAT grams	CHOLEST. mg	CARBOHYD. grams	SODIUM mg	PROTEIN grams
Fingerfoods (cont.):						
Taquitos: 5 piece	365	16	35	40	470	16
7 piece	510	22	50	56	650	22
Sauces: Sweet & Sour	40	<1	<1	11	160	<1
BBQ	45	<1	0	10	300	0
Seafood Cocktail	30	<1	0	7	200	<1
Mexican Food: Guacamole	55	5	0	2	130	1
Salsa	10	<1	0	2	130	0
Taco	190	11	20	16	400	8
Super Taco	290	17	35	21	760	12
Side Dishes:						
French Fries: Small	220	12	10	27	160	2
Regular	350	19	15	43	260	3
Jumbo	440	24	15	54	330	4
Onion Rings	380	23	30	39	410	5
Sesame Breadsticks	70	2	<1	12	110	2
Tortilla Chips	140	6	<1	18	130	2
Desserts & Beverages:						
Hot Apple Turnover	410	24	15	45	350	4
Cheesecake	310	17	60	29	210	8
Double Fudge Cake	290	9	20	49	260	4
Orange Juice	80	0	0	20	0	1
Milk, lowfat	120	5	20	12	120	8
Milk Shakes: Average	320	7	25	55	240	10
Coca-Cola (classic)	145	0	0	36	15	0
Ramblin' Root Beer	175	0	0	46	20	0
Sprite	145	0	0	36	45	0
Dr. Pepper	145	0	0	37	20	0

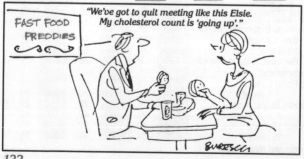

"We've got to quit meeting like this Elsie.
My cholesterol count is 'going up'."

FAST FOOD FREDDIES

BURRESCH

122

KENTUCKY FRIED CHICKEN	CALORIES	FAT grams	CHOLEST. mg	CARBOHYD. grams	SODIUM mg	PROTEIN grams
3-Piece Dinners: Average						
(Includes mash. potato/coleslaw)						
Original Recipe	890	51	260	49	2140	58
Extra Tasty Crispy	1120	70	280	58	2320	64
Lite 'n Crispy	785	44	185	n.a.	1600	n.a.
2-Piece Dinners:						
Original (w. pot./coleslaw)	655	37	175	40	1605	40
Extra Tasty Crispy	810	50	190	47	1720	44
Lite 'n Crispy	585	32	125	n.a.	1240	n.a.
2-Piece Snack: (w. biscuit)						
Original	695	40	175	44	1695	58
Extra Tasty Crispy	853	54	190	50	1815	44
Lite 'n Crispy	630	36	120	n.a.	1360	n.a.
Original Recipe Chicken:						
Wing	180	12	65	6	370	12
Drumstick	145	8	65	4	275	13
Centre Breast	285	15	90	9	670	27
Side Breast	270	16	75	11	735	20
Thigh	295	20	125	11	620	18
Extra Tasty Crispy Chicken:						
Wing	255	19	65	9	420	12
Centre Breast	340	20	115	12	790	33
Side Breast	345	22	80	14	750	22
Thigh	405	30	130	14	690	20
Drumstick	205	14	70	6	325	14
Lite 'n Crispy Chicken: Thigh	245	17	80	n.a.	385	n.a.
Side Breast	205	12	55	n.a.	420	n.a.
Centre Breast	220	12	55	n.a.	415	n.a.
Drumstick	120	7	50	n.a.	195	n.a.
Kentucky Nuggets & Sauces:						
Kentucky Nuggets: 6 nuggets	270	18	70	12	840	18
Sauces: Barbeque; Mustard	35	1	0	7	450	<1
Sweet 'n Sour	60	1	0	13	150	0
Honey	50	0	0	12	<15	0
Other Items:						
Hot Wings, 6 pieces	375	24	150	18	675	22
Colonel's Chicken Sandwich	480	27	45	39	1060	21
Chicken Littles Sandwich	170	10	20	14	330	6
Buttermilk Biscuit, one	235	12	1	28	655	4
Mashed Potato & Gravy	70	2	0	12	340	2
French Fries	245	12	2	31	140	3
Corn-on-the-Cob	175	3	0	32	20	5
Cole Slaw	120	7	5	13	195	1

LITTLE CAESAR

	CALORIES	FAT grams	CHOLEST. mg	CARBOHYD. grams	SODIUM mg	PROTEIN grams
Single Slice:						
Cheese Pizza	170	6	10	20	290	9
Pepperoni Pizza:						
Gr. Peppers/On./Mshr.	190	7	15	20	340	10
Meals:						
Pizza w. Gr. Peppers/Onion/						
Mushr. & Tossed Salad	640	22	40	76	1720	34
Cheese Pizza w. Toss. Salad	600	21	35	73	1600	30
Sandwiches:						
Ham & Cheese	520	21	45	55	1050	28
Tuna Melt	700	37	65	58	830	34
Italian Sub	590	28	60	55	1230	29
Vegetarian	620	30	55	58	1000	30
Salads: Individual Serving						
Antipasto	170	9	40	12	1150	10
Greek	140	8	25	8	1080	8
Tossed	80	2	0	11	750	4

LONG JOHN SILVER'S

	CALORIES	FAT grams	CHOLEST. mg	CARBOHYD. grams	SODIUM mg	PROTEIN grams
Fish Items:						
Fish & Fryes: 2 pieces	660	30	60	68	1120	30
3 pieces	810	38	85	77	1630	42
Fish & More	800	37	70	88	1390	31
Fish Dinner, 3 pieces	960	44	100	97	1890	43
Shrimp, Fish &						
Chicken Dinner	840	40	80	89	1450	31
Fish & Chicken	870	46	70	91	1540	35
Catfish Fillet Dinner	860	42	65	90	990	28
Homestyle Fish Dinner: 3 pc.	880	42	75	97	980	28
4 pc.	1010	50	90	106	1180	35
6 pc.	1260	64	130	124	1590	49
Chicken Dinners:						
Chicken Plank Dinner: 3 pc.	830	39	55	88	1340	31
4 pc.	940	44	70	94	1660	39
Breaded Items:						
Shrimp Feast: 13 pieces	880	41	90	110	1320	19
21 pieces	1070	51	125	130	1790	25
Homestyle Fish S'wich Platter	870	38	55	108	1110	26

Continued Next Page

LONG JOHN SILVERS (CONT.)	CALORIES	FAT grams	CHOLEST. mg	CARBOHYD. grams	SODIUM mg	PROTEIN grams
Miscellaneous:						
Seafood Platter	970	46	70	109	1540	30
Shrimp & Fish Dinner	770	37	80	85	1250	25
Clam Dinner	980	45	15	122	1200	21
Batter Fried Items:						
Shrimp Dinner: 6 pieces	740	37	90	82	1110	18
9 pieces	860	45	125	88	1470	24
Salads:						
Seafood Salad	270	7	90	36	670	16
Garden Salad	170	9	5	13	380	8
Ocean Chef Salad	250	9	80	19	1340	24
Baked Seafood:						
Cod	150	<1	135	<1	140	34
Cod Supreme	190	4	135	3	250	34
Cod Delight	180	1	135	4	390	35
Shrimp Scampi	160	7	205	7	660	15
Accompaniments:						
Rice Pilaf	250	3	0	52	660	5
Vegetables	120	6	<5	16	95	4
Cole Slaw	140	6	15	20	260	1
Side Salad, without dressing	20	0	0	5	20	1
Breadstick	110	3	0	18	120	3
Condiments:						
Catsup, 1 packet	15	<1	n.a.	3	170	<1
Seafood Sauce, 1 packet	45	1	0	8	530	<1
Tartar Sauce, 1 packet	80	3	<5	13	80	<1
Malt Vinegar, 1 packet	2	<1	n.a.	0	20	<1
Sweet 'n Sour Sauce, 1 pkt.	60	<1	0	13	125	<1
Honey Mustard Sauce, 1 pkt.	60	<1	0	13	170	<1
Ranch Dressing, 1 packet	140	3	<5	27	350	<1
Bleu Cheese Dressing, 1 pkt.	120	2	<5	22	380	2
Reduced Calorie Italian Dressing, 1 packet	18	1	<5	2	670	<1
Sea Salad Dressing, 1 pkt.	140	7	<5	20	260	<1
Club Crackers, 1 package	35	2	n.a.	5	85	<1
Children's Meals:						
1 Fish, Fryes & 1 Hushpuppy	440	20	30	49	590	16
2 Planks, Fryes & 1 Hushpuppy	510	24	30	52	730	20
1 Fish, 1 Plank, Fryes & 1 Hushpuppy	550	26	45	55	910	24

McDONALD'S	CALORIES	FAT grams	CHOLEST. mg	CARBOHYD. grams	SODIUM mg	PROTEIN grams
Burgers & Sandwiches:						
Big Mac	560	32	100	42	950	25
Cheeseburger	310	14	55	31	750	15
Filet-O-Fish	440	26	50	38	1030	14
Hamburger	260	10	35	31	500	12
McChicken	490	29	45	40	780	19
McD.L.T.	580	37	110	36	990	26
McLean Deluxe	320	10	60	35	670	22
with Cheese	370	14	75	35	890	24
Quarter Pounder	410	21	85	34	660	23
Quarter Pounder w. Cheese	520	29	120	35	1150	28
Test Items (Some States Only):						
Chicken Breast (Grilled) S/wich	250	4	50	30	740	24
Chicken Fajitas	185	8	35	20	310	11
Chicken McNuggets:						
Chicken McNuggets, 6-pack	270	15	55	17	580	20
Barbeque Sauce	50	1	0	12	340	0
Honey Sauce	45	0	0	11	0	0
Hot Mustard Sauce	70	4	5	8	250	1
Sweet & Sour Sauce	60	0	0	14	190	0
French Fries: Small	220	12	10	26	110	3
Medium French Fries	320	17	10	36	150	4
Large French Fries	400	22	15	46	200	6
Shakes, Sundaes, Cookies:						
Apple Pie	260	15	5	30	240	2
Milkshakes: Vanilla	290	1	10	60	170	11
Chocolate	320	2	10	66	240	12
Strawberry	320	1	10	67	170	11
Frozen Yogurt Cones	100	1	5	22	80	4
Frozen Yogurt Sundae:						
Strawberry	210	1	5	49	95	6
Hot Fudge	240	3	5	50	170	7
Hot Caramel	270	3	15	59	180	7
McDonaldland Cookies	290	9	0	47	300	4
Chocolaty Chip Cookies	330	16	5	42	280	4
Soft Drinks (with Ice):						
Coca-Cola; Sprite, 12 fl.oz	140	0	0	38	15	0
16 fl.oz	190	0	0	50	20	0
22 fl.oz	260	0	0	70	25	0
Diet Coke, 12 fl.oz	1	0	0	0	30	0
Orange Drink, 12 fl.oz	130	0	0	33	10	0

McDONALD'S (CONT.)	CALORIES	FAT grams	CHOLEST. mg	CARBOHYD. grams	SODIUM mg	PROTEIN grams
Salads:						
Chef Salad	230	13	130	7	490	20
Garden Salad	110	7	85	6	160	7
Chunky Chicken Salad	140	3	80	5	230	23
Side Salad	60	3	40	3	85	4
Croutons	50	2	0	7	140	1
Bacon Bits	16	1	0	0	95	1
Salad Dressings — Per Pkg:						
Bleu Cheese, 2½ oz	350	35	30	6	750	3
Ranch, 2 oz	330	35	20	5	520	1
1000 Island, 2½ oz	390	38	40	12	500	1
Lite Vinaigrette, 2 oz	60	2	0	8	300	1
Red French Red. Calorie, 2 oz	160	8	0	21	440	<1
Peppercorn, 2½ oz	400	44	35	3	425	1
Breakfast Items:						
Burritos (Some States Only)	280	17	135	21	680	12
Egg McMuffin	290	11	225	28	740	18
Hotcakes with Butter & Syrup	410	9	20	74	640	8
Scrambled Eggs	140	10	400	1	290	12
Pork Sausage	180	16	50	0	350	8
English Muffin with Butter	170	5	10	27	270	5
Hashbrown Potatoes	130	7	10	15	330	1
Biscuit with Biscuit Spread	260	13	1	32	730	5
Sausage	440	29	50	32	1080	18
Sausage & Egg	520	35	275	33	1250	20
Bacon, Egg & Cheese	440	26	255	33	1230	17
Sausage McMuffin	370	22	65	27	830	16
Sausage McMuffin & Egg	440	27	265	28	980	28
Danish & Breakfast Muffins:						
Apple Danish	390	18	25	51	370	6
Iced Cheese Danish	390	22	45	42	420	7
Cinnamon Raisin Danish	440	21	35	57	430	6
Raspberry Danish	410	16	25	61	310	6
Apple Bran Muffin	190	0	0	46	230	6
Milk, Juices & Cereals:						
Milk, 8 fl.oz	120	5	20	12	130	8
Orange Juice	80	0	0	18	0	1
Grapefruit Juice, 6 fl.oz	80	0	0	18	0	1
Cheerios	80	1	0	14	210	6
Wheaties	90	0	0	19	220	2

MACHEESMO MOUSE	CALORIES	FAT grams	CHOLEST. mg	CARBOHYD. grams	SODIUM mg	PROTEIN grams
Chicken Burrito	545	10	110	76	655	37
Chicken Burrito Dinner	810	10	110	135	915	46
Combo Burrito	600	11	125	78	840	47
Combo Burrito Dinner	865	11	125	137	2000	55
Vegetarian Burrito	600	7	20	112	750	23
Vegetarian Burrito Dinner	865	7	20	170	1010	31
Chicken Majita	705	9	130	121	785	36
Famouse #5	585	5	20	111	635	23
Vegetarian Plate	530	5	0	110	430	12
Chicken with Green Salad	380	6	130	53	500	28
Chicken Tacos	295	6	80	31	255	25
Chicken Taco Dinner	560	8	80	89	515	33
Vegetarian Tacos	295	6	20	45	265	16
Vegetarian Taco Dinner	560	6	20	103	525	24
Chili Tacos	315	8	65	33	425	28
Chili Taco Dinner	580	8	65	91	685	36
Chicken Salad, large	610	15	120	84	750	36
small	325	7	75	45	390	21
Veggie Taco Salad, large	650	13	20	11	670	20
small	380	8	10	66	425	10
Salad w. Mari. Veg., large	55	1	2	11	130	1
small	30	1	2	5	85	1
Cheese Quesadilla	340	13	40	35	535	21
Chicken Quesadilla	405	15	100	35	575	34
Nacho Grande	705	38	75	61	625	31
Bean & Cheese Enchiladas	405	8	30	63	450	20
Bean & Cheese Ench. Dinner	670	8	30	121	710	28
Chicken Enchiladas	330	10	90	35	400	26
Chicken Enchilada Dinner	600	10	90	93	660	34
Kid's Plate	280	5	20	45	330	14
Kid's Plate with Chicken	350	7	80	45	360	28
Side Orders: Beans	215	0	0	42	120	11
Boss Sauce	30	0	0	8	140	0
Enchilada Sauce	5	0	0	1	65	0
Cheese	80	5	20	1	180	8
Chicken	105	3	90	0	45	20
Chili	135	3	65	3	300	24
Chips	395	17	0	56	30	5
Corn Tortilla	130	0	0	29	10	3
Flour Tortilla	160	2	0	32	140	4
Whole Wheat Tortilla	160	2	0	30	130	6
Guacamole	200	5	0	38	220	0
Mexican Cheese	100	8	25	0	280	7

MACHEESMO MOUSE (CONT.)

	CALORIES	FAT grams	CHOLEST. mg	CARBOHYD. grams	SODIUM mg	PROTEIN grams
Side Orders (cont.):						
Mini Corn Tortilla	160	0	0	36	13	4
Mixed Greens	0	0	0	0	20	0
Rice	275	0	0	64	300	5
Sour Cream	55	5	10	1	20	1
Vegetables	43	0	0	11	80	0
Yogurt, nonfat	15	0	1	2	20	2

MRS WINNER'S CHICKEN & BISCUITS

	CALORIES	FAT grams	CHOLEST. mg	CARBOHYD. grams	SODIUM mg	PROTEIN grams
Per Serving:						
Baked Beans	150	<1	1	31	450	5
Biscuit	245	5	<1	45	500	4
Chicken: Baked Fillet	120	2	35	<1	360	10
Breaded Sandwich	205	10	35	12	1000	19
Fillet Sandwich	380	7	30	45	540	12
Salad	585	8	5	39	875	9
Salad Sandwich	315	6	<5	33	600	10
Cole Slaw	190	16	<5	9	560	1
Country: Fried Steak	220	14	5	<1	200	12
Ham	60	1	15	<1	570	4
Mashed Potatoes with Gravy	150	3	<5	22	830	3
Potato Fries	225	9	<5	27	220	6
Sausage Patties	200	10	10	<1	400	6
Seafood Salad	555	9	5	41	760	5
Steak Sandwich	430	11	20	43	650	11
Tossed Salad	6	0	<5	1	440	1

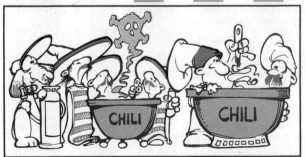

PIZZA HUT

	CALORIES	FAT grams	CHOLEST. mg	CARBOHYD. grams	SODIUM mg	PROTEIN grams
Pan Pizza (Medium):						
Cheese, 2 slices	490	18	35	57	940	30
Pepperoni	540	22	40	62	1130	29
Supreme	590	30	50	53	1360	32
Super Supreme	560	26	55	53	1450	33
Thin 'n Crispy (Medium):						
Cheese, 2 slices	400	17	35	37	870	28
Pepperoni	410	20	45	36	990	26
Supreme	460	22	40	41	1330	28
Super Supreme	465	21	55	44	1340	29
Hand Tossed (Medium):						
Cheese, 2 slices	520	20	55	55	1280	34
Pepperoni	500	23	50	50	1270	28
Supreme	540	26	55	50	1470	32
Super Supreme	560	25	55	54	1650	33
Personal Pan Pizza:						
Pepperoni, 1 whole	675	29	55	76	1330	37
Supreme, 1 whole	650	28	50	76	1310	33

PONDEROSA

Steaks & Meats:
(Figures based on charbroiled meat. Weights are raw weights.)

	CALORIES	FAT grams	CHOLEST. mg	CARBOHYD. grams	SODIUM mg	PROTEIN grams
Chopped Steak: 4 oz serving	230	15	75	0	n.a.	21
5½ oz serving	310	20	100	0	n.a.	29
Hot Dog, 1½ oz	145	13	25	0	n.a.	5
New York Strip, 8 oz steak	370	16	140	0	n.a.	51
Porterhouse, 12 oz steak:						
with ¼" fat	730	53	200	0	n.a.	60
w/out fat (lean only)	440	22	160	0	n.a.	55
Rib Eye, 5 oz steak	330	24	90	0	n.a.	27
Sirloin: 7 oz steak (w/¼" fat)	360	22	125	0	n.a.	39
w/out fat (lean only)	240	12	90	0	n.a.	32
5 oz steak, with ¼" fat	260	16	90	0	n.a.	28
w/out fat (lean only)	180	9	70	0	n.a.	24
Sirloin Tips, 5 oz	210	10	80	0	n.a.	28
T-bone, 8 oz steak (w/¼" fat)	370	27	100	0	n.a.	30
w/out fat (lean only)	220	11	80	0	n.a.	28

Note: Above figures are approximate only
– calculated by author.
(Following figures supplied by Ponderosa)

PONDEROSA (CONT.)	CALORIES	FAT grams	CHOLEST. mg	CARBOHYD. grams	SODIUM mg	PROTEIN grams
Fish: Bake 'R Broil, 5 oz	230	13	50	10	330	19
Baked Scrod, 7 oz.	120	1	65	0	80	27
Broiled: Halibut, 6 oz	170	2	60.	0	70	35
Salmon, 6 oz	190	3	60	3	70	37
Swordfish, 6 oz	270	9	80	0	0	44
Trout, 5 oz	230	4	110	1	50	29
Fish, fried, 3 oz	190	9	15	17	170	9
Fish Nuggets, 1 piece	30	2	5	2	52	2
Shrimp, fried, 7 pieces	230	1	105	31	610	21
Mini Shrimp, 6 pieces	50	0	20	6	125	4
Potatoes: Baked, 7 oz	145	0	0	33	5	4
French Fried, 3 oz	120	4	5	17	40	2
Mashed, 4 oz	60	0	20	13	190	2
Sauces: BBQ Sauce, 2 Tbsp	50	0	0	10	500	0
Sweet & Sour, 2 Tbsp	35	0	0	8	80	0
Tartar, 2 Tbsp	85	11	10	11	480	0
Side Items:						
Breaded Cauliflower, 4 oz	115	1	0	23	445	4
Breaded Onion Rings, 4 oz	215	9	0	30	620	3
Breaded Zucchini, 4 oz	100	1	0	18	585	3
Gravy: Brown/Turkey, 2 oz	25	1	0	4	200	1
Italian Breadsticks, each	100	1	0	19	200	4
Tortilla Chips, 1 oz	150	8	0	16	80	3
Macaroni & Cheese, 4 oz	70	2	5	18	320	3
Potato Wedges, ½ cup	130	6	n.a.	16	170	3
Rice Pilaf, 4 oz	160	4	20	26	450	4
Rolls: Dinner, each	185	3	0	33	310	5
Sourdough, small	110	1	0	22	230	4
Sauce: Cheese, 2 oz	50	2	5	6	355	1
Spaghetti, 2 oz	110	4	0	17	520	2
Spaghetti; Pasta Shells, 2 oz	75	0	0	16	0	2
Stuffing, 4 oz	230	11	20	27	800	6
Desserts:						
Banana Pudding, 4 oz	200	0	0	25	110	2
Canned Peaches, 4 oz	70	0	0	18	10	0
Mousse: Chocolate, 4 oz	310	18	0	28	70	10
Spiced Apples, rings, 4 oz	100	0	0	24	20	0
Toppings: Chocolate, 2 oz	180	1	0	49	75	1
Strawberry, 2 oz	140	1	0	47	60	0
Whipped, 2 oz	160	13	0	10	30	0
Strawberries, 2 oz	15	0	0	3	60	0
Yogurt: Fruit, 4 oz	115	1	5	23	70	4

QUINCY'S FAMILY STEAKHOUSE

	CALORIES	FAT grams	CHOLEST. mg	CARBOHYD. grams	SODIUM mg	PROTEIN grams
Dinner Items:						
Sirloin: Large	850	70	n.a.	0	240	50
Regular	650	54	n.a.	0	205	38
Petite	445	37	n.a.	0	120	26
Sirloin Club	285	10	n.a.	0	160	44
T-Bone, extra thick	1610	159	n.a.	0	390	71
Sirloin, extra thick	890	73	n.a.	0	280	52
Ribeye, extra thick	865	78	n.a.	0	300	40
Filet, extra thick	330	12	n.a.	0	160	51
Ribeye Steak	665	60	n.a.	0	205	31
T-Bone Steak	1045	95	n.a.	0	220	43
Sirloin Tips, 1 order	235	9	n.a.	0	115	37
Chopped Steak	465	34	n.a.	0	95	40
Luncheon Chopped Steak	350	25	n.a.	0	70	30
Country Style Steak with Mushroom Sauce	290	19	17	315	18	
Chicken Strips, 4 pieces	320	15	n.a.	4	n.a.	39
Catfish Filets, 2 pieces	310	12	n.a.	19	100	26
Shrimp, 7 pieces	250	12	n.a.	11	205	22
Burgers:						
Chili Cheeseburger	920	54	n.a.	46	1100	57
¼ lb Hamburger	405	19	n.a.	32	285	25
¼ lb Hamburger w. Cheese	450	23	n.a.	32	430	28
Side Dishes:						
Steak Fries, 1 order	425	21	n.a.	56	90	7
Baked Potato without Butter	180	1	n.a.	41	10	5
Barbeque Beans, 1 order	295	13	n.a.	43	1100	9
Texas Toast w.out Butter, 1 sl.	75	1	n.a.	14	145	2
Country Style Roll	70	1	n.a.	14	135	2
Corn Bread, 1 piece	180	6	n.a.	28	265	4
Chili w. Beans, 1 order	345	16	n.a.	32	1380	20
Miscellaneous:						
Margarine, 1 oz	205	22	n.a.	1	270	1
Green Beans, 1 order	40	1	n.a.	7	500	2
Cole Slaw, 1 order	60	5	n.a.	4	75	1
Peppers & Onions, 1 order	80	5	n.a.	8	10	1
Mushroom Sauce, 1 order	30	1	n.a.	5	365	1
Soups:						
Vegetable Beef Soup	80	2	n.a.	10	1045	5
Clam Chowder	200	14	n.a.	15	1185	6
Cream of Broccoli Soup	195	14	n.a.	13	1045	3

RAX

	CALORIES	FAT grams	CHOLEST. mg	CARBOHYD. grams	SODIUM mg	PROTEIN grams
Sandwiches:						
Roast Beef: Large	570	35	35	41	1170	22
Regular	320	11	35	33	970	20
Small	260	14	20	21	560	12
Grilled Chicken	440	19	50	36	1050	24
BBC (Beef/Bacon/Chicken)	720	49	135	40	1875	30
Philly Beef & Cheese	470	22	50	44	1345	25
Turkey Bacon Club	670	43	85	41	1880	29
Double WB, plain	440	24	50	33	570	20
BBQ	420	14	25	53	4665	21
Fish	460	17	1	58	935	14
Ham & Swiss	430	23	35	42	1735	23
French Fries & Potatoes:						
French Fries: Regular	260	13	5	33	70	2
Large	390	20	5	50	105	3
Potatoes: Plain	270	1	1	60	70	8
with Margarine	370	11	1	60	170	8
with Sour Cream	400	11	1	65	150	11
Cheese (3 oz) & Bacon	780	28	25	110	910	22
Cheese (3 oz) & Broccoli	760	26	10	112	490	19
Pre-Packed Salads:						
Garden Salad, no Dressing	160	11	275	4	360	12
Chef Salad, no Dressing	230	14	320	4	1050	22
Mexican Bar:						
Cheese Sauce: Regular, 4 oz	480	19	10	66	415	11
Nacho, 4 oz	535	25	10	65	215	11
Refried Beans, 4 oz	135	5	2	18	420	7
Sour Topping, 4 oz	150	12	1	6	90	3
Spanish Rice, 4 oz	100	1	1	22	505	3
Taco Sauce, 4 oz	35	1	1	7	920	1
Taco Shells, 1 shell	40	2	1	6	55	1
Tortillas, 1 tortilla	110	2	1	19	285	3
Pasta Bar:						
Alfredo Sauce, 4 oz	90	3	10	13	80	2
Chicken Noodle Soup, 8 oz	90	1	25	18	90	5
Cream of Broccoli Soup, 8 oz	115	5	1	14	500	2
Pasta Shells, 4 oz	190	4	1	30	5	8
Pasta/Vegetable Blend, 4 oz	115	5	1	14	15	5
Rainbow Rotini, 4 oz	205	5	2	34	10	7
Spaghetti, 4 oz	160	5	1	26	1	4
Spaghetti Sauce, 4 oz	90	1	1	22	725	1
Spag. Sauce w. Meat, 4 oz	170	9	1	14	480	8

RED LOBSTER

	CALORIES	FAT grams	CHOLEST. mg	CARBOHYD. grams	SODIUM mg	PROTEIN grams

Fish:

Per Lunch Portion (5 oz raw wt.)
(For **Dinner Portion** of 10 oz,
double the figures.)

Prepared with No Added Fat
Add extra for butter sauce.
(1 tsp = 30 cals/3g fat/30mg sodium)

	CALORIES	FAT grams	CHOLEST. mg	CARBOHYD. grams	SODIUM mg	PROTEIN grams
Catfish	170	10	85	0	50	20
Cod (Atlantic)	100	1	70	0	200	23
Flounder	100	1	70	1	95	21
Grouper	110	1	65	0	70	26
Haddock	110	1	85	2	180	24
Halibut	110	1	60	1	105	25
Mackerel	190	12	100	1	250	20
Monkfish	110	1	80	0	95	24
Ocean Perch (Atlantic)	130	4	75	1	190	24
Pollock	120	1	90	1	90	28
Red Rockfish	90	1	85	0	95	21
Red Snapper	110	1	70	0	140	25
Norwegian Salmon	230	12	80	3	60	27
Sockeye Salmon	160	4	50	3	60	28
Lemon Sole	120	1	65	1	90	27
Swordfish	100	4	100	0	140	17
Tilefish	100	2	80	0	60	20
Rainbow Trout	170	9	90	0	90	23
Yellowfin Tuna	180	6	70	0	70	32
Shellfish:						
King Crab Legs, 16 oz	170	2	100	6	900	32
Snow Crab Legs, 16 oz	150	2	130	1	1630	33
Calamari, breaded and fried	360	21	140	30	1150	13
Langostino, 5 oz	120	1	210	2	410	26
Maine Lobster, 18 oz	240	8	310	5	550	36
Rock Lobster, 1 tail, 13 oz	230	3	200	2	1090	49
Calico Scallops, 5 oz	180	2	115	8	260	32
Deep Sea Scallops, 5 oz	130	2	50	2	260	26
Shrimp, 8-12 pcs., 7 oz	120	2	230	0	110	25
Steaks & Chicken:						
Sirloin Steak, 8 oz	350	15	150	0	110	51
Strip Steak, 9 oz	560	40	150	0	115	47
Hamburger, 1/3 lb	410	28	130	0	115	37
Filet Mignon, 8 oz	350	16	140	0	105	47
Rib Eye Steak, 12 oz	980	82	220	0	150	56
Skinless Chicken Breast, 4 oz	140	3	70	0	60	26

ROY ROGER'S

	CALORIES	FAT grams	CHOLEST. mg	CARBOHYD. grams	SODIUM mg	PROTEIN grams
Breakfast Items:						
Crescent Sandwich: Regular	400	27	150	25	860	13
with Bacon	730	30	150	26	1030	15
with Sausage	450	29	170	26	1290	20
Egg & Biscuit Platter: Regular	395	27	280	22	730	17
with Ham	440	29	300	22	1150	24
Pancake Platter: w/Syr./Butt.	450	15	50	72	840	8
with Ham	505	17	75	72	1260	14
with Sausage	610	30	95	72	1160	14
Burgers & Sandwiches:						
Bacon Cheeseburger	580	39	100	25	1530	32
Cheeseburger	565	37	95	27	1400	30
Hamburger	455	28	75	27	500	24
RR Bar Burger	610	39	110	28	1820	36
Roast Beef	315	10	55	29	780	27
Roast Beef with Cheese	425	19	80	30	1700	33
Large Roast Beef	360	12	75	30	1050	34
with cheese	465	21	95	30	1950	40
Chicken & Chicken Nuggets:						
Breast	410	24	120	17	610	32
Breast & Wing	605	36	160	25	900	42
Drumstick	140	8	40	5	190	12
Thigh	295	20	85	12	400	20
Chicken Nuggets, 6 pieces	265	17	50	n.a.	676	n.a.
Potatoes: Hot Topped, plain	210	0	0	48	65	6
with Bacon 'n Cheese	395	22	35	33	780	17
with Broccoli 'n Cheese	375	18	20	40	520	14
with Oleo	275	7	0	48	160	6
with Sour Cream/Chives	410	21	30	48	140	7
w. Taco Beef 'n Cheese	465	22	40	45	720	22
Miscellaneous: Biscuit	230	12	5	26	570	4
French Fries: Regular	270	13	40	32	160	4
Large	355	18	55	43	220	5
Cole Slaw, regular	110	7	5	11	260	1
Potato Salad, regular	105	6	5	11	700	2
Desserts & Beverages:						
Brownie	265	11	10	37	150	3
Danish Apple	250	11	15	32	250	5
Hot Fudge Sundae	335	12	25	53	180	7
Strawberry Sundae	215	7	25	33	100	6
Shakes: Chocolate	360	10	40	61	290	8
Strawberry	315	10	40	49	260	8

SHAKEY'S

	CALORIES	FAT grams	CHOLEST. mg	CARBOHYD. grams	SODIUM mg	PROTEIN grams
Pizzas (12"): 1 Slice (1/10th Pizza)						
Cheese only: Thin Crust	135	5	15	13	320	8
Thick Crust	170	5	15	22	420	7
Homestyle Pan	305	14	20	31	590	14
Onion/Olives/Mushrooms:						
Thin Crust	125	5	10	14	315	7
Thick Crust	160	4	15	22	420	9
Homestyle Pan	320	15	20	32	650	15
Saus. Pepperoni: Thin Crust	165	8	15	13	395	9
Thick Crust	205	8	20	22	425	11
Homestyle Pan	375	20	25	31	680	17
Saus. Mushroom: Thin Crust	140	6	15	13	335	8
Thick Crust	180	6	15	22	420	10
Homestyle Pan	340	17	25	31	680	16
Pepperoni: Thin Crust	150	7	15	13	400	8
Thick Crust	185	6	15	22	420	10
Homestyle Pan	345	15	25	31	740	16
Shakey's Special: Thin Crust	170	9	15	13	475	13
Thick Crust	210	8	20	22	420	13
Homestyle Pan	385	21	30	32	880	18
Other Items:						
Spaghetti w/Meat Sce/Garlic Brd.	940	33	n.a.	134	1900	26
15 Piece Potatoes	950	36	n.a.	120	3700	17
Shakey's Super Hot Hero	810	44	n.a.	67	2690	36
Hot Ham & Cheese	550	21	n.a.	56	2135	36
5-Piece Fried Chicken & Pot.	1700	90	n.a.	130	5330	97
3-Piece Chicken & Potatoes	945	56	n.a.	51	2290	57

SIZZLER

	CALORIES	FAT grams	CHOLEST. mg	CARBOHYD. grams	SODIUM mg	PROTEIN grams
(Approximate figures only)						
Sizzler Steak (9½ oz raw wt.)	500	30	170	0	n.a.	55
Sirloin Steak (7 oz raw wt.)	360	22	120	0	n.a.	39
Strip Sirloin (13 oz)	690	42	240	0	n.a.	75
Steak, lunch/Combin. (5¼ oz)	280	17	100	0	n.a.	30
Bacon-wrapped Filet	540	40	180	0	n.a.	46
Lemon Herb Chicken	160	4	80	0	n.a.	31
Hibachi Chicken	260	15	85	0	n.a.	27
Shrimp, broiled, 2 skewers	135	3	200	1	n.a.	26
Shrimp Fry (4 oz)	250	12	200	11	n.a.	22
Snapper/Halibut, broiled, lunch	150	4	70	1	n.a.	27
Dinner portion (7½ oz raw)	200	6	95	1	n.a.	37

STEAK 'N SHAKE	CALORIES	FAT grams	CHOLEST. mg	CARBOHYD. grams	SODIUM mg	PROTEIN grams
Steakburgers & Sandwiches:						
Steakburger	275	7	60	33	425	18
with Cheese	355	13	80	33	660	23
Super	375	12	100	33	445	30
Super with Cheese	450	18	120	33	680	35
Triple	475	17	160	33	470	43
Triple with Cheese	625	30	180	34	935	52
Ham Sandwich	450	22	n.a.	37	1860	29
Grilled Cheese Sandwich	250	13	20	24	610	9
Grilled Chicken Sandwich	510	22	85	53	1150	26
Other Items: French Fries	210	10	10	28	300	3
Chili & Oyster Crackers	335	14	n.a.	37	1160	16
Chili Mac & 4 Saltines	310	12	n.a.	34	1300	15
Chili 3 Ways & 4 Saltines	410	16	n.a.	45	1730	19
Baked Beans	175	4	0	27	655	9
Lett./Tom. Salad/1oz 1000 Isl.	170	15	15	7	225	1
Chef Salad	315	18	120	6	1580	41
Cottage Cheese, ½ cup	95	4	20	3	200	12
Desserts: Apple Danish	390	24	30	35	350	6
Brownie	260	12	10	39	165	3
Cheesecake	370	11	60	61	295	7
Cheesecake w/Strawberries	385	11	60	65	295	7
Pies: Apple	405	18	40	61	480	4
Cherry	335	14	30	48	270	6
Apple, A La Mode	550	25	80	76	525	4
Cherry, A La Mode	475	22	70	63	315	6
Sundaes: Brownie Fudge	645	35	30	81	260	7
Hot Fudge Nut	530	34	60	51	120	5
Strawberry	330	22	50	29	80	2
Vanilla Ice Cream	215	12	40	23	70	1
Shakes & Drinks:						
Floats: Coca-Cola	515	17	0	76	230	16
Orange	500	17	0	74	225	16
Lemon	555	19	0	82	250	18
Root Beer	530	17	0	78	240	17
Freezes: Lemon	550	25	0	69	215	15
Orange	515	24	0	63	200	14
Hot Chocolate	685	19	50	129	670	17
Shakes: Chocolate	610	38	100	57	180	13
Strawberry	650	40	100	62	190	16
Vanilla	620	38	100	58	180	13

(Cholesterol Figures — Estimate only)

SUBWAY

	CALORIES	FAT grams	CHOLEST. mg	CARBOHYD. grams	SODIUM mg	PROTEIN grams
6" Subs:						
Cold Cut Combo	425	20	80	41	1110	23
Spicy Italian	520	31	65	41	1510	21
BMT	490	27	65	41	1570	22
Subway Club	345	11	40	41	1350	22
Tuna	550	36	40	40	750	18
Seafood & Crab	490	28	30	47	930	15
Seafood & Lobster	470	26	25	47	1040	14
Meatball	455	22	45	48	1010	21
Steak & Cheese	385	16	40	42	780	20
Turkey Breast	320	10	35	41	1230	20
Roast Beef	345	11	35	42	1140	21
Ham & Cheese	325	14	35	40	850	19
Veggies & Cheese	265	14	10	40	530	10

**Note: Figures based on Italian Roll.
For Honey Wheat Roll (6"),
add 15 cals, 1g Fat, 30mg Sodium.**

	CALORIES	FAT grams	CHOLEST. mg	CARBOHYD. grams	SODIUM mg	PROTEIN grams
Footlong Subs:						
Cold Cut Combo	855	40	160	82	2220	46
Spicy Italian	1045	63	130	83	3020	42
BMT	980	55	130	83	3140	44
Subway Club	690	22	85	83	2710	45
Tuna	1100	72	85	81	1500	36
Seafood & Crab	985	57	55	94	1960	29
Seafood & Lobster	945	53	55	94	2080	28
Meatball	915	44	90	96	2020	42
Steak & Cheese	765	32	80	84	1560	40
Turkey Breast	645	19	65	82	2460	40
Roast Beef	690	23	75	84	2290	42
Ham & Cheese	645	18	70	80	1710	38
Veggies & Cheese	535	18	20	86	1070	20

**Note: Figures based on Italian Roll.
For Honey Wheat Roll (Footlong),
add 30 cals, 2g Fat, 60mg Sodium.**

	CALORIES	FAT grams	CHOLEST. mg	CARBOHYD. grams	SODIUM mg	PROTEIN grams
Fixin's:						
Standard: Tomato	15	0	0	3	0	1
Cheese, 2 slices, 0.8 oz	85	7	20	1	340	4
Olives	15	2	0	0	200	0
Oil	40	5	0	—	0	—
Additional: Mustard	15	1	0	1	200	1
Mayonnaise	100	10	5	0	30	0
Hot Peppers	5	0	0	1	1	0

SUBWAY
(CONT.)

	CALORIES	FAT grams	CHOLEST. mg	CARBOHYD. grams	SODIUM mg	PROTEIN grams
Salads:						

Regular Salad has same meat/cheese and fixin's as Footlong (+ extra lettuce). **Small Salad** has half amount of meat/cheese in regular salad.

	CALORIES	FAT grams	CHOLEST. mg	CARBOHYD. grams	SODIUM mg	PROTEIN grams
Cold Cut Combo: Small	305	25	80	12	910	18
Regular	505	37	160	14	1820	33
Spicy Italian: Small	400	33	70	12	1140	16
Regular	700	60	140	14	2280	30
B.M.T.: Small	370	30	65	12	1200	17
Regular	635	52	130	14	2400	30
Subway Club: Small	225	13	40	12	990	17
Regular	345	19	85	14	1980	32
Tuna: Small	430	37	40	11	380	13
Regular	755	68	85	12	760	23
Seafood & Crab: Small	370	30	30	18	610	10
Regular	640	54	55	25	1230	16
Seafood & Lobster: Small	350	28	30	18	670	9
Regular	600	50	55	25	1340	15
Turkey Breast: Small	200	11	35	12	860	15
Regular	300	16	65	14	1720	27
Roast Beef: Small	220	10	38	13	770	16
Regular	340	20	75	15	1550	29
Ham & Cheese: Small	200	12	35	11	850	14
Regular	300	18	70	12	1710	25
Veggies & Cheese: Regular	190	14	20	12	330	7
Salads & Salad Dressings:						
Blue Cheese	320	28	25	14	580	2
Thousand Island	250	24	20	10	510	0
Lite Italian	25	1	1	4	950	0
French	265	20	1	20	460	0
Creamy Italian	255	26	10	5	550	0
Cookies & Snack Items:						
Cheese Popcorn	150	9	0	14	180	3
Doritos	140	7	0	18	250	2
Fritos; Potato Chips	150	10	0	16	220	1
Cheetos	160	10	0	16	330	1
Cookies: Average	200	9	n.a.	27	90	2
Soda: Pepsi Cola	155	0	0	41	1	0
Diet Pepsi	8	0	0	0	10	0
Lemon-Lime Slice	150	0	0	38	15	0
Mand. Orange; Mountain Dew	170	0	0	44	15	0

TACO BELL	CALORIES	FAT grams	CHOLEST. mg	CARBOHYD. grams	SODIUM mg	PROTEIN grams
Burritos:						
Bean Burrito: Red Sauce	355	10	10	55	880	13
Green Sauce	350	10	10	52	760	13
Beef Burrito: Red Sauce	405	17	55	39	1050	22
Green Sauce	400	17	55	37	920	22
Burrito Supreme: Red Sauce	415	17	30	46	920	17
Green Sauce	410	17	30	45	795	18
Double Beef Burrito:						
Supreme Red Sauce	455	21	55	41	1055	23
Supreme Green Sauce	450	21	55	40	930	23
Miscellaneous:						
Tostada: Red	240	11	15	26	595	9
Green	235	11	15	25	470	9
Enchirito: Red	380	20	55	31	1240	20
Green	370	20	55	28	990	19
Cinnamon Crispas	260	15	1	27	125	3
Pintos & Cheese: Red	190	9	15	18	640	9
Nachos	345	18	10	37	400	7
Nachos Bellgrande	650	35	35	60	995	22
Mexican Pizza	575	36	50	39	1030	21
Tacos:						
Taco	185	10	30	10	275	10
Taco Bellgrande	355	23	55	17	470	18
Taco Light	410	28	55	18	590	19
Soft Taco	230	12	30	18	515	12
Soft Taco Supreme	275	16	30	19	515	12
Super Combo Taco	285	16	40	21	460	14
Taco Salad (with Salsa)	940	61	80	63	1660	36
without Shell	520	31	80	30	1430	30
w/out Shell or Salsa	500	31	80	26	1055	29
Chicken Taco	215	10	45	18	550	13
Steak Taco	220	11	15	18	420	14
Sauces:						
Taco Sauce, packet	2	0	0	0	125	0
Salsa	20	0	0	3	375	1
Ranch Dressing	235	25	35	1	570	2
Jalapeno Peppers	20	0	0	4	1370	1
Sour Cream	45	4	0	1	n.a.	1
Pico De Gallo	5	0	0	1	85	0
Guacamole	35	2	0	3	110	0
Mexi Melt	265	15	40	19	690	13

WENDY'S

	CALORIES	FAT grams	CHOLEST. mg	CARBOHYD. grams	SODIUM mg	PROTEIN grams
Sandwiches:						
Plain Single	340	15	65	30	500	24
Single with Everything	420	21	70	35	890	25
Wendy's Big Classic	570	33	90	47	1085	27
Jr. Hamburger	260	9	34	33	570	15
Jr. Cheeseburger	310	13	35	33	770	18
Jr. Bacon Cheeseburger	430	25	50	32	835	22
Jr. Swiss Deluxe	360	18	40	34	765	18
Kids' Meal Hamburger	260	9	35	32	570	15
Kids' Meal Cheeseburger	300	13	35	33	770	18
Grilled Chicken Fillet	100	3	55	<1	330	18
Grilled Chicken Sandwich	340	13	60	36	815	24
Chicken Breast Fillet	220	10	55	11	400	21
Chicken Sandwich	430	19	60	41	725	26
Chicken Club Sandwich	505	25	70	42	930	30
Fish Fillet Sandwich	460	25	55	42	780	18
¼ lb Hamburger Patty	180	12	65	<1	210	19
Sandwich Toppings:						
American Cheese Slice	70	6	15	<1	260	4
Bacon	30	3	5	<1	100	2
Ketchup	15	<1	0	4	145	<1
Mayonnaise	90	10	10	<1	60	<1
Mustard	4	<1	0	<1	45	<1
Pickles	2	<1	0	<1	200	<1
Honey Mustard	70	6	5	4	170	<1
Tartar Sauce	120	14	15	<1	115	<1
Potatoes, Chili & Nuggets:						
French Fries: Small, 3.2 oz	240	12	0	33	145	3
Large	310	16	0	43	190	4
Biggie Fries	450	23	0	62	270	6
Chili, regular, 9 oz	220	7	45	23	750	21
Chicken Nuggets: 6 pieces	280	20	50	12	600	14
9 pieces	420	30	75	18	900	21
Nugget Sauces: Barbeque	50	<1	0	11	100	<1
Honey	45	<1	0	12	1	<1
Sweet & Sour	45	<1	0	11	55	<1
Sweet Mustard	50	1	0	9	140	<1
Hot Baked Potatoes: Plain	270	<1	0	63	20	6
Bacon & Cheese	520	18	20	70	1460	20
Broccoli & Cheese	400	16	0	58	455	8
Cheese	420	15	10	66	310	8
Chili & Cheese	500	18	25	71	630	15
Sour Cream & Chives	500	23	25	67	125	8

Continued Next Page.

WENDY'S (CONT.)

	CALORIES	FAT grams	CHOLEST. mg	CARBOHYD. grams	SODIUM mg	PROTEIN grams
Salads & SuperBar:						
Prepared Salads: Chef Salad	180	9	120	10	140	15
Garden Salad	100	5	0	9	110	7
Taco Salad	660	37	35	46	1110	40
Salad Dressings:						
Per 1 Tbsp (½ ladle)						
(*)2 oz packet. Multiply by 3.6						
Blue Cheese(*)	10	10	10	<1	105	<1
Celery Seed	70	6	5	3	65	<1
French(*)	60	6	0	4	180	<1
French, Sweet Red	70	6	0	5	125	<1
Hidden Valley Ranch(*)	50	6	5	<1	95	<1
Italian Caesar	80	9	5	<1	140	<1
Italian, Golden	45	4	0	3	250	<1
Salad Oil, 2 Tbsp	250	28	0	0	0	0
Thousand Island(*)	70	7	5	2	105	<1
Wine Vinegar	2	0	0	<1	5	<1
Red. Cal. Bacon/Tom.	45	4	0	3	190	<1
Reduced Calorie Italian	25	2	0	2	185	<1
Superbar – Mexican Fiesta:						
Cheese Sauce, 2 oz	40	2	1	5	305	1
Picante Sauce, 2 oz	20	<1	0	4	5	<1
Refried Beans, 2 oz	70	3	1	10	215	4
Rice, Spanish, 2 oz	70	1	1	13	440	2
Taco Chips, 1½ oz	260	10	0	40	20	4
Taco Meat, 2 oz	110	7	25	4	300	10
Taco Sauce, 1 oz	15	<1	1	3	140	<1
Taco Shells, each	45	3	0	6	45	<1
Tortilla Flour, 1¾ oz	110	3	0	19	220	3
Superbar – Pasta:						
Alfredo Sauce, 2 oz	35	1	1	5	300	1
Fettucini, 2 oz	190	3	10	27	5	4
Garlic Toast, each	70	3	1	9	65	2
Pasta Medley, 2 oz	60	2	1	9	5	2
Rotini, 2 oz	90	2	1	15	1	3
Spaghetti Sauce, 2 oz	30	<1	1	7	345	<1
Spag. Meat Sauce, 2 oz	60	2	10	8	315	4
Garden Spot Salad Bar:						
Applesauce, chunky, 1oz	20	<1	0	6	1	<1
Bacon Bits, ½ oz	40	2	10	<1	350	5
Breadsticks, each	30	1	0	5	30	1
Broccoli, 1½ oz	10	0	0	2	10	1
Cantaloupe, 2 pcs., 2 oz	20	0	0	5	5	<1

WENDY'S (CONT.)

	CALORIES	FAT grams	CHOLEST. mg	CARBOHYD. grams	SODIUM mg	PROTEIN grams
Garden Salad Bar (cont.):						
Cheddar Chips, 1 oz	160	12	5	12	445	3
Cheese, imitation, 1oz	90	6	1	1	125	6
Chicken Salad, ¼ cup	120	8	1	4	215	7
Chow Mein Noodles, ½ oz	75	4	0	8	60	1
Cole Slaw, 2 oz	70	5	5	8	130	<1
Cottage Cheese, 3½ oz	110	4	15	3	425	13
Croutons, ½ oz	60	2	0	8	155	2
Eggs, hard cooked, ¾ oz	30	2	90	<1	25	3
Garbanzo Beans, 1 oz	45	1	0	8	5	3
Green Peas, 1 oz	20	0	0	4	30	1
Honeydew Melon, 2 oz	20	0	0	5	5	<1
Jalapeno Peppers, ½ oz	2	0	0	<1	190	<1
Olives, black, 1 oz	35	3	0	2	245	<1
Parmesan Cheese, 1 oz	130	9	20	1	525	12
Imitation Parmesan, 1 oz	80	3	1	4	410	9
Pasta Salad, ¼ cup, 2 oz	35	<1	0	6	120	2
Peaches, 2 oz	30	0	0	8	5	<1
Pepperoni, sliced, 1 oz	140	12	35	2	435	5
Pineapple, chunks, 3½ oz	60	0	0	16	1	<1
Potato Salad, ¼ cup, 2 oz	125	11	10	6	90	<1
Puddings, 2 oz	90	4	1	12	70	<1
Red Peppers, 1 oz	120	4	0	15	5	5
Seafood Salad, ¼ cup, 2 oz	110	7	1	7	455	4
Sour Topping, 1 oz	60	5	0	2	30	<1
Sunflower Seeds/ Raisins, 1 oz	140	10	0	6	5	5
Three Bean Salad, 2 oz	60	<1	0	13	15	1
Tuna Salad, ¼ cup, 2 oz	100	6	1	4	290	8
Turkey Ham, ¼ cup, 2 oz	70	2	30	<1	550	10
Watermelon, 2 pce., 2 oz	20	0	0	4	1	<1
Desserts & Beverages:						
Frosty Dairy Dessert: Small	400	14	50	59	220	8
Medium	520	18	65	77	290	11
Chocolate Chip Cookie	275	13	15	40	256	3
Cola, small, 8 oz	100	0	0	25	10	0
Diet Cola, small, 8 oz	1	0	0	<1	20	0
Lemon-Lime Soft Drink, small	100	0	0	24	20	0
Hot Chocolate, 6 oz	110	1	1	22	115	2
Lemonade, 8 oz	90	0	0	24	1	0
Milk, Chocolate, 8 oz	160	5	15	24	140	7
Milk, 2%, 8 oz	110	4	20	11	115	8

WHATABURGER

	CALORIES	FAT grams	CHOLEST. mg	CARBOHYD. grams	SODIUM mg	PROTEIN grams
Burgers:						
Whataburger	580	24	70	58	1090	32
Whataburger & Cheese	670	33	95	58	1470	35
Whataburger Jnr.	305	13	30	31	680	14
Whataburger Jnr. & Cheese	350	18	40	30	920	17
Justaburger	265	11	25	28	540	12
Justaburger & Cheese	310	15	35	28	780	15
Whatacatch	475	27	35	43	720	14
Whatacatch & Cheese	520	31	45	43	960	17
Sandwiches:						
Whatachicken Sandwich	670	32	70	61	1460	35
Egg Omelette Sandwich	310	15	190	29	700	14
Mexican:						
Fajita Taco	300	11	55	27	1070	23
Taquito	310	18	220	17	710	18
Taquito & Cheese	355	22	230	17	950	22
Potato and Egg Taquito	310	14	75	35	470	11
Potato & Egg Taq. & Cheese	360	19	85	35	710	13
Miscellaneous:						
French Fries: Small	220	12	1	25	30	4
Regular	330	18	1	37	45	5
Onion Rings	225	13	1	23	410	4
Apple Pie	235	12	1	30	260	3
Blueberry Muffin	265	13	0	34	185	3
Oat Bran Muffin	250	9	0	42	380	5
Pecan Danish	270	16	10	28	420	5
Orange Juice, 6 oz	85	0	0	20	2	1
Vanilla Shake, small	320	9	35	50	170	9

WHITE CASTLE

	CALORIES	FAT grams	CHOLEST. mg	CARBOHYD. grams	SODIUM mg	PROTEIN grams
Cheeseburger	200	11	50	15	360	8
Sandwiches: Chicken	185	7	80	11	500	8
Fish (w/out Tartare)	155	4	80	20	200	6
Sausage	200	12	80	13	400	7
Sausage & Egg	320	17	280	13	650	13
Hamburger	160	8	40	14	250	6
French Fries	300	15	15	37	200	2
Onion Chips	330	13	10	28	600	4
Onion Rings	245	16	10	26	550	3

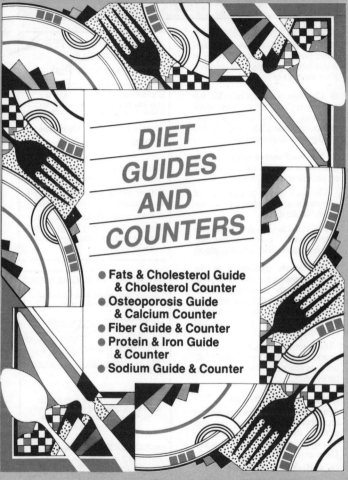

DIET GUIDES AND COUNTERS

- Fats & Cholesterol Guide
  & Cholesterol Counter
- Osteoporosis Guide
  & Calcium Counter
- Fiber Guide & Counter
- Protein & Iron Guide
  & Counter
- Sodium Guide & Counter

Supplement to:
Allan Borushek's Pocket Calorie & Fat Counter
© 1991 Allan Borushek

NOTES ON CHOLESTEROL

● **Cholesterol** is a white waxy substance produced mainly by our liver. It is also found in animal food products. Plant foods have no cholesterol.

● **Cholesterol is essential to life.** It is part of every body cell and is the building block for vitamin D, sex hormones, and bile acids which help in the digestion of dietary fats.

● **The body makes sufficient cholesterol for its needs** and does not rely on cholesterol in the diet.

The body usually produces less of its own cholesterol when there is cholesterol in the diet.

Fats in the diet influence blood cholesterol levels — even more than dietary cholesterol. (See following pages)

● **Too much cholesterol in the blood increases the risk of atherosclerosis** — the thickening and narrowing of arteries that can reduce or block blood flow to the heart muscle, brain, eyes, kidneys, sex organs and other body parts.

This in turn increases the risk of heart attack, stroke, blindness, kidney failure, impotence and other blood circulatory problems.

OTHER RISK FACTORS

Apart from high blood cholesterol levels, **other lifestyle factors** can also increase the risk of atherosclerosis (through damage to the arteries). These include:

- ● **High Blood Pressure**
- ● **Tobacco Smoking**
- ● **Obesity**
- ● **Diabetes (uncontrolled)**

BLOOD CHOLESTEROL LEVELS
— Check Your Risk —

Cholesterol Level (mg per deciliter)	Risk of Heart Attack
Below 200	Desirable
200-239	Borderline High
240 & Above	High Risk

● **Over 50% of American adults** have above desirable blood cholesterol levels.

● **Know your cholesterol level,** particularly if there is a family history of heart disease or stroke. If high, see your doctor for advice.

ARTERY WITH ATHEROSCLEROSIS

Artery is clogged with cholesterol and fatty deposits

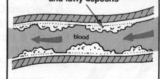

blood

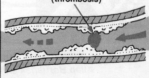

BLOOD CLOT (thrombus) can form on roughened atherosclerotic surface and block blood flow (thrombosis)

POSSIBLE EFFECTS OF ATHEROSCLEROSIS IN ARTERIES AROUND THE BODY

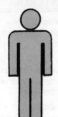

Brain - Stroke

Eyes - Loss of Sight

Heart - Angina Pain
      - Heart Attack

Kidneys - Kidney Failure

Intestines - Cramp, Pain

Sex Organ - Impotence

Legs - Pain on Walking
      - Gangrene

- Atherosclerosis can begin early in life and progress into adulthood.
- No problems may occur until an artery is over 50% blocked. There are usually no warning signs.

CHECK-LIST FOR HEALTHY ARTERIES & BLOOD-FLOW

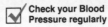 **Check your Blood Pressure regularly**

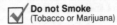 **Do not Smoke** (Tobacco or Marijuana)

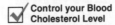 **Control your Blood Cholesterol Level**

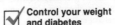 **Control your weight and diabetes**

 Exercise regularly

 Learn to manage stress and anger

WHERE CHOLESTEROL COMES FROM

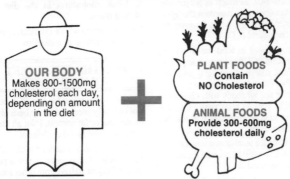

OUR BODY
Makes 800-1500mg cholesterol each day, depending on amount in the diet

+

PLANT FOODS
Contain NO Cholesterol

ANIMAL FOODS
Provide 300-600mg cholesterol daily

- The body makes sufficient cholesterol for its own needs. It does not rely on cholesterol in the diet.
- Fats in the diet can influence blood cholesterol levels as much as dietary cholesterol itself. (Extra notes — see next page.)

EFFECTS OF DIET ON BLOOD CHOLESTEROL

For most people, diet is the most important factor which affects our blood cholesterol level (BCL). Hereditary elevations affect few people. The most important dietary factors are:

● Fats and Oils: The amount and type of fat has the greatest influence on BCL — more so than the actual amount of cholesterol in the diet.

Saturated fats (mainly in fatty meats, butter and high-fat dairy products) tend to raise blood cholesterol.

Mono- and polyunsaturated fats (mainly in plant seeds and oils, nuts, avocados, olives and oily fish) tend to lower BCL and/or other blood fats.

Note: While monounsaturated fats (e.g. in olive and canola oils, avocados) do not lower BCL as much as polyunsaturated fats/oils, they maintain the 'good' cholesterol (HDL), while lowering the 'bad' cholesterol (LDL).

● Cholesterol in food has a variable response on BCL from person to person. For most, it depends on the types of fats and fiber eaten at the same meal.

While not all foods with cholesterol (e.g. fish, yogurt) need raise BCL, it is prudent to limit cholesterol in the diet to 300mg daily.

Note: Even if a meal contains no cholesterol, BCL can still be raised if the meal is high in saturated fat.

● Fiber: Certain types of fiber may lower BCL — particularly the soluble fiber of fruits, vegetables, dried beans and peas, oat bran and psyllium. Rice bran, nuts and seeds are also effective.

HINTS TO CONTROL BLOOD CHOLESTEROL

1. Maintain a healthy weight.
If overweight, lose weight. Plan meals carefully. Exercise regularly.

2. Avoid high-fat foods.
Look for lower fat alternatives. Trim fat off meats and poultry. Limit all types of fats and oils. Use low-fat cooking.

3. Reduce saturated fat intake.
Avoid butter, lard, fatty meats, high-fat dairy products. Use polyunsaturated margarines and oils, and olive or canola oils, in controlled amounts as part of a low-fat diet.

4. Eat more fresh fruit, vegetables, wholegrain breads and cereals.
Introduce regular vegetarian dishes with dried beans, (including baked beans), lentils and chick peas.

5. Limit cholesterol in the diet to 300mg daily.

Note: For extra advice on dietary planning, seek referral to a dietitian.

IT IS THE TOTAL DIET THAT COUNTS

The effect of any one food on BCL cannot be totally predicted on the basis of its cholesterol or fat content. (Not all saturated fats raise blood cholesterol.)

One must also consider the effects of other dietary components within a particular food, or indeed from other foods eaten at the same meal.

Most persons can expect a low-fat/low-cholesterol diet to lower their blood cholesterol levels by 10-20%.

REDUCING DIETARY FATS

● **Fats in the diet** are essential for good health, but too much fat can be unhealthy. Fat is a concentrated source of calories (1 gram fat = 9 calories; 1 gram protein/carbohydrate = 4 calories).

● **Excess fats contribute to obesity** and a subsequent greater risk of heart disease, high blood pressure, diabetes, gall stones and other problems.

● **Even without obesity**, a high-fat diet increases the risk of cancer of the breast and colon, and atherosclerosis.

● **Dietary fat is more readily converted** and stored as body fat, compared to carbohydrate and protein. Thus, a low-fat diet is best for weight control.

FINDING HIDDEN FAT

Detecting fat in food is difficult. The taste of fat is hidden by other flavors and textures.

EXAMPLES — Grams of Fat

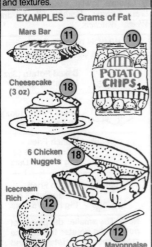

Mars Bar — 11
Potato Chips — 10
Cheesecake (3 oz) — 18
6 Chicken Nuggets — 18
Icecream Rich — 12
Mayonnaise 1 Tbsp — 12

RECOMMENDED FAT INTAKE

● **Americans consume too much fat.** Around 40% of total calories is consumed as fat. A range of 20-30% is considered much healthier (equivalent to 22-33 grams fat/1000 calories).

MAXIMUM DESIRABLE FAT INTAKE

	FAT	%Fat Cals
1200 Calories —	30g	(22.5%)
1500 Calories —	40g	(24%)
2000 Calories —	60g	(27%)
2500 Calories —	80g	(29%)
3000 Calories —	100g	(30%)

Note: At lower calorie levels, the percent of fat calories should decrease to allow for protein calories (which have nutritional priority).

PERCENTAGE OF CALORIES FROM FAT (% Fat Calories)

Knowing the percent fat calories of foods may be useful in spotting high-fat foods.

However, it is **not** implied nor even recommended that you eat only those foods less than 20-30% fat calories. Some higher fat foods such as avocados, nuts and seeds, are nutritious and can even help to lower blood cholesterol. **Moderation** is the aim ... **not elimination.**

Formula for percent fat calories:

$$\frac{\text{Grams of Fat/Serving} \times 9}{\text{Total Calories/Serving}} \times \frac{100}{1}$$

Example: Mars Bar (11g fat; 240 cals)
Percent of Calories from Fat

$$= \frac{11 \times 9}{240} \times \frac{100}{1} = 41\%$$

— HINTS TO REDUCE FAT & CHOLESTEROL —

Meats & Poultry

● **Choose** lean cuts of meat with little marbling. **Choose** the white meat of chicken and turkey, and extra lean ground beef. **Avoid** organ meats.

● **Trim all visible fat** from meat, and remove the skin from poultry.

● **Eat modest portions** (3-4 oz ckd) of meat, poultry or fish. Add extra beans, lentils, vegetables, potatoes, rice.

● **Avoid** high-fat meat products; e.g. salami, bacon, sausage, frankfurters. **Choose** lean luncheon meats (90% or more fat-free).

● **Broil or bake. Avoid** frying. Allow casseroles to cool and skim off any surface fat.

Fish & Seafoods

● **Choose** fresh or frozen fillets, canned fish (in water pack). Limit shrimp and squid (higher in cholesterol).

● **Avoid** fried fish, frozen fish in batter, canned fish in oil.

Eggs & Egg Substitutes

● **Limit** egg-yolks to 3 weekly. **Avoid** if blood cholesterol is very high.

● Egg-whites and egg substitutes (e.g. *Egg Beaters*) are suitable.

Fats & Oils

● Use **minimal amounts** of all types of fat and oil. All are high calories.

● **Avoid** butter, lard, dripping, ghee, margarine (other than polyunsaturated). **Avoid** coconut oil and hydrogenated palm oil products. (Plain palm oil does not raise blood cholesterol.)

● **Choose** fat-reduced polyunsaturated or canola margarines. Use polyunsaturated oils or monounsaturated oils (e.g. *Canola*, olive) in moderation.

Salad Dressings

● **Limit** mayonnaise, and oil dressings. **Choose** low-oil or no-oil dressings (e.g. *Hidden Valley Ranch, Kraft Free, Pritikin*). Note: Oil in dressing is polyunsaturated.

Milk & Dairy Products

● **Choose** lowfat and skim milk; and yogurts. **Avoid** full-cream milk, cream, Half & Half, coffee creamers.

● **Choose** lowfat and fat-reduced cheeses; (e.g. cottage, part-skim ricotta. Cheese substitutes with no cholesterol can still be high in fat.

● **Icecream: Choose** lowfat ice milks, frozen yogurt, sorbet, sherbet and ices. **Limit** regular icecream to a small serving. **Avoid** rich high-fat icecreams.

Frozen Entrees & Meals

● **Choose** lowfat varieties, such as *Lean Cuisine, Healthy Choice* and *Weight Watchers.*

WHICH IS THE BEST FAT-SAVING CHOICE?

 Baked Potato (3oz) Nil Fat/65 Cals

 Roast Potato (3oz) 8g Fat/155 Cals

 French Fries (Large Cut) 3 oz 12g Fat/220 Cals

 French Fries (Small Cut) 3 oz 15g Fat/275 Cals

Note: The smaller the pieces of potato, the greater the surface area exposed to fats/oils; and the greater the fat and calories.

— HINTS TO REDUCE FAT & CHOLESTEROL —

Breads, Bagels & Crackers

● All breads are **suitable** as well as pita, bagels, English muffins and rice cakes. **Avoid** croissants, sweet rolls, danish pastry and doughnuts. **Avoid** fat-soaked toast and garlic bread.

● **Choose** lowfat crackers such as graham, saltines, matzo, bread sticks, rye crispbreads and zweiback. **Avoid** cheese or butter crackers.

Breakfast Cereals, Pasta, Rice

● Most cold and hot cereals are low in fat with nil cholesterol. **Avoid** granola made with hydrogenated oils.

● **Choose** plain pasta or rice. **Avoid** dishes made with cream, butter or cheese sauces. **Limit** egg noodles.

Fruits & Vegetables

● **Choose** all types. **Limit** olives and avocado if overweight. (**Avocados** contain no cholesterol. Their fat and fiber can help lower blood cholesterol.) Use mashed avocado on bread in place of fat.

● **Choose** dried beans, lentils, chick peas, baked beans.

● **Avoid** french-fried potatoes and regular potato salad. **Avoid** vegetables made in butter, cream or sauce.

● **Avoid** deli-style salads made with high-fat dressings.

Snacks, Cookies & Candy

● **Avoid** high-fat snacks such as potato chips, corn/tortilla chips, *Chee-Tos, Cheez Balls,* buttered popcorn, chocolate and carob bars.

● **Choose** plain popcorn, lowfat cookies and muffins, hard candy, jelly beans, fruit rolls and frozen fruit bars/popsicles.

● **Choose** fresh and dried fruits, vegetables. **Limit** nuts and seeds.

● **Choose** lowfat vegetable or noodle soups. *Cup-A-Soup* is also suitable.

Desserts/Sweets

● **Avoid** high-fat desserts, e.g. fruit pies, pastries, cheesecake, cheese board.

● **Choose** fresh fruits, fruit salad, low-fat custard, yogurt, frozen yogurt, sorbet. Use yogurt in place of cream.

Cooking Methods

● **Choose** cooking methods that require minimal fat or oil; e.g. microwaving, broiling, steaming, baking. **Use** non-stick pans and sprays (e.g. *Pam*).

● **Adapt** recipes to use minimal fat and oil.

Fast-Foods

● **Deli's: Choose** sandwiches/bread-rolls, pitas with lowfat fillings and plain salad. **Limit** meat/cheese to small portions. **Avoid** high-fat deli salads. **Choose** plain salads and fresh fruit.

● **Chicken & Fish: Avoid** deep-fried chicken or fish, BBQ chicken with fat and skin, chicken nuggets. **Choose** broiled or baked chicken breast without fat or skin.

● **Hamburgers: Choose** medium size or lowfat (e.g. *McLean*). **Avoid** bacon. Have a side salad (without dressing).

● **Pizzas: Avoid** sausage/pepperoni. **Choose** vegetarian topping and modest quantity of cheese. Eat a moderate serving. Eat extra salad and fruit.

● **French Fries: Avoid** french fries, fried onion rings. **Choose** whole roast potatoes, salad, coleslaw, bean salad, corn, peas.

● **Desserts: Avoid** apple pie, danish, choc-chip cookies. **Choose** lowfat muffins (e.g. *McDonald's*). **Avoid** regular shakes, sundaes. **Choose** lowfat milk, lowfat shakes (e.g. *McDonald's*), frozen yogurt, fruit salad, orange juice.

CHOLESTEROL COUNTER

MEATS, POULTRY

	CHOL (mg)
Average all types	
Lean Meat: Raw, 4 oz	70
Cooked, 4 oz (from 5-6 oz raw)	95
Fatty Meat: Raw, 4 oz	80
Cooked, 4 oz (from 5-6 oz raw)	105
Fat: thick strip, 2 oz	35

(Note: While lean meat and fat have similar amounts of cholesterol, choose lean meat to limit fat intake.)

Chicken: (roasted; with or without skin)	
White meat, 4 oz	95
Dark meat, 4 oz	105
Turkey: Light meat, 4 oz	85
Dark meat, 4 oz	100
Organ Meats:	
Liver: Chicken, ½ cup	440
Beef, fried, 4 oz	550
Kidneys, beef, 3 oz	330
Brains, beef, pan-fried, 3 oz	1700
Tongue, lamb's, ½ cup, 4 oz	150
Bacon: cooked, 3 slices, ¾ oz	16
Sausages: Frankfurter, 1½ oz	23
Pork Link, 1 oz	11
Bologna, 2 sl, 2 oz	30
Salami, 2 sl., 2 oz	37
Luncheon Meats: Hams, 2 oz	30
Average all types, 2 oz	30

FISH & SHELLFISH

Fish Fillets, average, cooked, 4 oz	70
Tuna/Salmon, canned, 3 oz	30
Scallops, 9 medium, 3 oz	30
Shrimp, raw, 3 oz (12 large)	130
Oysters, raw, 6 med., 3 oz	45
Lobster; Crab, raw, 3 oz	80
Fish Sticks, 3 sticks	80
Cod Liver Oil, 1 Tbsp, ½ oz	75

EGGS

Chicken, 1 large egg	215
Omelet, 2 eggs, plain	450
Egg Yolk, 1 large	215
Egg White	0
Egg Substitutes (*Egg Beaters*)	0

MILK, YOGURT, CHEESE

	CHOL (mg)
Milk: Whole, 1 cup, 8 fl. oz	33
2% fat, 1 cup	18
Skim, 1 cup	55
Buttermilk, 1 cup	10
Soymilk, 1 cup	0
Yogurt: Nonfat, 8 oz	<5
Lowfat, plain/flavored, 8 oz	<20
Cheese: Natural/Hard, aver., 1 oz	25-30
Cream Cheese, 1 oz	30
Process Cheese, aver., 1 oz	15
Cheese Spreads, aver., 1 oz	20
Cottage, lowfat, 4 oz	5
creamed, 4 oz	17
Ricotta, part-skim, 4 oz	25
whole milk, 4 oz	60
Cheese Dips, average, 1 oz	<10

ICECREAM & FROZEN DESSERTS

Icecream, regular, ½ cup	30
rich (16% fat), ½ cup	45
Ice Milk, hard, ½ cup	10
Frozen Yogurt, Sherbet, ½ cup	<10
Fruit Ice/Popsicle, *Tofutti*	0

FATS, OILS, DRESSINGS

Butter: 2 Tbsp, 1 oz	60
Butter Blend, 2 Tbsp	10
Lard, Beef Tallow, 2 T., 1 oz	25
Margarine: all types	0
Oils, vegetable	0
Mayonnaise, 1 Tbsp	<10
Salad Dressings, French, Italian	0
Blue Ch., Creamy, Thousand Isl, 1T	<5
Coleslaw, 1 Tbsp	<10
Cream: Heavy, Whipping, 2 T., 1 oz	40
Light/Coffee, 2 T, 1 oz	20
Half & Half; Sour, 2 T., 1 oz	10
Pressurized, whipped, ¼ cup	10
Non-dairy topping	0
Creamers (e.g. *Coffee Mate*)	0

FROZEN ENTREES/MEALS

Lean Cuisine:	
Beef/Chicken/Fish base	80-100
Vegetable/Pasta/Rice base	25-50
French Bread Pizzas	20-40
Pasta Salads	20-70
Healthy Choice, average	40-60
Morton Dinners, average	35-60
Patio Mexican Dinners, average	30-40
Weight Watchers, average	50-70
Pizzas, per serving	35-45

FAST-FOODS
See Fast-Foods Section

	CHOL (mg)
BREAD, CEREALS	
Bread, Bagels, average all types	0
Breakfast Cereals, Oatmeal, Granola	0
SPAGHETTI, PASTA, NOODLES, RICE	
Macaroni/Pasta, plain	0
Spaghetti, canned, w/meatballs, 1 c.	20
Spaghetti Sauce, meatless	0
meat flavored, ½ cup	<5
Egg Noodles, ckd, 1 cup	50
Rice, plain	0
Fried Rice, w/egg/shrimp/pork, 1 cup	60
COOKIES, CAKES, SWEETS	
Cookies, average, 1 pce	<5
Croissant	15
Doughnut, average	20
Muffin, average	25
Pancakes, 3 x 4″	50
Waffle, 7″	100
Apple Pie, 1 serving	<10
Lemon Meringue Pie (⅛ of 9″ pie)	140
Cheesecake, 4 oz	120
Pecan Pie, frozen (⅛ of 9″ pie)	30
Pound Cake, 1 slice	60
Angel Food Cake	0
Gelatin	0
Chocolate Mousse, ½ cup	30
Custard, egg, ½ cup	230
SNACKS, CANDY	
Beef Jerky, average, 1 oz	20
Cheetos, cheese-flavored	0
Corn Chips, Tortilla Chips	0
Crackers: cheese-filled, each	5
Peanut Butter filled, each	0
Chocolate, 1 oz	5
Hard Candy, Life Savers, Gum, Carob	0
Granola Bars, Pretzels	0
Popcorn, plain/microwave	0
Potato Chips	0
FRUIT, VEGETABLES, NUTS, SEEDS	0
Avocado, Olives	0
French Fried Potatoes	<10
Dried Beans & Peas, Tofu	0
Baked Beans in Tom. Sce	0
Veges w/Cheese/Cream Sce	10-30
BEVERAGES	
Coffee, Tea, Soda, Beer, Wine, Alcohol	0

BENEFITS OF FISH OILS

Eating fish regularly (several times weekly) may benefit our heart and general health.

Fish oils are rich in **omega-3 fatty acids** (E.P.A. and D.H.A.). They are highly polyunsaturated fats that may lessen the risk of both atherosclerosis and unwanted blood clots (thrombosis).

They can also decrease triglyceride blood fats, and lessen the inflammation of arthritis and psoriasis.

Although fish contains cholesterol, the oil in fish **prevents** any increase in blood cholesterol — providing the fish is not fried in animal or hydrogenated vegetable fats.

As little as **0.5-1 gram/day** of omega-3 f.a's may be beneficial.

Plant Sources: Some omega-3 f.a.'s are found in kale, purslane, green beans, walnuts, soybeans, linseed, soybean lecithin, tofu, seaweed, canola oil, wheatgerm oil.

OMEGA-3 FATTY ACIDS IN FISH (Per 4 oz, Raw)

High Content (Approx. 2g)
Herring, Mackerel, Sablefish, Sardines
Salmon (Chinook), Trout (lake), Tuna

Medium Content (1-2g)
Anchovy, Bluefish,
Salmon (Pink/Red/Coho/Chinook)

Fair Content (0.4-1g)
Bass, Catfish, Cod, Grouper, Hake, Halibut, Kingfish, Mullet (striped), Perch (White/Yellow), Pollock, Shark, Trout (Rainbow), Tuna (Skipjack), Crab, Oysters, Blue Mussel, Shrimp, Squid

Least (Less than 0.4g)
Eel, Flounder, Haddock, Ocean Perch, Pike, Red Snapper, Sole, Swordfish, Lobster, Clams.

OSTEOPOROSIS GUIDE

CALCIUM'S ROLE IN THE BODY

Calcium plays a vital role in nerve and muscle function, clotting of blood, enzyme regulation, insulin secretion and overall bone strength. Bones and teeth store 99% of the body's calcium.

The calcium level in blood is kept at a steady level by the continual exchange of calcium between blood and bone. When insufficient calcium is obtained from food the body draws calcium out of the bones.

This bone loss over a period of years may lead to **osteoporosis — thinning of the bones** (literally 'porous bones').

The bones may become weak, brittle and easy to fracture, particularly the bones of the wrist, hips and spine. Loss of height and curvature of the spine may also result, as may periodontal disease — the deterioration of the jaw bones that support the teeth.

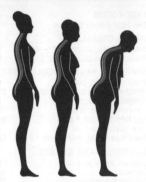

As osteoporosis progresses after menopause, vertebrae may collapse causing spine to curve and shoulders to hunch.

COMMON IN WOMEN

Women are particularly vulnerable to osteoporosis (1 in 4 by age 60). They have about **30% less bone than men** and also a greater bone loss after menopause due to a decrease in estrogen hormone levels.

Unless dietary calcium needs are adequate during pregnancy and breastfeeding, calcium bone reserves will be drawn upon and the bones will be even more susceptible to osteoporosis. By the time a woman reaches her eighties she can have lost up to two thirds of her skeleton.

Slender framed people with less bone are at a greater risk of osteoporosis — particularly women after the menopause.

CAUSES OF OSTEOPOROSIS

The major factors associated with the bone loss of osteoporosis appear to be:

- hormone changes of menopause
- insufficient calcium in the diet
- insufficient exercise.

Other contributing factors may include: excess alcohol, excess phosphorus (from meats and soft drinks), caffeine, insufficient vitamin D, prolonged use of aluminium containing antacids, and smoking.

RECOMMENDED DAILY INTAKE OF CALCIUM (mg)		
Infants:	0-6 mths	**360mg**
	6-12 mths	**540mg**
Children:	1-10 yrs	**800mg**
	10-12 yrs	**1200mg**
Teenagers:	13-18 yrs	**1200mg**
Adults:	19+ yrs	**800mg**
Women: Pre-menopausal		**1000mg**
Menopausal (beginning)		**1200mg**
Post-menopausal		**1500mg**
Pregnancy/Breast-feeding:		
	10-18 yrs	**1600mg**
	19+ yrs	**1200mg**

IMPORTANCE OF EARLY PREVENTION

Gradual loss of bone usually begins in the thirties after maximum bone mass is reached. The stronger the bones at that time, the less trouble is likely to occur later. **There are often no symptoms of bone loss** and 30-40 years may pass before the first fracture occurs. The earlier that prevention or treatment begins, the greater the benefit. The key to prevention is to build strong, dense bones.

Young women may lessen the risk by eating high-calcium foods and taking regular exercise. This helps to increase the density and strength of bones.

Hormone therapy as well as calcium supplements and exercise, may help to retard osteoporosis. Your doctor will advise you.

Note: While **dietary calcium cannot reverse age-related bone loss**, it may help to slow down the process.

DIETARY SOURCES OF CALCIUM

Milk, yogurt and cheese are the richest sources of calcium. **Canned fish** with edible bones (salmon, tuna, sardines) are high in calcium. **Tofu** (soybean curd), green vegetables such as **broccoli** and cabbage, and **dried beans** are also good sources.

Dieters and others concerned with fat and cholesterol may still consume lowfat and nonfat dairy products. Skim milk and lowfat milk and yogurt contain as much calcium as whole milk.

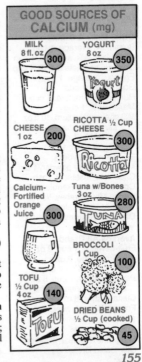

GOOD SOURCES OF CALCIUM (mg)

MILK 8 fl. oz — 300

YOGURT 8 oz — 350

CHEESE 1 oz — 200

RICOTTA ½ Cup CHEESE — 300

Calcium-Fortified Orange Juice — 300

Tuna w/Bones 3 oz — 280

BROCCOLI 1 Cup — 100

TOFU ½ Cup 4 oz — 140

DRIED BEANS ½ Cup (cooked) — 45

EXTRA NOTES

- Persons who have difficulty eating sufficient calcium-rich foods should consider a **calcium supplement**. People with kidney stones should check with their doctor before significantly increasing calcium intake. Drink plenty of water to flush the kidneys. Take calcium with a meal for best absorption.

- **Excess calcium** (over 3000 mg daily) can interfere with iron absorption.

- Once body calcium needs have been met **extra amounts of calcium give no extra benefit.** For example, bones are not further strengthened.

- Factors which **decrease calcium absorption** or retention include: excess protein, fat and salt; too little vitamin D; too little exercise; smoking; hormonal changes of menopause.

CALCIUM COUNTER

Daily Calcium Requirements — See Previous Page.
Calcium Counter figures are rounded off for ease of use.

MILK & MILK DRINKS	Calcium (mg)
Milk, Fluid:	
Whole, 1 cup, 8 fl.oz	30
1 glass, 6 fl.oz	220
Lowfat, 1 cup, 8 fl.oz	300
Skim, 1 cup, 8 fl.oz	300
Hi-Calcium (Borden), 1 cup	1000
Viva, w. extra Calcium, 1 cup	500
Condensed Milk, sweet, 1 fl.oz	110
Evaporated Milk, Skim, 1 fl.oz	90
Whole/Lowfat, 1 fl.oz	80
Dry/Powder, Whole, ¼ cup	290
Skim/Nonfat, ¼ cup	380
Other Milks & Drinks	
Buttermilk, average, 1 cup	300
Chocolate Milk, average, 1 cup	300
Cocoa/Chocolate w. Milk, 1 cup	300
Eggnog, average, 1 cup	300
Goat's Milk, 1 cup	320
Human Milk, mature, 1 cup	80
Malted Milk, 1 cup	350
Milkshakes: Medium, 10 fl.oz	280
Large, 15 fl.oz	450
Soybean Milk, 1 cup	60
Dry/Powder, 1 oz	80
Milk Drink Powders	
Malted Milk, dry powder, 1 oz	80
Chocolate, Instant, 3 Tbsp	10
Cocoa Powder: Regular, 1 Tbsp	10
Cocoa Mix: Hershey, ⅓ cup	40
Alba High Calcium, 1 envel.	320
Other Beverages: Page 160.	

YOGURT	Calcium (mg)
Average All Brands	
Fruit-flavored, 1 cup, 8 oz	350
Small Cup, 6 oz	250
4½ oz Cup	230
Plain: Average, 1 cup, 8 oz	350
Dannon, Nonfat/Lowfat, 8 oz	430
Custard-style, 6 oz	200
Frozen Yogurt, aver., ½ cup	100

FATS/OILS	Calcium (mg)
Butter, Lard, Fats	Negl
Margarine, Regular/Imitation	Negl
Oils, Salad Dressings	Negl

CREAM	Calcium (mg)
Average: Unwhipped, 1 Tbsp	15
Whipped, 1 heaping Tbsp	15
Half & Half, 1 Tbsp	15
Non-dairy Creamers, 1 tsp	Negl

ICE CREAM/ICE MILKS	Calcium (mg)
Ice Cream, regular, 1 scoop	65
½ cup	90
Premium, 1 serve, 4 oz	150
Soft Serve, ½ cup	120
Ice Milk, average, ½ cup	100
Sherbet, average, ½ cup	50
Fruit Sorbet	0
Sundae, regular, 6 fl.oz	200
Tofu Ices, average, ½ cup	10

CHEESE: Per 1 oz (1¼" cube)	Calcium (mg)
Natural, Hard: Average 1 oz	200
Process Cheese: Aver. 1 oz	150
Single-wrapped, ¾ oz	120
Cheese Substitutes: Aver. 1 oz	200
Specific Cheeses: Blue, 1 oz	150
Brie	50
Camembert	110
Cheddar	200
Cottage Cheese, ½ cup	60
Cream Cheese, e.g. Philadelphia	20
Dorman's Light, average 1 oz	200
Edam, Gouda	200
Feta	140
Gruyere	290
Kraft Light Naturals, aver.	250
Light-Line (Borden), singles	200
Monterey	210
Mozzarella, average	170
Muenster	200
Parmesan, grated, 1 Tbsp	70
Processed, average	160
Provolone	210
Ricotta, lowfat, ½ cup	330
Swiss	270
Cheese Dishes: Souffle, 4 oz	240
Macaroni & Cheese, 1 cup, 8 oz	150
Ham & Cheese Crepes, 8 oz	350
Quiche, 1 serve, 6 oz	200

EGGS	Calcium (mg)
1 large Egg	30
Scrambled, w. Milk	50
Omelet, w. Cheese (½ oz)	120

FISH & SEAFOODS
Canned Fish:

Salmon, with bones, 3 oz	190
Sardines, with bones, 3 oz	300
Tuna, with bones, 3 oz	280
If bones discarded, 3 oz	40
Fresh Fish: cooked, aver. 4 oz	35
Lobster, cooked, 4 oz	60
Mussels/Oysters, (10), 4 oz	95
Crabmeat, cooked, 4 oz	50

MEATS & POULTRY

Average all types, cooked, 4 oz	20

SOUPS: Average all types

No Milk or Cheese added	30
with Milk, ½ cup, 1 serve	180

SAUCES

Average all kinds, 1 Tbsp	10
Cheese/White Sauce, 2 Tbsp	40

SPICES & HERBS

Average all types, 1 tsp	5-20

BREAD, BAGELS

Bread: White, 1 slice	30
Wholewheat, Rye, 1 slice	30
Bagels, average	30
Buns/Rolls: Small	40
Large	90
Muffins, average	40
Pita, 6½″ diameter, 2 oz	50
Tortillas, Corn, 1 oz	40

BREAKFAST CEREALS
Ready To Eat:

Average all types, 1 oz	20
with ½ cup Milk	170
Hot Type, cooked:	
Corn (Hominy) Grits, 1 cup	Negl
Cream of Wheat, 1 cup	50
Malt-O-Meal, 1 cup	5
Oatmeal/Rolled Oats:	
Regular, non-fortif., 1 cup	20
Instant, fortified, 1 pkt	100

Note: Cereals are a good medium for calcium-rich milk (150 mg/½ cup).

FLOURS, GRAINS, PASTA	Calcium (mg)
Wheat Flour: All-purpose, 1 cup	20
Self-rising, 1 cup	330
Whole-wheat, 1 cup	50
Carob Flour, 1 cup, 3½ oz	360
Corn meal, 1 cup, 4 oz	20
Soybean Flour, 1 cup, 3 oz	170
Grains, Barley, Rice, average:	
Cooked, 1 cup	15
Macaroni, Noodles, cookd, 1 cup	15
Macaroni & Cheese, aver., 1 cup	150
Pasta, Spaghetti, average:	
Cooked, 1 cup	15
Lasagne, average, 1 serve	300
Spaghetti w. Meat Sce, 1 serve	20
with 1 Tbsp Parmesan	90

SUGAR & SYRUPS

Sugar: White	0
Brown, 1 Tbsp	10
Syrups: Per 2 Tbsp, 1 oz	
Choc., Thin type, 2 Tbsp	5
Fudge type, 2 Tbsp	40
Molasses: Light, 2 Tbsp	70
Blackstrap, 2 Tbsp	270
Table Syrup, 2 Tbsp	0

HONEY, JAM, JELLY
Contain neglible calcium.

COOKIES & CAKES

Cookies: Aver. all types, 1 only	5
Crackers, average, 1 only	5
Cake:	
Plain, average, 2 oz	40
Carrot Cake with Icing	45
Cheesecake, 1 piece	80
Fruitcake, 1 piece	40
Croissants, average, 2 oz	20
Danish Pastry, average, 2 oz	60
Donuts, average, 2 oz	20
Muffins: Regular, aver. 1½ oz	40
English Muffins, 2 oz	90
Pancakes, 4″ diam. aver., 1 oz	40
Pies:	
Apple/Fruit, average, 5 oz	20
Custard Pie, average, 5 oz	140
Pecan Pie, 1 piece, 5 oz	70
Pumpkin Pie, 1 piece, 5 oz	80
Waffles, 7″ diam. average	160

CALCIUM COUNTER (CONT)

DESSERTS	Calcium (mg)
Custard, average, ½ cup	150
Gelatin, plain w. water, ½ cup	2
Puddings: Canned, aver., 5 oz	80
Dry Mix, made w. milk, ½ cup	150
Rice Pudding: ½ cup	120
Snack Can, 5 oz	60
Pancakes, 4″ diam., 2	120

CANDY	
Chocolate: Milk	
Plain/Fruit, 1 oz	50
with Almonds, 1 oz	65
Kit Kat Wafer, 1½ oz	80
Mars Bar	80
Milky Way Bar, 2 oz	60
Carob Bar, average, 2 oz	220
Plain Candy, uncoated, 1 oz	Negl
Jelly Beans, M'shmallow, 1 oz	Negl

SNACKS	
Breakfast Bars (Carnation)	20
Corn Chips, 1 oz	40
Granola Bars, average	30
Popcorn, 1 cup	Negl
Potato Chips, 1 oz	10
Tortilla Chips, 1 oz	40

NUTS & SEEDS (Shelled)	
Almonds, 12-15 nuts, ½ oz	40
Brazil Nuts, 4 medium, ½ oz	30
Cashews, 6-8 nuts, ½ oz	5
Coconut, fresh, ½ oz	5
Filberts (Hazelnuts), ½ oz	40
Macadamias, 6 medium, ½ oz	10
Peanuts, raw, 1 oz	25
Seeds: Pumpkin, 1 oz	15
Sesame, 1 Tbsp	10
Sunflower, 1 oz	30
Tahini, 1 Tbsp, ½ oz	20
Walnuts, 1 oz	20

BEVERAGES	
Beer, Cider, Wine, 1 glass	8
Spirits, 1 fl.oz	0
Coffee, Tea	Negl
Soft Drinks, regular/low cal.	Negl
Fruit Ades, Punches	Negl
Water: Tap, average, 1 cup	5
Perrier, 1 glass, 6 oz	20

FRUIT	Calcium (mg)
Fresh Fruit:	
Average all types, 1 serve	20
Apple, 1 medium	10
Avocado, 1 medium	20
Banana, 1 medium	10
Orange, 1 medium	50
Pear, 1 medium	20
Rhubarb, cooked, ½ cup	170
(calcium largely not available to body)	
Dried Fruit: Average, 1 oz	20
Figs, 3 medium, 2 oz	80
Fruit Juice: Average, 1 cup	25
Orange Juice, calcium fortified (e.g. Citrus Hill Plus Calcium, Minute Maid), 1 cup, 8 fl.oz	300

VEGETABLES	
Average all types, ½ cup	20
1 cup	40
Higher Calcium Content:	
Beans, dried: cookd, ½ cup	50
Baked/Refried Beans, ½ cup	60
Broccoli, chopped, 1 cup	100
Chickpeas, boiled, ½ cup	40
Collards, cooked, 1 cup	150
Dandelion Greens, cooked, 1 cup	150
Kale, 1 cup	130
Mustard Greens, 1 cup	100
Potato, plain, 1 large	20
Au Gratin, 1 cup	200
Mashed w/Milk, 1 cup	60
Spinach, cooked, ½ cup	120
Soybeans, cooked, ½ cup, 3 oz	90

TOFU, MISO, TEMPEH	
Tofu: Hinoichi, regular, 4 oz	140
Nasoya, firm, 4 oz	100
Soft (Hinoichi/Nasoya), 4 oz	190
Silken (Mori Nu), 4 oz	40

CALCIUM SUPPLEMENTS	
Caltrate 600, 1 tablet	600
Cal-Sup, 1 tablet	300
Citracal, 1 tablet	200
Mature Essentials, 1 tablet	600
Os-cal, 1 tablet	500
Ostal, 1 tablet	500
Postare Calcium, 1 tablet	600
Shaklee (Non-chewable), 1 tab.	400
Tums, 1 tablet	200

FROZEN ENTREES/MEALS

	Calcium (mg)
Budget Gourmet Light:	
Chicken Au Gratin; Linguini	100
Cheese Ravioli; Lasagne	250
Cheese Lasagne w/Vegetables	300
Healthy Choice: Chick. Parmig.	100
Chicken & Pasta Divan	150
Fettucini Alfredo; Lasagne	100
Le Menu: Beef Sirloin/Strogan.	100
Manicotti, Cheese (Entree)	400
Chicken Florentine/Parmigiana	150
Light Style: Turkey Dinner	100
Chicken Cacciatore	100
3-Cheese Stuffed Shells	150
Lean Cuisine:	
Chse. Cannelloni; Z'cchini Lasag.	300
Enchanadas: Beef/Bean; Chick.	150
Filet of Fish: Divan	200
Florentine; Jardiniere	150
Lasagne/Meat; Rigatoni Bake	200
Salisbury Steak; Turkey Dijon	150
French Pizzas: Extra Cheese	500
Chse., Deluxe, Pepper., Saus.	250
Nasoya: Vegetable Lasagne	150
Stuffed Shells (2); Manicotti (2)	160
Mexican Enchil.; Shells Provenc.	200
Stouffers: Tortellini (Cheese Alfr.)	
Ch. Enchiladas; Veg. Lasagne	600
Chicken Divan; Ham & Asparag.	200
Chick. Enchil.; Tortell./Tom. Sce	300
Lasagne; Fiesta Lasagne	250
Swanson: Beef Enchiladas	150
Entrees: Lasag., Macaroni & Ch.	450
Salisbury Steak	250
Scalloped Potatoes & Ham	300
Weight Watchers: Beef Enchil.	250
Chicken a la King; Brd. Chicken	150
Chicken Fettucini; Veal Patty	200
Filet of Fish Au Gratin	150
Broccoli/Cheese Baked Potato	300
Cheese Enchiladas Ranchero	500
Ch. Manicotti; Pasta Rigati/Prim.	300
Lasagne w. Meat Sce/Garden	400
Pizza: Cheese; Pepperoni; Saus.	400
French Bread: Average	400

FAST FOODS, RESTAURANTS

	Calcium (mg)
Chicken: Grilled/BBQ, ¼ chicken	20
Battered & Fried, 2 pieces	80
Nuggets, 6-pack	20
Sandwich, McChicken	140
Croissant Sandwich: Plain	40
with Cheese, 1 oz	240
Fish Sandwich: no Cheese	60
with Cheese	140
Filet-O-Fish	170
Fish, fried, 2 pieces	20
French Fries: Small Serving	10
Hamburgers: Aver. all outlets	
Regular, no Cheese	120
Cheeseburger: Regular	200
Big Mac	250
Mc D.L.T.; McLean w/cheese	230
Quarter Pounder w/Cheese	300
Egg McMuffin	260
Hot Dog: Plain	60
with Cheese	150
Mexican: Burrito	120
Enchilada	300
Nachos, regular	200
Taco, regular	140
Taco (Bell) Salad	400
Pizza: Average all types	
Medium (12"), 2 slices	250
Double Cheese, 2 slices	350
Large (16"), 2 slices	350
Double Cheese, 2 slices	500
Pizza Hut, Medium:	
Cheese, 2 slices	650
Meat, 2 slices	520
Potato: Plain, baked, 8 oz	20
Stuffed w. Cheese Topping	100
with Cheese Filling	300
Sandwiches: Average	
no Cheese	60
with 1 oz Cheese	260
with 2 oz Cheese	460
Subway: 6" S/wich, average	100
Tuna, 6"; Tuna Salad (sm.)	100
Salads, small, average	100
Salads: Chef, regular	300
Coleslaw, small	20
Milkshakes, average	330

INTRODUCTION

● **Fiber** is the general term for those parts of **plant** food that we cannot digest. It is **not** found in foods of animal origin (meat, dairy products).

● Fiber promotes intestinal health, bowel regularity, can benefit diabetes and blood cholesterol levels, and may help prevent colon cancer. High fiber foods also assist weight control.

● Most Americans do not eat enough fiber — on average only 15 grams/day (women, 12g; men, 18g) — instead of a **healthier 25 to 35 grams/day.**

● Fiber-rich whole-foods usually **increase the nutrient content** of the whole diet — especially if high-fat rich foods are replaced.

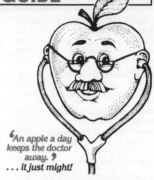

'*An apple a day keeps the doctor away.*'
. . . it just might!

TYPES OF FIBER

Plant foods contain a mixture of different fibers in varying proportions. Fibers are divided into **2 categories** based on their solubility in water. Both types are beneficial.

(a) **Insoluble fibers** (cellulose, hemi-celluloses, lignin) make up the structural parts of plant cell walls. The **best sources** are wheat bran, corn bran, rice bran, whole-wheat cereals and breads, dried beans and peas, nuts, seeds and the skins of fruits and vegetables.

These fibers absorb many times their own weight of water. They create a soft bulk and hasten the passage of waste products through the intestines.

They promote **bowel regularity**, and aid in the prevention and treatment of uncomplicated forms of **constipation, diverticulosis and hemorrhoids.**

The risk of **colon cancer** may also be reduced by fiber's diluting effect of potentially harmful substances.

TYPES OF FIBER (CONT)

(b) **Soluble fibers** (pectin, gums, mucilages) are found mainly within plant cells. **Best sources:** fruits and vegetables, psyllium, oat bran, barley, dried beans and peas and flax seed.

These fibers form a **gel** which slows both stomach emptying and the absorption of sugars from the intestines. This helps to control **blood sugar** levels and lessens the amount of insulin required — of particular benefit to persons with **diabetes.**

Weight control is also aided by the slower emptying of the stomach and the feeling of fulness provided by soluble fiber. (Also see notes opposite)

Some soluble fibers can lower **blood cholesterol** by their binding action on bile acids. (Bile acids, a break-down product of cholesterol produced in the body, help to emulsify and break up fats in the intestines. Bile acids are normally reabsorbed by the body and reform cholesterol. Some fibers bind bile acids and excrete them. More body cholesterol must then be broken down to supply bile acids.)

Note: Rice bran, while not high in soluble fiber can lower blood cholesterol.

FIBER & WEIGHT CONTROL

Fiber can assist weight control in several ways. **Fiber-rich foods** such as fresh fruit and vegetables, potatoes and whole-wheat bread **contain few calories** for their large volume (due to their low-fat, high water content).

Their bulk **fills the stomach** and satisfies appetite much earlier than fiber-depleted foods. The **extra chewing time** also contributes to satiety, and gives the stomach time to register a feeling of fulness. Excessive calories are less likely to be consumed.

Fiber-depleted foods and drinks are more concentrated in calories; e.g. fats, sugar, candy, soft drinks, fruit juices, alcohol. They **require little or no chewing.** Large amounts with excessive calories can be consumed before appetite is satisfied.

Example: Whereas one fresh apple might satisfy our appetite, an apple juice drink with the equivalent sugars and calories of 2-3 apples does little to satisfy appetite.

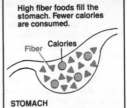

High fiber foods fill the stomach. Fewer calories are consumed.

Fiber   Calories

STOMACH

Low fiber foods are more concentrated in calories. More food must be eaten to fill the stomach

Calories   Fiber

STOMACH

EFFECTS OF REMOVING FIBER FROM FOOD

2-3 pieces of fresh fruit produces 1 glass of fruit juice.
The removal of fiber concentrates the sugar and calories.

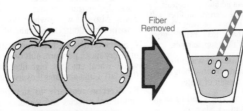

Fiber Removed

FRESH FRUIT
- High Fiber
- Low Calorie Density
- Long Eating Time
- Satisfies Hunger
- Sugar Slowly Absorbed
- Less Insulin Required

FRUIT JUICE
- Negligible Fiber
- High Calorie Density
- No Eating Time (Drink)
- Does Not Satisfy Hunger
- Sugar Quickly Absorbed
- More Insulin Required

FIBER GUIDE — CONSTIPATION

Constipation can reasonably be defined as a failure to have a bowel movement at least every second day — and just as importantly, without straining or pain.

Typically, stools are too hard, too narrow, and too small . . . *sinkers* rather than *floaters*.

The **main cause** is simply lack of dietary fiber. Other contributing factors include insufficient fluids, too little exercise, emotional stress, gastro-intestinal diseases, lack of proper dentition to chew high-fiber foods, and some medications (e.g. some antacids, antidepressants, tranquilizers).

Note: Check with your doctor to rule out any underlying medical problem — especially if you have a change in bowel habits in middle-age or later years.

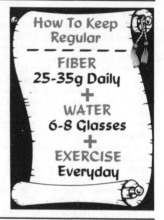

How To Keep Regular

FIBER 25-35g Daily

+

WATER 6-8 Glasses

+

EXERCISE Everyday

HINTS TO INCREASE FIBER & AVOID CONSTIPATION

1. **Breakfast** is an important contributor to daily fiber intake. Eat high-fiber breakfast cereals (bran-based cereals, oatmeal etc.). Add 1-2 tablespoons of unprocessed wheat bran if required.

Dried fruits, chopped nuts, and seeds are also excellent additions to cereals. **Note:** A **gradual** increase in fiber will prevent bloating, gas or pain. Persons intolerant to bran may benefit from psyllium-based fiber supplements.

2. **Drink 6-8 glasses of water or fluid daily.** Fiber works by absorbing many times its own weight of water.

3. **Eat whole-wheat bread or bran-enriched bread.** 1 slice of whole-wheat bread has more fiber than 3 slices of white bread.

4. **Enjoy fruit as fresh fruit** with skins rather than as fruit juice. Enjoy **wholemeal pasta, brown rice, nuts and seeds.**

5. **Eat more vegetables, salads and legumes** — especially dried beans, baked beans, lentils, potatoes with skins, avocado, broccoli, brussel sprouts, cabbage, carrots, celery, and peas.

6. **Add wheat or rice bran** to soups, casseroles, yogurt, desserts, cookies, cakes. Also use whole-wheat flour in place of white flour. Use nuts and seeds.

7. **Snack** on fresh or dried fruits, carrot or celery sticks, popcorn, nuts or seeds, whole-wheat crackers, high-fiber bars (low-fat). Limit amounts if overweight.

8. **Exercise regularly** to strengthen abdominal muscles and stimulate the gut; e.g. walking, swimming, cycling.

9. **Avoid indiscriminate and regular use of harsh laxatives.** They can over-stimulate the intestinal muscles and may make normal bowel activity impossible. It may take several weeks to restore normal bowel function.

FIBER
(g)

RECOMMENDED FIBER INTAKE
25-35 Grams/Day

BREAKFAST CEREALS	FIBER (g)
Breadshop: Oat Bran, 1/3 cup, 1 oz	4
Triple Bran, 1 oz	6.5
Nectar-Sweet Granolas, 1 oz	3
Health Valley: Per 1 oz	
Amaranth Cereal, 1/2 cup	4.2
Corn Flakes (Fat Free), 3/4 cup, 1 oz	4
Crisp Brown Rice, 3/4 cup	2
Fiber 7 Flakes (Reg./w. Raisins), 1/2 c.	3.7
Fruit & Fitness Cereal, 1/2 cup	5.3
Granola (Fat Free), 1/4 cup, 1 oz	2.5
Healthy Crunch (No Fat Added), 1/4 cup	3.5
Lites/Fruit Lites: Corn/Rice, 1/2 cup	0.4
Wheat, 1/2 cup, 1/2 oz	1.5
Oat Bran Flakes, all types, 1/2 cup	3.7
Orangeola, (No fat Added) 1/4 cup, 1 oz	3
Real Oat Bran Crl. (No Fat Added), 1/4 c.	4
Sprouts 7, w/Raisins, 1/4 cup, 1 oz	4.7
10 Bran Cereal (Fat Free), 3/4 c. 1 oz	5
General Mills: Cheerios, 1 1/4 cup, 1 oz	2
Clusters, 1/2 cup	3
Crispy Wheats 'N Raisins, 3/4 cup, 1 oz	2
Fiber One, 1/2 cup, 1 oz	13
Raisin Oat Bran, Total, Wheaties, 1 oz	3
Oatmeal Swirlers, 1 serving	2
Kellogg's (Per 1 oz): All-Bran, 1/3 cup	10
All-Bran w/Extra Fiber, 1/2 cup	14
Bran Buds (w/Psyllium), 1/3 cup, 1 oz	11
Bran Flakes (2/3 c.) Raisin Br., (3/4 c)	5
Common Sense Oat Bran, 1/2 cup	3
Corn Flakes, Frt. Loops, Honey Smacks	1
Special K, Cocoa/Rice Krispies, 1 c	0
Heartwise; Nutri-grain (Rais. Br), 2/3 c	5
Nutri-grain (Wheat/Almond Rais.) 2/3 c	3
Mueslix, 2/3 cup	3
Nabisco: 100% Bran, 1/2 cup, 1 oz	10
Shredded Wheat, 2 bisc.	6
Nature Valley: Average, 1/3 cup, 1 oz	1
Quaker (& Brands): Per 1 oz	
Cap'n Crunch (3/4 c) Cr. Nut Oh!s (1 c)	1
Crunchy Bran, 2/3 cup, 1 oz	5
Life Cereal (2/3cup); Oat Squares (1/2 cup)	2.5
Oat Bran (Quaker & Mothers), 1/3 cup	4.2
Oatmeal, average, 1 packet	2.7
100% Natural Cereals, aver., 1/4 cup	1.8
Puffed Rice, 1 cup, 1/2 cup	0.2
Puffed Wheat, Popeye Crunch, 1 c.	1
Sun Country Granola, 1/4 cup	1.8

BREAKFAST CEREALS (Cont)	FIBER (g)
Post: Alpha Bits, Corn flakes, 1 oz	0
Bran Flakes (Natural), 3/4 cup, 1 oz	5
Fruit & Fibre, 1 1/4 oz	5
Granola (Hearty), Fruity Pebbles	0
Grape-Nuts Brand/Flakes, 1 oz	3
Honey Bunches of Oats, 1 oz	1
Oat Flakes, 1 cup, 1 oz	2
Smurf Magic, Super Golden, 1 oz	0
Ralston: Fruit Muesli, 1/2 cup, 1 1/2 oz	3
Multi-Bran Chex, 2/3 cup, 1 oz	4
Wheat Chex, 2/3 cup, 1 oz	2

BRANS & SUPPLEMENTS	
Oat Bran: 1 Tbsp (level)	0.8
1/3 cup, (5 1/3 Tbsp), 1 oz	4.2
Rice Bran: 1/3 cup, 1 oz	6
Wheat Bran, unprocessed: 1 Tbsp	1.6
2 Tbsp (level), 1/4 cup	3.2
1/4 cup/4 Tbsp, 1/2 oz	6.4
1/2 cup, 1 oz	13
Corn Germ: 1/4 cup, 1 oz	5
Wheat Germ: 1/4 cup, 1 oz	3
Psyllium Seed Husks, 2 Tbsp	8
FiberSonic (Matol), 1 packet, 1.35 oz	11
Metamucil, 1 dose	3.4

HOT CEREALS, OATMEAL	
Bulgur (cracked wheat), ckd, 1 cup	8
Cream of Wheat, ckd, 2/3 cup	1
Hominy Grits, dry, 3 Tbsp, 1 oz	1.2
Kashi (Breakfast Pilaf), 5 oz	5
5 Bran Kashi, 1/2 envelope	16
Oatmeal, uncooked, 1/3 cup, 1 oz	2.7
cooked, 2/3 cup,	2.7

SAMPLE FOOD QUANTITIES TO OBTAIN 35g FIBER

	Fiber
Bkfst. Cereal (higher-fiber)	(5g)
+ 4 slices whole-wheat Bread	(6g)
+ 3 servings fresh Fruit	(9g)
+ 1 medium Potato (w/skin) **or** 1 cup Brown Rice **or** 1/2 cup whole-wheat Pasta	(4g)
+ 3-4 servings Veges/Salad	(6g)
+ 1 cup Bean Soup **or** 1 cup Baked Beans **or** 1/2 cup Corn/Peas/Lentils **or** 1 1/4 oz Almonds (natural)	(5g)

FOODS WITH NIL FIBER
- Dairy Products (Milk, Cheese, etc.)
- Meats, Poultry, Fish, Eggs
- Fats/Oils, Sugar/Syrups

(Only foods of plant origin contain fiber.)

BREADS & CRACKERS

	FIBER (g)
Bread: White, 1 slice, 1 oz	0.7
Whole-wheat, 1 slice, 1 oz	1.5
Whole-grain, 1 slice, 1 oz	2
Rye, Pumpernickel, 1 oz	1.5
Bagel/Roll/Bun, 1 medium, 2 oz	1.5
Pita, whole-wheat, 5″ pocket	4.5
Crackers: Graham, average, 2	1.4
Saltine, 4 crackers	0.3
Crispbreads (Rye), average, 2	4
Matzo, 1 board, 1 oz	1
Rice Cakes, average, 1 cake	0.3
Tortilla: Regular, 6″	0.5
Whole-wheat, 6″	1.3

BARLEY, PASTA, RICE & FLOURS

	FIBER (g)
Barley, pearled, raw, ¼ cup, 1.7 oz	5
Rice: White, ckd, 1 cup, 7 oz	1.6
Brown, cooked, 1 cup	3.2
Rice-A-Roni, average, 1 cup	1.5
Spaghetti/Noodles, cooked, 1 cup	2
Whole-wheat, cooked, 1 cup	7
Amaranth (Health Valley), 1 cup	9
Flour: All-purpose, 1 cup, 4 oz	<1
Whole-wheat, 1 cup	10
Cornmeal, stone ground, 1 cup	8
Carob Flour, 1 cup, 3½ oz	11
Soymeal, defatted, 1 cup	14

FROZEN ENTREES & DINNERS

Average All Brands — Per Serving

Potato/Pasta base, average	4-6
Vegetable base, average	3
Meat/Chicken base, average	2-3
Pizzas, ¼ large, average	3

SOUPS

Chicken Noodle, 1 cup	<0.5
Tomato Soup, average, 1 cup	<1
Vegetable Soup, average, 1 cup	3
Health Valley — Per 7½ oz serving:	
Black Bean Soup	16
Chunky Vegetable Chicken	4
Green Split Pea Soup	14.5
5-Bean Vegetable; Lentil	10
Minestrone Soup	12.5
Mushr. Barley; Potato; Vegetable	8
Fat Free Range: Average, 1 cup	3

FAST-FOODS & RESTAURANTS

	FIBER (g)
Hamburgers: Small, average	1.5
Large/Whopper, average	2.5
Hot Dog, regular	1.5
French Fries: Small serving, 2½ oz	2.5
Regular/Medium, 3½ oz	3.5
Chicken Nuggets, 6-pack	<0.5
Chicken Sandwich, average	2
Taco, average	4
Sundaes, Shakes, Soft Drinks	0
Arby's: Baked Potato w/Broccoli	7
Roast Beef Sandwich	1.5
Denny's: Chef's/Tuna Salad	3
Dennyburger (w/fries/salad)	5
The Club	6
Grilled Chicken S/wich	4
Domino's (Pizza): Veggie, 2 sl. (16″)	8
Pepperoni, 2 slices (16″)	4.5
Cheese, Deluxe, Saus./Mushr., 2 sl.	7
McDonald's: McLean, ¼ Pounder	1.5
McD.L.T.	2
Egg McMuffin	1.3
Salads (Chef/Garden/Chicken)	3
Pizza Hutt: (Per 2 slices, Medium)	
Pan Pizza: Cheese, Pepperoni	5
Supreme	7
Thin'n Crispy: Supreme	5
Hand-Tossed, average	7
Personal Pan Pizza, 1 whole	9
Subway: 6″ S/wich, white roll	2.5
w/Honey Wheat Roll	3.2
Footlong, w/Wheat Roll	6.4
Salads, average	2

CAKES, COOKIES, SNACK BARS

Apple/Fruit Pie, 1 piece	2
Cake, w/plain flour, 1 piece	1
w/whole-wheat flour, 1 piece	3
Carrot Cake, 1 piece	2
Cookies, Oatmeal, (3 small/1 large)	3
Donuts	0
Fruit Cake, 1 piece	3
Fi-Bar (Natural Nectar), 1 bar	4
Figs Bars, 2	1.3
Granola Bars, average	1
Health Valley: Fat-Free Fruit Bars	3.7
Oat Bran Jumbo Fruit Bars	7
Fat-Free Cookies, 2	2
Fat-Free Fruit Muffins, 1	5
Muffins, Oat Bran (2 small/1 large)	5
Meal On The Go (Provesta), 1½ oz	4
Pathway Bars (Matol): Matola Bars	11
Crunchy Oat & Peanut Granola	8

CHOCOLATE, CHIPS, POPCORN	FIBER (g)
Chocolate, Hard Candy, Cheese Balls	0
Chocolate with nuts/fruit, 2 oz bar	1
Mars Bar	1
Cheese Balls/Curls/Twists	0
Potato Chips, Corn Chips, 1 oz	1
Popcorn, 3 cups	2
Pretzels, Twists, 6	1

NUTS, SEEDS

Almonds: Natural, 25 kernels, 1 oz	4
Blanched (skins removed), 1 oz	3
Cashews, Filberts, Pecans, 1 oz	1.7
Peanuts, Mixed Nuts, Coconut, 1 oz	2.5
Peanut Butter, 2 Tbps, 1 oz	1.8
Pistachio Nuts, dried, shelled, 1 oz	3
Walnuts, Black/English, dried, 1 oz	1.5
Seeds: Amaranth, 2½ Tbsp, 1 oz	3.5
Flax Seeds, 3 Tbsp, 1 oz	6
Quinoa Seeds, 3 Tbsp, 1 oz	2.7
Psyllium Seed Husks, 5 Tbsp, 1 oz	20
Sesame Seeds, whole, 1 oz	3
Sesame Butter/Tahini, 2 Tbps, 1.1 oz	3
Sunflower kernels, ¼ cup, 1 oz	4.4
Teff Seeds, 1 oz	3.8

FRUIT — FRESH

Apples: Early season, 1 medium, 6 oz (whole)	
with skin + core	5.5
with skin, no core	4.5
without skin, no core	3.7
Late season, 1 med. 6 oz, w/skin, no core	3
Apricots, 2 medium, 4 oz	2
Avocado, average, ½ medium	3
Banana, 1 medium, 6 oz (w/skin)	2
Blueberries, raw, ½ cup, 5 oz	4.4
Cherries, sweet, raw, 10 fruits, 2½ oz	1.5
Grapefruit, average, ½ 8½ oz	1
Grapes, 1 med. bunch, seedless, 7 oz	3
Kiwifruit, 1 medium, 3 oz	3
Mango, 1 medium, 11 oz (whole)	1.6
Melons, cantaloup, 4 oz (edible)	1
Nectarine, 1 medium, 4 oz	1.8
Olives, average all types, 7 jumbo, 2 oz	1.5
Oranges: 1 medium (7-8 oz w/skin),	
5½ oz (peeled)	3.8
Passionfruit, 2 medium, 2½ oz	5
Peaches, 1 large, 6 oz	2
Pears, raw, 1 medium, 6 oz	4.5
Pineapple, 1 slice, 3 oz	1.8
Plums, 2 medium, 6 oz	2.8
Strawberries, 6 medium/3 large, 2 oz	1.5
Watermelon, 4 oz (edible)	0.5

FRUIT — DRIED, JUICE	FIBER (g)
Dried Fruit: Apricots, 8 halves, 1 oz	2.2
Dates (3 med.); Raisins (2 Tbps), 1 oz	1.5
Figs, 2 medium, 1.4 oz	3.5
Prunes, 4 medium, 1 oz	2
Fruit Juice: Orange/Apple etc, 1 gl.	<0.5
Prune Juice, 5 oz	1.4
Carrot Juice, 8 oz	1.8

VEGETABLES

Asparagus, 4 spears	2
Bean Sprouts, ½ cup, 2¼ oz	1.5
Beans: Snap/Green, ½ cup, 2½ oz	2
Baked Beans in tom sce, ½ c, 4½ oz	10
Dried Beans, ckd, average, ½ cup	7
Beets, ckd, slices, ½ cup, 3 oz	1.5
Broccoli, cooked, ½ cup, 3 oz	2.2
Brussels Sprouts, ckd, ½ cup, 3 oz	3.5
Cabbage: White, ckd, ½ cup, 2½ oz	1
Red, ckd, ½ cup, 2½ oz	2
Carrots, 1 medium (7½"), ½ c., 3 oz	2.7
Cauliflower, cooked, ½ cup, 3 oz	2.8
Celery, raw, diced, ½ cup, 2½ oz	1
Chick Peas (Garbanzos), ckd, ½ c. 3½ oz	6
Corn, kernels, ckd, ½ cup, 2½ oz	2.5
Cream-style, ½ cup, 4½ oz	1.5
Cucumber/Lettuce/Mushrooms, 2 oz	0.5
Eggplant, raw, sliced, ½ cup	2.5
Lentils, cooked, ½ cup, 3½ oz	4
Onions, 1 medium, 4 oz	1.8
Spring Onions, chop., ¼ cup, 1 oz	0.7
Peas: Green, ½ cup, 3 oz	5
Cowpeas (Black-eyed), ckd, ½ c.	10
Split Peas, ckd, ½ cup, 4½ oz	6.5
Peppers, sweet, raw, 1 large, 3½ oz	1.5
Potatoes: 1 medium, with skin, 5 oz	4
without skin	2
½ cup, mashed, 3½ oz	1.5
French Fries, 3 oz serving	3
Spinach, cooked, ½ cup, 3 oz	2
Squash: Summer, ckd, 3 oz	1.2
Winter, cooked, 3 oz	2.4
Tomatoes: 1 medium, 5 oz	2
Tomato Sauce, 1 cup	0.3
Frozen: Mixed Veges, ckd, ½ cup	2
Soybean Products: Miso, ½ c., 5 oz	7.7
Tempeh, 1 piece, 3 oz	2
Tofu, 4 oz	1.4
SALADS: Side Salad, average	1
Bean Salad, ½ cup	5
Coleslaw, ½ cup	1
Potato Salad, ½ cup	2

165

GENERAL NOTES

● Protein has many important body functions. It builds and repairs muscle, and is the basis of our body's organs, hormones, enzymes and antibodies.

● Protein is also an emergency fuel in the absence of sufficient carbohydrate and fats. For this reason, **weight loss** should be gradual so as to preserve protein levels in muscle, the heart and other body organs.

● It is easy to obtain sufficient protein in our diet — even a vegetarian diet. Plant proteins are not inferior to animal proteins.

Only small amounts of animal foods (lowfat) need be eaten, if at all desired.
Note: Infants require some form of milk in the diet to obtain sufficient protein and calories.

● When changing to a **vegetarian diet,** include soybeans, lentils, tofu, nuts, and wholegrain breads and cereals. Milk, yogurt, cheese and eggs greatly enhance nutrient intake.

PROTEIN & MUSCLE

● Although muscles are built of protein, protein is not a special fuel for working muscle cells…carbohydrates and fats are.

In fact, a diet high in protein (and fat) with little carbohydrate, can significantly reduce the performance of an athlete involved in endurance sports. **Carbohydrate** is the best fuel for muscles used for long periods of exercise.

● Any **extra protein** required by athletes and body-builders, can easily be obtained from the extra food eaten to satisfy hunger and energy needs — even allowing an excessive 120g protein daily for a 170 lb athlete (0.7g/lb body wt; twice the R.D.A.).

● Remember, **excess protein** in food will not build bigger muscles. It is converted and stored as fat. Excess protein can also strain the kidneys which excrete the waste products of protein metabolism.

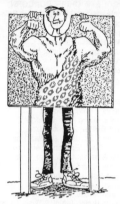

Protein needs are easily met with sensible eating.
Athletes who eat enough food for their energy needs, can obtain sufficient protein.

RECOMMENDED DAILY PROTEIN INTAKE (grams)		
(Figures in brackets — Recommended amount of protein/lb of ideal body wt.)		
Infants: 0-6 mths	13g	(1g/lb)
6-12 mths	14g	(0.7g/lb)
Children: 1-3	16g	(0.6g/lb)
4-6	24g	(0.5g/lb)
7-10	28g	(0.5g/lb)
Males: 11-14	45g	(0.45g/lb)
15-18	59g	(0.4g/lb)
19-24	58g	(0.36g/lb)
25+	63g	(0.4g/lb)
Females: 11-14	46g	(0.45g/lb)
15-18	44g	(0.37g/lb)
19-24	46g	(0.36g/lb)
25+	50g	(0.36g/lb)
Pregnancy:	60g	
Breast-feeding:	65g	
(Note: Above figures allow for a large safety margin for most persons.)		

● **Iron deficiency** is one of the most common nutritional deficiencies in women. The risk is increased in dieters who do not eat well-balanced meals. Chronic shortage of iron leads to **anemia**.

● **Women** between 11 and 50 years of age are at greater risk because of the monthly loss of menstrual blood. Pregnancy, growth, and endurance sports also demand extra iron.

● In **red blood cells,** iron combines with protein to form **hemoglobin** (Hb) — the red pigment which carries oxygen in the blood. A lack of iron limits the production of Hb and hence the amount of vital oxygen delivered to body cells.

Note: A **blood test** will tell you whether your Hb and iron stores (ferritin) are adequate. (Iron stores can be low even when Hb is normal.)

● **Iron absorption** is enhanced by vitamin C-containing veges/salad/fruit eaten with the meal. Small amounts of meat, fish or poultry help to absorb iron from vegetables.

Iron absorption is **lessened** by tea (tannin) drunk within 1 hour of a meal; and by excessive bran fiber and calcium supplements.

● For **infants** to 1 year, use iron-fortified milk/soy formula if not breast-feeding. Introduce iron-fortified baby cereals at 4-6 mths. (Note: Iron deficiency in children (even without anemia), can result in lethargy, irritability, repeated infections, and development problems.)

IRON SUPPLEMENTS

● **Most people** can obtain adequate iron from their diet. A **wide variety** of animal and plant foods contain iron. (See Counter.)

● An **iron supplement** is recommended for women with heavy menstrual blood losses, during pregnancy, endurance athletes with low blood ferritin (iron stores), and for persons with diagnosed anemia.

● **Dieters** may also benefit from a multi-vitamin/mineral supplement with iron. Excess iron (above 70mg daily) can be toxic.

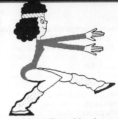

A nutritious diet with adequate iron is important — particularly for women and athletes.

ANEMIA SYMPTOMS

Anemia reduces the amount of oxygen carried in the blood. The body tissues become oxygen-starved and produce the following symptoms:

● Pale skin.
● Excessive tiredness or fatigue.
● Breathlessness.
● General feeling of malaise and irritability.
● Always feel cold.
● Decrease in attention span.

(**Note:** Other medical conditions may also cause similar symptoms. Check with your doctor.)

RECOMMENDED DAILY INTAKE OF IRON (mg)

Infants:	IRON
0-6 mths:	
Breast-fed	— 1mg
Bottle-fed	— 3-6mg
6-12 mths	— 6-10mg
Children: 1-11	— 10mg
Males: 11-18	— 12mg
19+	— 10mg
Females: 11-50	— 15mg
51+	— 10mg
Pregnancy:	— 30mg
Breast-feeding:	— 15mg

MEAT

	Pro (g)	Iron (mg)
Steak: Average all cuts, lean (no fat)		
Small (4 oz raw/3 oz ckd)	23	2.3
Medium (6 oz raw/4¼ oz ckd)	34	3.4
Large (10 oz raw/11¼ oz ckd)	57	5.7
Roast Beef: Lean, 2 slices, 3 oz	24	2.5
Grnd. Beef Patty, lean, ckd, 3 oz	21	2
Lamb Chop, broiled, 3 oz	22	1.5
Liver, cooked, 3 oz	23	5.5
Veal Cutlet, 1 medium	23	1
Pork, cooked, lean, 3 oz	24	1
Bacon, 3 medium slices	6	0.3
Ham, roasted, 2 pieces, 3 oz	18	1
Ham, luncheon, 2 slices, 1½ oz	7	0.3
Pastrami (Osc.Mayer) 3 sl., 1¾ oz	10	1.3
Sausages: Bologna, 2 sl., 2 oz	7	1
Braunschweiger, 2 sl., 2 oz	8	5.3
Pork link, thick, 2 oz	6	0.4
Frankfurter, 1½ oz	5	0.5
Salami, hard, 3 slices, 1 oz	7	0.5

CHICKEN/TURKEY

Chicken, ckd: Brst. portion, 3 oz	27	1
Leg/Thigh, lean, 3 oz	24	1
½ Whole Chicken	60	2.5
Drumstick, 1 medium, 3 oz	12	0.6
Turkey, cooked: Light meat, 3 oz	24	2
Dark meat, lean, 3 oz	24	2

FISH

Finfish — Per 4 oz, cooked		
Cod, Flounder/Sole, Pollock	28	0.5
Catf., Haddock, Halibut, M/Mahi	28	1.3
Ocn. Perch, Swordf., Or. Roughy	28	1.3
Canned Fish: Tuna, Light, 3 oz	25	1.5
White, 3 oz	23	0.5
Salmon, pink, 3 oz	17	0.7
Salmon, red, 3 oz	17	1
Sardines, 3 whole (3″), 1¼ oz	9	1
Anchovies, 1 can, 1½ oz	13	2
Shellfish: Crabmeat, 3 oz	17.5	0.7
Clams, raw, 4 lge/9 sml, 3 oz	11	12
Crayfish, cooked, 3 oz	20	2.7
Lobster, cooked, 3 oz	17	0.5
Oysters, raw, 6 medium, 3 oz	7	5
Scallops, 2 lge/5 small, 1 oz	5	0.1
Shrimp, raw, 6 large, 1½ oz	8.5	1
Fish Products:		
Fish Sticks, 4 sticks	10	0.5
Fish Portions, in batter, 4 oz	13	0.6
Gefilte Fish, 1 med. ball, 2 oz	8	1

EGGS (USDA rev. 1989)

	Pro (g)	Iron (mg)
1 Large Egg, whole	6	0.7
Egg Yolk	3	0.7
Egg White	3	0
Omelet: Plain, 2 eggs	13	1.4
Ham & Cheese	17	3
Egg Substitutes (liquid):		
Eggbeaters, 1 egg equiv.	4.5	1
Scramblers, ¼ cup, 2 oz	6	0.7

MILK & DAIRY PRODUCTS

Milk, Whole/Lowfat/Skim:		
1 cup, 8 fl.oz	8	0.1
1 pint, 20 fl.oz	19	0.3
Chocolate Milk, 1 cup	8	0.6
Thick Shake, Chocolate, 10 oz	9	1
Vanilla, 10 oz	11	0.3
Soymilk (fortified), aver., 1 cup	7	1
Yogurt: Plain, 6 oz	10	0.1
Fruit flavors, 6 oz	8	0.3
8 oz	11	0.5
Icecream: Rich, ½ cup	2	0
Regular, vanilla, ½ cup	2.5	0
Sherbet, ½ cup	1	0
Custard, baked, ½ cup	7	0.5

CHEESE

Hard Cheeses, average, 1 oz	7	0.2
4 oz	28	0.8
Cottage Cheese, ½ cup	13	0.3
Ricotta, part skim	14	1

BREAD, BAGELS, BISCUITS

Bread (with enriched flour):		
1 slice, 1 oz	2	1
4 slices, 4 oz	8	4
4 thick slices, 6 oz	12	6
Bagel, plain, 2 oz	6	1.5
Biscuits, 1 oz	2	0.7
Pita Bread, 1 pita, 1½ oz	4	1
Pumpernickel, 1 slice, 1 oz	3	1

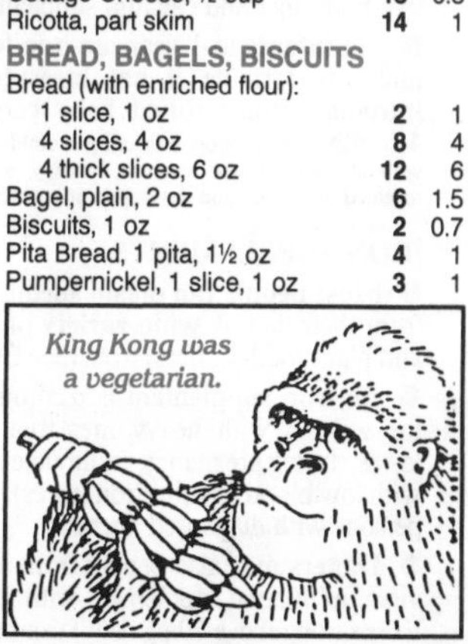

King Kong was a vegetarian.

PROTEIN & IRON COUNTER

BREAKFAST CEREALS	Pro (g)	Iron (mg)
Hot Type, cooked:		
Bulgur, cooked, 1 cup, 5 oz	9	2
Oatmeal: Reg., non-fortif., 1 cup	6	1.5
Instant, fortified, aver., 1 pkt	4	6
Quaker, reg. w/Cin. Spice	4	8
Quaker Extra, all flavors	4	18
Total, all types, 1 pkt	4	18
Corn/Hominy Grits: Reg., 1 cup	3	1.5
Quaker: Reg., 3 Tbsp, 1 oz	2	0.8
Instant White, 1 packet	2	8
Cream of Wheat, 1 cup	4	10
Ready-To-Eat: *(Per 1 oz Serving)*:		
Arrowhead, (ready-to-eat):		
Average, all varieties, 1 oz	3	1
General Mills: Body Buddies, 1 c.	2	8
Cheerios, regular, 1¼ cups	4	8
Cocoa Puffs, 1 cup	1	4.5
Corn Flakes, 1 cup	2	8
Fiber One, ½ cup	2	4.5
Kix, 1½ cups; Kaboom (1 c.)	2	8
Total, regular, 1 cup	3	18
Wheaties, 1 cup	3	4.5
Granola: Home-made, ½ c., 2 oz	7	7
Health Valley: Orangeola, ¼ c.	5	1.4
Amaranth w/Bananas, ½ cup	4	1
100% Organic: C/Flakes, ½ c.	3	4
Other variet., ½ cup	3	1
Real Oat Bran, ¼ cup	5	1.4
Sprouts 7, ¼ cup	3	1
Kellogg's, All Bran, ⅓ cup	4	4.5
Big Mixx, ½ cup	2	4.5
Bran Flakes, ⅔ cup	3	18
Cocoa Krispies, ¾ cup	1	2
Corn Flakes, 1 cup	2	2
Just Right, ⅔ cup	2	18
Nutrigrain Raisin Bran, 1 cup	4	18
Raisin Bran, ¾ cup, 1½ oz	3	18
Rice Krispies	2	2
Shredded Wheat, all types	2	8
Special K, 1 cup	6	4.5
Nature Valley: All varieties, ⅓ c.	2	0.7
Nectar-Sweet Granola (Breadshop)		
Calif. Or. Crm; Honey G/Nuts	3	3.5
Supernatural/Super Cereal	3	2.7
Other varieties	3	1
Quaker: Crunchy Bran, ⅔ cup	2	8
Oat Squares, ½ cup, 1 oz	4	6
100% Natural Cereal, ¼ c.	3	1
Puffed Rice/Wheat, 1 c., ½ oz	1	0.5
Shredded Wheat, 2 bisc.	4	1

CEREALS (CONT.)	Pro (g)	Iron (mg)
Ralston: Almond Delight, ¾ cup	2	2
Corn Chex, 1 cup, 1 oz	2	8
Rice Chex, 1 cup, 1 oz	1	8
Wheat Chex, ⅔ cup	3	8
Fruit Muesli, ½ cup, 1½ oz	4	4

BRANS & WHEATGERM		
Oat Bran, raw, 2 Tbsp	2	0.5
⅓ cup, 1 oz	6	1.5
Rice Bran, raw, 2 Tbsp	1	1
Wheat Bran, unproc., 2 Tbsp	1	1
Wheat Germ, ¼ cup, 1 oz	8	2.5
2 Tbsp, ½ oz	4	1.3

GRAINS & FLOURS		
Amaranth, 1 cup, 3½ oz	10	3
Barley, ½ cup, 3½ oz	8	2
Buckwheat Flour, dark, 1 cup	11.5	2.7
light, 1 cup	6	1
Carob Flour, 1 cup	5	3
Corn Flour, 1 cup, 4 oz	9	2
Corn Meal, enriched, 1 cup	11	3.5
Millet, wholegrain, 1 cup, 3½ oz	10	7
Rye Flour, dark, 1 cup, 4½ oz	21	6
light, 1 cup, 3½ oz	10	1
Soy Flour, full fat, 1 cup, 3 oz	32	5.5
Wheat Flour, white, enriched:		
All purpose, 1 cup, 4½ oz	13	6
Wholegrain, 1 cup, 4¼ oz	16	5

PROTEIN & DIET POWDERS/SUPPS.		
Ensure, 8 fl.oz	9	2.3
Joe Weider Super Protein, 1 oz	9	7.2
Nature's Best Prot. Shake, 11 fl.oz	20	2
90-Plus Protein, 1 oz	23	3.6
Pathway Shake (Matol), 2 scoops	12	5.4
Slim-Fast: Reg./Ultra, 1 oz	5	6.3
Sustagen, 8 fl.oz	27	4.5
YEAST: Brewer's, dry, 1 Tbsp	3	1.5

INFANT/BABY FOODS	Pro (g)	Iron (mg)
Infant Formula Milk:		
(Made up — Per 5 fl.oz)		
Enfamil/Gerber/Similac:		
Regular/Low Iron	2.2	0.2
With Iron	2.2	1.8
Isomil/Nursoy/ProSobee	3	1.8
Baby Cereals, average all brands		
Dry, 4 Tbsp, ½ oz	1	7
Jars (w/fruit), 4½ oz	1	7

RICE, SPAGHETTI

	Pro (g)	Iron (mg)
Rice, brown/white, average 1 cup, cooked, 6½ oz	5	1
Spaghetti/Macaroni/Noodles (enriched) cooked, 1 cup, 4½ oz	7	2
Canned: in Tomato Sce, ½ cup	2	0.5
w/Meatballs, 1 cup, 8 oz	9	2

SOUPS

With Noodles/Vegetables, 1 cup	3	0.5
With Meat/Beans/Peas, 1 cup	8	1.5

FRUIT

Fresh/Canned:

Average all types, 1 serving 1 medium/2 small fruit	1	0.5
Avocado, ½ medium	2	1

Dried Fruit:

Apricots, 8 halves, 1 oz	1	1.3
Dates, 6 dates, 2 oz	1.5	0.7
Figs, 3 medium figs, 2 oz	2	1.3
Prunes, 5 medium, 1½ oz	1	1
Raisins, 1 oz	1	0.7
Fruit Juice, average, 1 cup	0.5	0.5
Prune Juice, 6 fl.oz	1	2.5
Tomato Juice, 6 fl.oz	0.5	1

VEGETABLES

Beans: Snap/green, ½ cup	1	0.8
Dried: Average all types, cooked, ½ cup	7	2.5
Baked Beans, ½ cup, 4½ oz	5	2
Bean Sprouts, mung, 1 cup	3	1
Broccoli, ¾ cup pieces, 4 oz	4	1.4
Cabbage; Cauliflower, 1 cup	1	0.6
Corn, ½ cup kernels, 3 oz	2.5	0.3
1 ear trimmed to 3½"	2	0.4
Lentils, cooked, ½ cup, 3½ oz	9	3.3
Mushrooms, raw, ½ cup sliced	0.5	0.5
Peas, green, ½ cup, 3 oz	4	1.2
Split Peas, cooked, 1 cup	16	2.5
Potatoes, cooked:		
1 medium, with skin, 5 oz	3.3	2
without skin, 4 oz	2.3	1
French Fries, 3 oz	3	1
Potato Salad, ½ cup	3.5	0.8
Pumpkin, ½ cup, mashed	1	0.7
Seaweed, kelp, 1 oz	<1	0.7
Spinach, cooked, ½ cup, 3 oz	2.7	3.2
Squash, ckd, all types, ½ cup	1	0.3
Tomatoes, 1 medium, 4½ oz	1	0.6
Vegetables, mixed, ckd, 1 cup	2.5	0.4
Soybeans, dry, ckd, ½ cup, 3 oz	14	4.4

TOFU, TEMPEH, MISO

	Pro (g)	Iron (mg)
Tofu, raw, firm, ½ cup, 4½ oz	10	1.5
Tempeh, ½ cup, 3 oz	16	2
Miso, ½ cup, 4¾ oz	16	4
Soybean Protein (TVP), 1 oz	18	3

CAKES, PASTRIES, PIES
(Made with enriched flour)

Carrot w/cream cheese frosting 1 piece, 3½ oz	4	1.3
Cheesecake, 1 piece, 3½ oz	5	0.5
Chocolate, 1 piece, 2 oz	2	2
Fruitcake, 1 piece, 1½ oz	2	1.2
Plain, 1 piece, 3 oz	4	1.2
Croissant, plain, 2 oz	5	2
Danish Pastry, 1 pastry, 2¼ oz	4	1.3
Doughnuts, average, 2 oz	4	1.2
Muffins, aver., 1 medium, 1½ oz	3	1
Pancakes, 4" diam., two, 2 oz	4	1
Pies: Fruit, 1 piece, 5½ oz	4	1.5
Pecan, 1 piece, 5 oz	7	4.5
Puddings, aver., ½ cup, 4½ oz	4	0.3
Waffles, 1 large, 2½ oz	7	1.5

COOKIES & CRACKERS

Cookies, average 4 cookies	2	1
Crackers: Graham, 2½" sq., two	1	0
Rice Cakes, average, one	1	0

SUGAR, HONEY, JAM

Sugar: White	0	0
Brown, 1 Tbsp	0	0.3
Molasses: Light/Medium, 1 Tbsp	0	1
Blackstrap, 1 Tbsp, ¾ oz	0	3
Corn Syrup, 1 Tbsp, ¾ oz	0	1
Honey, Jams, Jelly	0	0.2

CANDY, CHOCOLATE, SNACK BARS

Candy, sugar-based	0	0
Chocolate: Plain, 2 oz bar	4	0.8
with Nuts, 2 oz bar	6	0.8
Carob, plain, 2 oz	6	0.7
Corn/Potato Chips, 1 oz	2	0.3
Granola Bars, average	2	0.5
Matoi, Pathway Bars: Matola	7	5.4
Oat & Peanut Bar	9	6.3
Meal On The Go, Orig. 3 oz	7	4.7
Peanut Bar (Planters), 1½ oz	7	0.7
Power Bars, 2¼ oz bar	10	2.7
Ultra Slim-Fast Bars	5	6.3

COFFEE, SODA

Coffee, Coffee Substitutes, 1 cup	0	0.1
Tea (all types); Soft Drinks/Soda	0	0
Hot Chocolate, 6 fl.oz	2	2.2

PROTEIN & IRON COUNTER

NUTS & SEEDS — Per 1 oz	Pro (g)	Iron (mg)
Almonds, shelled, 20-25 nuts	6	1
Brazil Nuts, 7-8 medium nuts	4	1
Cashew Nuts, 12-16 nuts	5	1.5
Coconut, raw, 1½ oz pce (2"x2½")	1	1
Filberts, 1 oz	4	1
Macadamias, 1 oz	2	0.5
Mixed Nuts, 1 oz	5	1
Peanuts, dry roasted, 40 nuts, 1 oz	6	0.6
Peanut Butter, 1 Tbsp	1	0.5
Pecans, 24 halves, 1 oz	2	0.5
Pumpkin Kernels, dry, hulled, 1 oz	7	4.2
Sesame Seeds, dry, 1 Tbsp	2	0.6
Sunflower Seeds, dried, hulled, 1 oz	6	2
Tahini, 1 Tbsp, ½ oz	2.5	1.4
Walnuts, 15 halves, 1 oz	4	0.7

BEER, WINE, SPIRITS

	Pro (g)	Iron (mg)
Beer, 12 fl.oz	1	0
Wines, red/white, 1 glass	0	0.4
Spirits	0	0

FAST-FOODS/HAMBURGERS

Note: See Fast-Foods Section for comprehensive protein counts.

	Pro	Iron
Arby's: Roast Beef S/wich, reg.	22	4
Giant Roast Beef S/wich	36	6
Chicken Breast Sandwich	23	3.5
Turkey Deluxe Sandwich	24	3
Fish Fillet Sandwich	22	3.5
Cashew Chicken Salad	34	3
Burger King: Whopper S/wich	27	5
Double Whopper w/Cheese	51	7
Hamburger/Deluxe	15	3
Bacon Double Cheeseburger	32	4
Chicken Sandwich	26	3.5
Fish Fillet	20	2.5
Carl's Jr: Famous Star H/burger	24	6
Super Star Hamburger	37	7
Chicken Club Sandwich	26	6
Roast Beef 'n Swiss	31	5.5
Domino's Pizza: Large (16"), 2 sl:		
Cheese, 2 slices	22	2.3
Pepperoni, Sausage/Pepp.	24	3
Vegi; Dble. Cheese/Pepp.	31	4.5
French Fries: Medium, 3½ oz	4.5	0.7
Hardee's: Big Deluxe Burger	27	5
Roast Beef, regular	15	4
Turkey Club	29	3
All Beef Hot Dog	11	3
Chef Salad	22	2
Chicken 'n Pasta Salad	27	9
Hot Dog, regular	9	1.5

Kentucky Fried Chicken:	Pro	Iron
2-Pce. Snack (Original)	45	4
3-Pce. Dinner (Original)	58	4
Kentucky Nuggets, 6	17	0.6
Colonel's Chicken Sandwich	21	1.3
Long John Silver's:		
Fish Dinner, 3 pces.	43	3.5
Chicken Plank Din., 3 pces.	31	5
Seafood Platter	30	4.5
McDonald's: Hamburger	12	2.3
Big Mac; McD.L.T.	25	4
Cheeseburger	15	2.3
Quarter Pounder	23	4
Filet-O-Fish	14	2
McLean Deluxe	22	3.6
McChicken	19	2.6
Chicken McNuggets	20	1
French Fries, small, 2½ oz	3	0.5
Medium, 3½ oz	4.5	0.7
Breakfast: Egg McMuffin	18	1.3
Hotcakes w/butter syrup	8	2
Sausage McMuffin w/egg	23	3.4
Chef Salad	21	1.5
Milkshake, chocolate	12	1
Pancakes: 3 pancakes	8	2
Pizza Hut: Medium, 2 slices		
Pan Pizzas, average	30	5.5
Thin 'n Crispy: Chse., Pepp.	28	3
Supreme	28	6
Hand Tossed: Pepperoni	28	5
Supreme	32	8
Personal Pan Pizzas, aver.	35	6.3
Subway: 6" Subs, average	22	2
Footlong Subs, average	44	4
Subway Club Salad, reg.	32	2
Sundaes, average	7	0.3
Taco Bell: Bean Burrito	13	3.5
Beef Burrito	22	3.7
Tostado	10	1.5
Enchirito; Nachos Bellgrande	20	3
Taco Bellgrande	18	2
Taco Light	19	2.5
Taco Salad w/shell	35	7
Chicken Taco	13	2
Steak Taco	14	3
Wendy's: Hamburger, w/extras	25	5.5
Wendy's Big Classic	27	6.3
Junior H/burger; Kid's Meal	15	3.5
Grilled Chicken Sandwich	24	3.5
Stuffed Potatoes: Broc./Chse.	8	2.7
Bacon & Cheese	20	4.3
Taco Salad	40	6.3

SALT, SODIUM & HYPERTENSION

● Sodium is a mineral element most commonly found in salt (sodium chloride). It also occurs naturally in much smaller amounts in animal and plant foods, and water — sufficient for our needs without having to add salt.

● **Small amounts of sodium** in our diet are needed to regulate and balance the amount of fluid in our tissues and blood. (Sodium acts like a sponge to attract and hold fluids in body tissues.) Sodium also helps our nerves and muscles to work properly.

(Potassium and magnesium also play important roles in these functions.)

● **Excess salt and sodium** in the diet is linked with an extra risk of developing high blood pressure (hypertension), which in turn greatly **increases the risk** of stroke, coronary heart disease, congestive heart failure, and kidney failure. (Note: Hypertension does **not** mean being overly tense or nervous.)

Heredity, obesity, excess alcohol, and lack of exercise also contribute greatly to hypertension.

KNOW YOUR BLOOD PRESSURE

About **1 in 3** American adults has hypertension, many of whom do not know. It is generally symptomless, so **have your blood pressure checked** annually — particularly if there is a family history of hypertension.

Untreated hypertension overworks the heart, promotes damage to the arteries with consequent speeding up of atherosclerosis, and damages nerves. The **earlier** it is detected, the sooner it can be brought under control — possibly without drug medication.

NORMAL BLOOD PRESSURE
Diastolic — Less than 85 mm Hg
Systolic — Less than 140 mm Hg

SALT-SENSITIVE PERSONS

Normally, our **kidneys** excrete excess dietary sodium. The thirst we feel after a salty meal is the body calling for more water to dilute the sodium, and enable the kidneys to flush out excess sodium.

However, 'salt-sensitive' persons (perhaps 1 in 2-3 adults) tend to retain excess sodium — above approximately 3000mg daily — instead of excreting it. They are more likely to develop hypertension; and would most benefit from sodium reduction.

While tests to identify salt sensitivity are not yet widely available, persons with a family history of hypertension should assume they are susceptible.

● Although not everyone will benefit from reducing sodium intake, **all** Americans are being asked to **moderate their salt and sodium intake** as a public health measure — particularly that so many do not know whether or not they have hypertension; and we do not know just who is salt-sensitive.

TREATING HYPERTENSION

If your blood pressure is high, **consult a doctor** about diet and medication. (You may be referred to a dietitian for more detailed dietary advice and meal planning.)

● **Mild to moderate hypertension** can often be treated simply by **reducing sodium intake, losing weight** if overweight, **limiting alcohol** to 2 drinks or less daily, and **exercising** regularly. Dealing with stress is also important.

● **Severe hypertension** must be treated by prescribed medication. However, salt restriction and the above actions will **improve** the success of drug therapy, and enable **smaller drug doses** to be prescribed.

SODIUM CONTENT OF SALT

Sodium is measured in milligrams (mg). Sodium accounts for only 40% of the weight of salt. Examples:

1 gram (1000mg) Salt = 400mg Sodium
1 teasp. Salt (6g) = 2.4g or 2400mg Sodium
1 Teaspoon Salt = 2400mg Sodium

SODIUM REQUIREMENTS

As little as 200 mg (milligrams) of sodium is required daily for normal living. (This is equivalent to the sodium in 1/10 teaspoon salt, or 2 slices of bread, or ¾ cup Cornflakes, or 1 oz cheddar cheese, or 2 cups of milk.

There is sufficient sodium present in naturally-occurring foods to meet our needs without adding extra salt.

Note: Persons engaged in prolonged strenuous work or exercise (especially in hot, humid weather), may lose sodium through heavy sweating. A little extra salt at mealtimes is usually sufficient to satisfy any extra need. Do not take salt tablets.

Infants: Breast milk or infant formula for the first 6 months provides adequate sodium. Most commercial baby foods now have acceptably low sodium levels.

SAFE SODIUM LEVELS

A maximum sodium intake of **3000mg per day** is recommended by the American Heart Association (for adults with normal blood pressure).

This is equivalent to the sodium in 1¼ teaspoons of salt. The average American consumes 4000-6000mg sodium/day, equivalent to 2-3 teaspoons of salt.

FINDING HIDDEN SODIUM

On average, only 1/3 of our sodium intake comes from the salt shaker. The other 2/3 is hidden in processed foods that have salt added during manufacture.

Additionally, **other sodium compounds** added to food or medicinals can contribute significant sodium; e.g. sodium bicarbonate (27% sodium), monosodium glutamate (MSG), sodium ascorbate, sodium nitrite, sodium citrate.

Foods HIGH in Sodium

- Bread (See note next page)
- Cheese, Butter, Margarine
- Pickles, Sauerkraut, Olives
- Condiments, Sauces
- Salad Dressings
- Canned vegetables/salads/beans
- Deli Salads (with dressing)
- Frozen/Packaged Meals/Entrees
- Soups: Canned/dry; bouillon cubes
- Meats: Ham, bacon, sausage, hot dogs, luncheon meats, smoked meats
- Canned Fish
- Seasoning Salts (e.g. garlic, celery)
- Snack Foods (potato chips, pretzels)
- Tomato Juice, V8 Vegetable Juice

Note: Antacids with sodium bicarbonate (e.g. Alka-Seltzer) are high in sodium.

Foods MODERATE in Sodium

- Meat, Fish, Poultry — Unprocessed
- Milk, Yogurt, Eggs
- Peanut Butter
- Breakfast Cereals (< 200mg/serving)
- Chocolate Candy, Fruit/Nut Bars
- Reduced Sodium Products

Foods LOW in Sodium

- Products labelled *Low Sodium,* or *Sodium Free*
- Fresh fruits and vegetables
- Canned & Dried Fruits
- Potatoes, Rice, Pasta (plain)
- Dried Beans & Lentils, Tofu
- Nuts & Seeds (unsalted)
- Corn & Popcorn (unsalted)
- Pepper, Spices, Herbs
- Jam, Honey, Syrup
- Chewing Gum
- Hard & Jelly Candy
- Coffee, Tea, Alcohol
- Fruit Juices, Water

Note: These hints are for normal healthy persons wishing to moderate their salt/sodium intake. Persons with hypertension may require more strict sodium reduction and should consult their doctor for guidance.

● **Watch the salt shaker.** Start with an easy 50% cut in sodium by using *Lite Salt (Morton)*. Then, gradually cut back until you require no salt, and can leave the salt shaker off the table.

Or, switch to a sodium-free herb-spice blend such as *Mrs Dash*.

Note: Potassium salt substitutes may not be suitable for some persons. If under medical supervision, check with your doctor.

● **Taste your food before salting.** Use the pepper shaker (small holes) for more controlled sprinkling of salt.

● When cooking, **use herbs and spices** in place of salt and seasoned salts. Garlic, onions, peppers, dry mustard, nutritional yeast, *Angostura Bitters,* lemon/citrus juices, or even a little wine all add extra flavor without the sodium.

Avoid use of garlic/onion/celery salts, MSG, soy sauce, tomato sauce, or regular bouillon cubes.

● **Steam or microwave vegetables** to retain natural flavors instead of boiling. Make your own **sauces** with extra herbs and spices in place of salt.

● **Make cereals, legumes, vegetables and fruit the major part** of your diet.

● **Check labels for sodium levels.** The following sodium descriptors may appear on labels:

Reduced Sodium: at least 75% less sodium than the original product.
Low Sodium: 140mg or less/serving
Very Low Sodium: 35mg or less/serving
Sodium Free: Less than 5mg per serving.

● **Choose low sodium and reduced sodium products** in place of regular salted products.

● **Use sodium reduced breads, butter and margarine.** Regular varieties contain up to 2% salt. This is considered high in view of their significant contribution to our diet.

● **Go easy on condiments and sauces** such as ketchup, mustard, soy sauce, salad dressings and spaghetti sauces; as well as bottled peppers. Look for low sodium varieties.

● **Avoid salty snack foods** such as potato chips, corn chips, salted nuts, pretzels and cheesy-flavored snacks.

Choose plain popcorn, unsalted nuts or seeds, and fresh or dried fruits.

● **Drinks: Avoid** canned tomato and vegetable juices unless they are 'no salt added' varieties.

Most **water** supplies are low in sodium (less than 5mg/cup). Drier areas such as Southern California can have up to 20mg sodium/cup; and the use of distilled water or a water filter may be warranted for persons on low sodium diets.

Do not use water softeners as they add sodium to the water.

Sodium in **soft drinks** and **bottled waters** varies from 2-50mg/cup. The terms *soda* and *soda pop* do not refer to the sodium content.

● **When eating out,** request dishes without added salt. Most fast-food items are high in sodium. Check the *Fast Foods Section* of this book.

● **Do not salt your children's food to your taste.**

● **Avoid antacids** with sodium bicarbonate (e.g. *Alka-Seltzer*). They are high in sodium.

Do not swallow **toothpaste** or mouth washes — most contain sodium. Rinse your mouth well.

SODIUM COUNTER

The American Heart Association recommends a sodium intake of LESS THAN 3000mg/day.

MILK & DAIRY PRODUCTS

	Sodium (mg)
Milk: Whole/lowfat/skim, aver. 1 cup, 8 fl.oz	120
Whole, low sodium, 1 cup	6
Choc. Milk (Hershey's), 1 cup	130
Human Milk, 8 fl.oz	40
Soy Milk, 8 fl.oz	30
Buttermilk, cultured, 8 fl.oz	250
Dry Powder, skim, ¼ cup, 1 oz	110
Yogurt: with fruit, aver., 8 oz	130
Cheese, Kraft: Cheddar, 1 oz	180
Swiss, 1 oz	40
Parmesan, 1 oz	450
Blue, 1 oz	330
Philadelphia Brand Cream	85
Process Chse., aver., 1 oz	430
Cottage Cheese, ½ cup, 4 oz	450
Ricotta Cheese, ½ cup, 4 oz	150

ICECREAM, FROZEN YOGURT

Icecream, average, ½ cup	50
Frozen Yogurt, ½ cup	50

FATS/OILS/CREAM

Butter/Margarine, reg., 2 T., 1 oz	230
Unsalted, reg., 2 T., 1 oz	<5
Mayonnaise, aver., 2 Tbsp., 1 oz	160
Molly McButter, 1 tsp	120
Oils/Lard/Dripping	0
Cream, average, 1 Tbsp	6
Coffee-Mate: Powdered, 1 tsp	2
Liquid, 1 Tbsp	5

EGGS

Whole, 1 large	70
Egg White, 1 large	50
Omelette, 2 egg, plain	220
w/cheese	400
Egg Beaters (Fleischmann's), ¼ c.	80

MEATS

Meat, average all types, cooked (Beef/Lamb/Veal/Pork), 4 oz	80
Corned Beef, cooked, 3 oz	800
Bacon, cooked, 2 slices, ½ oz	270
Ham, 3 oz	1100

CHICKEN & TURKEY

Chicken, cooked, unsalted, 4 oz	80

SAUSAGES & MEATS

	Sodium
Bologna, 1 oz	280
Frankfurter, 2 oz	640
Ham, chopped, ¾ oz slice	290
Liverwurst (Braunschweiger), 1 oz	320
Pepperoni, 5 slices, 1 oz	570
Salami, cooked, 1 oz	350
dry/hard, 1 oz	600
Sausage, 1 oz link	220
Pork, 2 oz patty	260
Turkey Roll, 1 oz	160

FISH:

Fresh Fish, average, plain Cooked, 4 oz (no bone)	60
Broiled w/butter, 4 oz	150
Breaded & fried, 4 oz	320
Fish fillets, bat.-dipped, 3 oz	350
Fish sticks, 1 oz stick	160
Gefilte Fish (w/broth), 1 pce, 1½ oz	220
Herring, pickled, 2 pces., 1 oz	260
Lobster, meat only, 4 oz	180
Oysters, fresh, 6 med., 3 oz	95
Salmon, canned, 3 oz	460
No Salt Added, 3 oz	65
Smoked fish, average, 3 oz	650
Tuna, canned, 3 oz	330
No Salt Added, 3 oz	40

ENTREES & MEALS

Frozen Entrees, average	600-900
Lean Cuisine, average	900
Right Course (Stouffer's), av.	580
Dinners, average	900-1200
Side Dishes, average	400-600
Pizza, frozen, ¼ large, 6 oz	800-1200
Microwave Cup Meals	900-1200
Cup O'Noodles, average	1500

FAST-FOODS

(For comprehensive listings - See: **Fast Foods Section**)

Cheeseburger	750
Hamburger: Regular	500
Large with cheese	1100
Fish/Chicken Sandwich	1000
French Fries, medium, 2½ oz	150
Chicken Dinner (3-piece)	2200
Chicken Nuggets w/Sce.	800
Hot Dog (Frankfurter)	800
Pizza, 2 medium slices	1200
Taco	400
Shake, chocolate	250

Continued Next Page

SODIUM COUNTER (CONT)

SOUPS	Sodium
Condensed, 1 cup, 8 oz	800-1000
Low Sodium	70
Chicken Noodle, 1 cup	900
Bouillon Cube, average	950
Cup-A-Soup, average	850
Lite, average	450
Soup Mixes, aver. 1 cup	900

CONDIMENTS, SAUCES, DRESSINGS

A-1 Sauce, 1 Tbsp	270
Barbecue Sauce, 1 Tbsp	130
Chili Sauce, 1 Tbsp	230
Ketchup, tomato, 1 Tbsp	180
Low Sodium, 1 Tbsp	20
Mayonnaise, 1 Tbsp	80
Mustard, 1 tsp	70
Pizza Sauce, ½ cup	700
Salad Dressings, 2 T., 1 oz	160-400
Spaghetti Sauce, ½ cup	500
Soy Sauce, 1 Tbsp	1000
Sweet & Sour, ¼ cup	250
Tabasco, 1 tsp	25
Vinegar, Lemon Juice, ½ cup	1
Worcestershire, 1 Tbsp	200
Tomato: Sauce, 1 cup	1200
Paste/Puree (salted), ½ c.	1000
No Salt Added, ½ cup	25

SALT & SALT SUBSTITUTES

Table Salt: 1 tsp, 6g	2400
Single serve packet, 1g	400
Lite Salt (Morton), 1 tsp, 6g	1200
Salt Substitute (Potassium), 1 tsp	<1
Garlic Salt, 1 tsp, 6g	1800
Seasoned or Sea Salt, 1 tsp, 5g	1600

SEASONINGS, HERBS & SPICES

Baking Powder, 1 tsp, 3g	340
Baking Soda (Sod. bicarb.) 1 tsp, 3g	810
Accent (Flavor Enhancer), 1 tsp	600
Chili Powder, 1 tsp, 3g	25
Herbs/Spices; Curry Powder	<1
Lemon Pepper (Lawry's), 1 tsp	340
Meat Tenderizer, 1 tsp, 5g	1750
MSG (Monosodium glutamate), 5g	500
Mrs Dash (Herb/Spice Blend), 1 tsp	0
Pepper, Mustard (dry), , 1 tsp	1
Vegit, 1 tsp	<5
Yeast, Nutritional, 1 Tbsp	<20
Stuffing Mixes, average., ½ cup	500

BREAKFAST CEREALS	Sodium (mg)
Kellogg's:	
All-Bran, ⅓ cup, 1 oz	260
Bran Flakes, ⅔ cup, 1 oz	220
Corn Flakes, 1 cup, 1 oz	290
Just Right, ⅔ cup, 1 oz	200
Shredded Wheat Squares, ½ cup, 1 oz	5
Health Valley Cereals, 1 serving	<10
Quaker: Crunchy Bran, 1 oz	320
100% Natural, 1 oz	15
Puffed Rice/Wheat, 1 oz	1
Cap'n Crunch, average, 1 oz	250
Total, 1 cup, 1 oz	140
Natural Valley, average, 1 oz	90
Oatmeal: Regular, ¾ cup	1
Instant (Quaker), ⅔ cup (1pkt)	270

BREAD, BAGELS, CRACKERS

Bread, average all types, 1 oz	140
Low sodium, 1 oz	10
Bagels, plain, 2 oz	200
Sara Lee, 3 oz	500
Biscuits, average, 1 oz	180
Bun/Roll, 1 medium, 1½ oz	200
Cracker, Saltine, 2	70
Low Salt (Premium), 2	45
Graham, 2	50
Croissant, average, 2 oz	280
Rice Cakes, average	<30
RyKrisp Crispbread, Sesame, 2	100

COOKIES, CAKES, DESSERTS

Cookies, average, 1 cookie	30
Baked Custard, ½ cup	100
Brownie, ¼ oz piece	75
Cake, average, 3 oz piece	250
Cinnamon Sweet Roll, 2 oz	250
Danish, Apple	220
Donut, average	150
Muffins, 1 medium, 2 oz	150
Sara Lee, average, 2½ oz	300
Pancakes, 3 x 4"	360
Pie, average ⅙ of 9" pie	300
Pudding, average, ½ cup	160
Jell-O (Mix), Instant, ½ cup	400
Waffles: Home-made, 7", 2½ oz	350
Frozen, average, 1¼ oz	260
Aunt Jemima, aver., 2½ oz	630

(< = less than) FRUIT & JUICES	Sodium (mg)
Fresh Fruit, aver., 1 serving	1
Dried/Canned Fruit, ½ cup	<5
Fruit Juice: Fresh, sqz'd, 6 fl.oz	<5
Commercial, aver., 6 fl.oz	20
Carrot Juice (Ferraro's), 8 fl.oz	230
Tomato Juice (Campbell's), 6 fl.oz	570
Low Sodium (No Salt Added)	20
V8 Vegetable (Campbell's), 6 fl.oz	600
No Salt Added, 6 fl.oz	45

VEGETABLES

Fresh/Frozen (No Salt Added), ½ Cup	
Asparagus, Bean Sprouts, Corn	<5
Cucumb., Gr. Beans, Mushr., Okra	<5
Onions, Potato, Pumpkin, Squash	<5
Broccoli, Cabbage, Cauliflower	<15
Peppers, hot chili, raw, 1	3
Tomato, 1 medium, 5 oz	10
Beets, Carrots, Celery, ½ cup	40
Spinach, Turnips, ½ cup, ckd.	40
Canned: Asparagus, 4 spears	300
Beans, baked in tom. sce.	450
Beets, ½ cup, 3 oz	240
Corn Kernels, ½ cup, 3 oz	190
Creamed, ½ cup, 4½ oz	330
Mushrooms w/butter sce, 2 oz	550
Peas, ½ cup, 3 oz	250
Sauerkraut, ½ cup, 4 oz	750

PICKLES, OLIVES

Olives, pickled: Green, 1 large	90
Ripe/black, 1 large	40
Pickles: Brd. & Butt., 4 sl., 1 oz	200
Dill, 1 pickle, 2½ oz	900
Sweet, 1 gherkin, ½ oz	130

SOYBEAN PRODUCTS

Miso (Soy Paste), ¼ cup, 2½ oz	2500
Soybean Protein Isolate, 1 oz	280
Tempeh, ½ cup, 3 oz	5
Tofu, average, ½ cup, 4 oz	<10
Silken (Mori-Nu)	
Firm, ½ box (5¼ oz)	50
Extra Firm, 5¼ oz	95

JAM, HONEY, SYRUPS

Jam/Jelly, 1 Tbsp	<3
Honey, Maple Syrup, 1 Tbsp	<2
Log Cabin Syrup, 1 fl.oz	35
Lite, 1 fl.oz	90

PEANUT BUTTER	Sodium (mg)
Peanut Butter, regular, 1 Tbsp	70
Unsalted, 1 Tbsp	1

SNACKS, NUTS

Cheese Balls/Curls, 1 oz	280
Corn/Tortilla Chips, aver., 1 oz	220
Granola Bars, aver., 1 bar	80
Nuts: Plain, unsalted, 1 oz	1
Lightly salted, 1 oz	80
Salted or Honey Roasted, 1 oz	160
Popcorn: Plain (unsalted), 1 cup	1
Flavored, average, 1 cup	60
Salt added, 1 cup	180
Potato Chips, plain, 1 oz	160
Flavored, average, 1 oz	250
Pretzels, regular, 3, 1 oz	450

CANDY, CHOCOLATE

Chocolate, milk, 1 oz	30
Carob Milk Bar, 1 oz portion	55
Fudge, chocolate, 1 oz	55
Candy Bars, average, 1½ oz	60
Hard Candy, Jelly Beans, 1 oz	<10
Licorice, 1 oz	30

BEVERAGES, ALCOHOL

Coffee (& Substitutes), Tea, 1 cup	1
Cocoa, dry, plain, 1 Tbsp	0
Mix, average, 1 envelope	120
Quik (Nestle), 2 tsp	35
Soft Drinks, average, 8 fl.oz	<30
Mineral Water, Perrier, 8 fl.oz	5
Water, average, 1 cup, 8 fl.oz	<5
Drier regions, 1 cup	20+
Alcohol: Beer, average, 12 fl.oz	<20
Wines, average, 4 fl.oz	<15
Spirits (distilled), 1½ fl.oz	1

SPORTS DRINKS (Fluid Replacement)

Breakthrough (Weider), 8 fl.oz	30
Exceed, made up, 8 fl.oz	50
Gatorade Thirst Quencher, 8 fl.oz	110
Max, 8 fl.oz	15

ANTACIDS (Per Tablet)

Alka-Seltzer: Efferv. (Gold Box)	310
Pain Reliever (Blue Box)	520
Rolaids Antacid: Regular	50
Sodium-Free	<1
Tums E-X (Sodium-Free)	<3
Sodium Bicarb. (27% sodium), 1g	270

INDEX (C—K)

179

INDEX (T—Z)

Feedback Welcome

For the betterment of future editions
of this book, your comments would be
greatly appreciated.

- Range of foods presented:
  Which foods and food categories still need to be
  included or expanded upon?

- Format and presentation:
  Is the book easy to use? What changes would you make
  in future editions?

- Diet Information Sections:
  Which diet information sections did you find useful?
  What other features would you like to see included?

- How successful were you?
  Weigh and measure yourself before and during your
  program. How did you progress? How has weight loss
  affected your lifestyle and relationships?

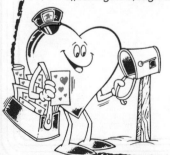

Please Write To:

Allan Borushek (Dietitian)
3001 Redhill Ave
The Esplanade, Suite 6-108
Costa Mesa, CA 92626

Notes